Evidence-Based Practices in Mental Health

Evidence-Based Practices in Mental Health

Debate and Dialogue on the Fundamental Questions

Editors

John C. Norcross, Larry E. Beutler,
and **Ronald F. Levant**

American Psychological Association • Washington, DC

Published by
American Psychological Association
750 First Street, NE
Washington, DC 20002
www.apa.org

To order
APA Order Department
P.O. Box 92984
Washington, DC 20090-2984

Tel: (800) 374-2721; Direct: (202) 336-5510
Fax: (202) 336-5502; TDD/TTY: (202) 336-6123
Online: www.apa.org/books/
E-mail: order@apa.org

In the U.K., Europe, Africa, and the Middle East, copies may be ordered from
American Psychological Association
3 Henrietta Street
Covent Garden, London
WC2E 8LU England

Typeset in Goudy by MacAllister Publishing Services, Indianapolis, IN

Printer: United Book Press, Inc., Baltimore, MD
Cover Designer: Naylor Design, Washington, DC
Project Manager: MacAllister Publishing Services, Indianapolis, IN

The opinions and statements published are the responsibility of the authors, and such opinions and statements do not necessarily represent the policies of the American Psychological Association.

Library of Congress Cataloging-in-Publication Data

Evidence-based practices in mental health : debate and dialogue on the fundamental questions / edited by John C. Norcross, Larry E. Beutler & Ronald F. Levant.
        p.   cm.
    Includes bibliographical references and index.
    ISBN 1-59147-290-3—ISBN 1-59147-310-1 (softcover)
    1. Evidence-based psychiatry.   I. Norcross, John C., 1957-   II. Beutler, Larry E.   III. Levant, Ronald F.

    RC455.2.E94E955 2005
    616.89—dc22

                                                                        2005004098

British Library Cataloguing-in-Publication Data
A CIP record is available from the British Library.

Printed in the United States of America
First Edition

To the American Psychological Association:
Large, diverse, and inclusive enough for all of us

CONTENTS

ABOUT THE EDITORS

John C. Norcross, PhD, ABPP, is Professor of Psychology and Distinguished University Fellow at the University of Scranton, a clinical psychologist in part-time practice, and editor of the *Journal of Clinical Psychology: In Session*. Author of more than 250 publications, Dr. Norcross has cowritten or edited 14 books, including *Psychotherapy Relationships That Work, Authoritative Guide to Self-Help Resources in Mental Health, Handbook of Psychotherapy Integration, Psychologists' Desk Reference,* and *Systems of Psychotherapy: A Transtheoretical Analysis.* He is past president of the International Society of Clinical Psychology and the American Psychological Association (APA) Division 29 (Psychotherapy). He currently serves on the Council of Representatives of the APA and on the board of directors of the National Register of Health Service Providers in Psychology. Dr. Norcross has received many professional awards, such as the APA's Distinguished Contributions to Education and Training Award, Pennsylvania Professor of the Year from the Carnegie Foundation, and election to the National Academies of Practice.

Larry E. Beutler, PhD, ABPP, is Distinguished Professor of Clinical Psychology at the Pacific Graduate School of Psychology, Professor of Homeland Security at the U.S. Navy Postgraduate School in Monterey, California, and a consulting professor of psychiatry and behavioral science at the Stanford University School of Medicine. Dr. Beutler is the former editor of the *Journal of Clinical Psychology* and the *Journal of Consulting and Clinical Psychology.* He is a fellow of the APA and the American Psychological Society. He is past president of the APA Division 12 (Society of Clinical Psychology), the APA Division 29 (Psychotherapy), and the (International) Society for Psychotherapy Research. He is the author of approximately 300 scientific papers and chapters and is the author, editor, or coauthor of 14 books on psychotherapy and psychopathology. Dr. Beutler is coeditor of a book on empirically defined principles of therapeutic change that is cosponsored by the APA Division 12 and the North American Society for Psychotherapy Research.

Ronald F. Levant, EdD, ABPP, is Professor of Psychology at Nova Southeastern University. Since earning his doctorate in clinical psychology and public practice from Harvard, Dr. Levant has been a psychologist in independent practice, a clinical supervisor in hospital settings, a clinical and academic administrator, and a faculty member. He has authored, coauthored, or coedited over 250 publications, including 14 books and 140 journal articles and book chapters. His books include *Between Father and Child, Masculinity Reconstructed, A New Psychology of Men, Men and Sex,* and *New Psychotherapies for Men.* Dr. Levant served as editor of the *Journal of Family Psychology* and is currently associate editor of *Professional Psychology: Research and Practice.* He served as president of the Massachusetts Psychological Association, president of the APA Division 43 (Family Psychology), cofounder of the Society for the Psychological Study of Men and Masculinity, two-term chair of the APA Committee for the Advancement of Professional Practice, member of the APA Council of Representatives, and recording secretary of APA. Dr. Levant is the 2005 president of the APA. One of his presidential initiatives is evidence-based practice in psychology.

CONTRIBUTORS

Michael E. Addis, PhD, Department of Psychology, Clark University, Worcester, MA

David O. Antonuccio, PhD, Department of Psychiatry and Behavioral Sciences, University of Nevada School of Medicine, Reno

Marna S. Barrett, PhD, Department of Psychiatry, University of Pennsylvania School of Medicine, Philadelphia

Larry E. Beutler, PhD, Pacific Graduate School of Psychology, Palo Alto, CA

Arthur C. Bohart, PhD, Department of Psychology, California State University, Dominguez Hills

Tom D. Borkovec, PhD, Department of Psychology, Pennsylvania State University, University Park

Laura S. Brown, PhD, Washington School of Professional Psychology, Argosy University, Seattle

Esteban V. Cardemil, PhD, Department of Psychology, Clark University, Worcester, MA

Louis G. Castonguay, PhD, Department of Psychology, Pennsylvania State University, University Park

Dianne L. Chambless, PhD, Department of Psychology, University of Pennsylvania, Philadelphia

Paul Crits-Christoph, PhD, Department of Psychiatry, University of Pennsylvania School of Medicine, Philadelphia

Robert J. DeRubeis, PhD, Department of Psychology, University of Pennsylvania, Philadelphia

Barry L. Duncan, PsyD, Institute for the Study of Therapeutic Change, Chicago, IL

Martin E. Franklin, PhD, Department of Psychiatry, University of Pennsylvania School of Medicine, Philadelphia

Leslie S. Greenberg, PhD, Department of Psychology, York University, Toronto, Ontario, Canada

Clara E. Hill, PhD, Department of Psychology, University of Maryland, College Park

Steven D. Hollon, PhD, Department of Psychology, Vanderbilt University, Nashville, TN

Ruth M. Hurst, MA, Department of Psychology, University of North Carolina at Greensboro

Brynne E. Johannsen, BS, Pacific Graduate School of Psychology, Palo Alto, CA

John F. Kihlstrom, PhD, Institute for the Study of Healthcare Organizations and Transactions, University of California, Berkeley

Neville J. King, PhD, Faculty of Education, Monash University, Victoria, Australia

Michael J. Lambert, PhD, Department of Psychology, Brigham Young University, Provo, UT

Ronald F. Levant, EdD, Center for Psychological Studies, Nova Southeastern University, Fort Lauderdale, FL

Lester B. Luborsky, PhD, Department of Psychiatry, University of Pennsylvania School of Medicine, Philadelphia

Stanley B. Messer, PhD, Graduate School of Applied and Professional Psychology, Rutgers University, Piscataway, NJ

Scott D. Miller, PhD, Institute for the Study of Therapeutic Change, Chicago, IL

Rosemery Nelson-Gray, PhD, Department of Psychology, University of North Carolina at Greensboro

John C. Norcross, PhD, Department of Psychology, University of Scranton, Scranton, PA

Rhoda Olkin, PhD, California School of Professional Psychology, Alliant International University, San Francisco

Thomas H. Ollendick, PhD, Department of Psychology, Virginia Polytechnic Institute and State University, Blacksburg, VA

Geoffrey M. Reed, PhD, Practice Directorate, American Psychological Association, Washington DC

Deacon Shoenberger, MA, Department of Psychology, University of Nevada, Reno

Louise B. Silverstein, PhD, Department of Psychology, Yeshiva University, Bronx, New York

William B. Stiles, PhD, Department of Psychology, Miami University, Oxford, OH

Shannon Wiltsey Stirman, MA, Department of Psychology, University of Pennsylvania, Philadelphia

George Stricker, PhD, The Derner Institute, Adelphi University, Garden City, New York

Stanley Sue, PhD, Department of Psychology, University of California, Davis

Greg Taliaferro, PhD, Cincinnati Psychoanalytic Institute, Cincinnati, OH

Bruce E. Wampold, PhD, Department of Counseling Psychology, University of Wisconsin—Madison

Jeanne C. Watson, PhD, Department of Adult Education and Counseling Psychology, University of Toronto, Ontario, Canada

Drew I. Westen, PhD, Departments of Psychology and Psychiatry, Emory University, Atlanta, GA

Nolan Zane, PhD, Department of Psychology, University of California, Davis

Evidence-Based Practices in Mental Health

PROLOGUE

JOHN C. NORCROSS, LARRY E. BEUTLER, AND RONALD F. LEVANT

Few topics in mental health are as incendiary, consequential, and timely as evidence-based practices. Yet, this multifaceted and complex topic has been reduced to simplistic and polarized arguments; regrettably, more heat than light has been shed on the topic. This book, designed primarily for mental health practitioners, trainers, and graduate students, addresses nine fundamental questions in the debate on evidence-based practices (EBPs). Each chapter centers on one particular question in the ongoing EBPs debate and consists of several focused position papers on that question. The position papers are followed by dialogues among the contributors on their respective points of convergence and contention.

In this brief introduction, we begin by describing the purpose and structure of *Evidence-Based Practices in Mental Health: Debate and Dialogue on the Fundamental Questions*. We then review the origins and controversies of EBPs in mental health. With these as the background, we place the nine pivotal questions in context.

PURPOSE AND STRUCTURE OF THE BOOK

Our abiding hope is that this book will explicate the central questions in this fiercely contested subject, will provide balanced positions on these polarizing questions, and will purge us of needless confusion and antagonism. In doing so, our aim is to underscore both the robust commonalities and the remaining contentions regarding EBPs in mental health.

The structure of the book follows directly from its purposes. Each chapter consists of position papers on a specific question followed by brief dialogues among the contributors. We recruited leading practitioners and researchers to contribute position papers. The papers were designed to be focused, persuasive pieces that advanced a particular perspective. The contributors were asked to use any combination of clinical experience, research findings, theoretical argument, and logical analysis to advance their positions. Contributors were free to take on a coauthor, and we requested them to keep diversity in mind when doing so. We sought contributor diversity not only in terms of gender, ethnicity, and sexual orientation but also in terms of theoretical orientation and representation across the practice–research continuum. Although many of the contributors were understandably tempted to comment upon multiple facets of the evidence-based debate, we asked them to limit themselves to the specific question posed in that chapter.

Contributors to a particular chapter then received the final drafts of the other contributors' position papers and were asked to comment briefly (1,000 words or less) on their respective points of agreement and remaining disagreements. We desired candid, vigorous, but respectful exchanges that illuminated both areas of convergence and remaining areas of contention. We specifically advised contributors that "the tone should be that of a respectful discourse among colleagues. Please do not exaggerate or mischaracterize other contributors' positions; we have plenty of substantive disagreement without resorting to unsavory rhetorical devices. And, of course, please refrain from any ad hominem attacks."

BRIEF HISTORY OF EMPIRICALLY SUPPORTED TREATMENTS AND EVIDENCE-BASED PRACTICES

Evidence-based practices, as is often said about clinical psychology (Boring, 1950), has a long past but a short history. The long past of EBPs entails hundreds of years of effort to base clinical practice on the results of solid, typically research, evidence. Starting with its separation from philosophy and Wilhelm Wundt's early laboratory experiments, psychology has always prided itself on its scientific roots and empirical rigor. Similarly, from Emil Kraeplin's diagnostic scheme to Benjamin Rush's initial empirical efforts, psychiatry has tried to distance itself from untested practices and to locate itself as a science of mind. From their very inceptions, mental health professions proclaim their allegiance to the methods and results of scientific research.

In medicine, analysts point to three landmarks on the road to EBPs (Leff, 2002). The first was the Flexner Report, which created a blueprint for medical education on the basis of a scientific and uniform curriculum. The second was medicine's first randomized clinical trial, which appeared in a 1948 issue of the *British Medical Journal*. The third landmark was the establishment of the Food and Drug Administration (FDA) and the related governmental organizations mandated to test the safety and effectiveness of health care interventions.

But the short past of EBPs in mental health traces back to the 1990s, originally in Great Britain and then gathering steam in the United States and around the globe. Foremost among these initiatives in psychology in the United States was the American Psychological Association (APA) Society of Clinical Psychology's (Division 12) Task Force efforts to identify empirically supported treatments (ESTs) for adults and to publicize these treatments to fellow psychologists and training programs. Since 1993, a succession of APA Division 12 Task Forces (now a standing committee) has constructed and elaborated a list of empirically supported, manualized psychological interventions for specific disorders on the basis of randomized, controlled studies that pass for methodological rigor (Chambless & Hollon, 1998; Chambless et al., 1996, 1998; Task Force on Promotion and Dissemination of Psychological Procedures, 1995). Oxford University Press published the influential *A Guide to Treatments That Work* (Nathan & Gorman, 1998), a volume that emanated from the work of a related Division 12 Task Force. Subsequently, ESTs were applied to children, adolescents, and older adults.

APA's Society of Clinical Psychology was not alone in developing and promoting statements on EBPs. The APA Division 17 (Society of Counseling Psychology) issued their own principles of empirically supported interventions (Wampold, Lichtenberg, & Waehler, 2002), and the APA Division 32 (Humanistic Psychology; Task Force, 1997) published guidelines for the provision of humanistic psychosocial services. The APA Division 29 (Psychotherapy) responded with a task force that identified empirically supported (psychotherapy) relationships or ESRs (Norcross, 2002).

Foremost among the evidence-based initiatives in psychiatry has been the American Psychiatric Association's practice guidelines. The organization has published a dozen practice guidelines on disorders ranging from schizophrenia to anorexia to nicotine dependence. Although not explicitly identified as "evidence-based," they and similar guidelines are similar in scope and intent: Use the best available knowledge to compile statements of "what works" or "best practices."

Interestingly, the APA itself has not promulgated practice guidelines or treatment guidelines for specific disorders. Instead, they have published "Criteria for Evaluating Treatment Guidelines" (APA, 2002) as well as "Criteria for Practice Guideline Development and Evaluation" (APA, 2002; and before that, a *Template for Developing Guidelines*, Task Force, 1995). A key feature of guidelines for APA is that they are aspirational in nature, unlike standards that are mandatory. In fact, APA policy requires that any guidelines note explicitly that they are not intended to be mandatory, exhaustive, or definitive. "APA's official approach to guidelines strongly emphasizes professional judgment in individual patient encounters and is therefore at variance with that of more ardent adherents to evidence-based practice" (Reed, McLaughlin, & Newman, 2002, p. 1042).

APA policy distinguishes between practice guidelines and treatment guidelines: The former consists of recommendations to professionals concerning their conduct, whereas the latter provides specific recommendations about treatments to be offered to patients. The evidence-based movement addresses both types, but primarily treatment guidelines.

Dozens of organizations are already synthesizing evidence and disseminating their respective lists of EBPs in mental health. One of the oldest is the Cochrane Collaboration (www.cochrane.org), founded in Great Britain and named in honor of Archibald Cochrane, a noted British epidemiologist. Another group modeled after the Cochrane Collaboration is the Campbell Collaboration (www.campbellcollaboration.org), named in honor of the American psychologist and methodologist. The American Psychiatric Association, National Association of Social Workers, and other professional organizations issue practice guidelines (see the National Guidelines Clearinghouse at www.guideline.gov). Several federal agencies, the Substance Abuse and Mental Health Services Administration (SAMHSA) and the Agency for Health Care Research and Quality among them, have specific centers or special initiatives devoted to the identification and transfer of EBPs in mental health.

All these initiatives and policies are attempting to address the larger societal context. The EBP movement is truly a juggernaut, racing to achieve accountability in medicine, psychology, education, public policy, and even architecture. The zeitgeist is to require professionals to base their practice, to whatever extent possible, on evidence. No profession can afford to sit on the sidelines; the movement will not magically disappear by avoiding it.

In fact, EBPs are already being defined for mental health practitioners. The APA Division 12's lists of ESTs have been referenced by a number of local, state, and federal funding agencies who are beginning to reimburse practitioners only for the use of these ESTs. Such lists are also being used by some managed care and insurance companies to control costs by restricting the practice of psychological health care.

All these efforts are part of a worldwide movement toward EBP in mental health. In Great Britain, for one example, a Guidelines Development Committee of the British Psychological Society authored a Department of Health (2001) document entitled *Treatment Choice in Psychological Therapies and Counselling: Evidence-Based Practice Guidelines*. In Germany, for another example, the federal government commissioned an expert report on the effectiveness of psychotherapy to guide the revisions of laws regulating psychotherapy (Strauss & Kaechele, 1998).

Although the desire to base clinical practice on solid evidentiary grounds is old and unanimous, the promulgation of specific practice guidelines and evidence-based treatments has been relatively recent and divisive.

Their introduction has provoked practice modifications, training refinements, and organizational conflicts. For better and for worse, insurance carriers and government policymakers are increasingly turning to ESTs, EBPs, and practice guidelines to determine which psychotherapies to approve and fund. Indeed, along with the negative influence of managed care, probably no issue is more central to clinicians than the evolution of EBP in mental health (Barlow, 2000).

CULTURE WARS OF EBPS

Language is powerful, as any mental health practitioner can readily attest. Freud famously remarked that words were once magic. Most social and professional controversies entail powerful meanings of words. What is *marriage*? What is the definition of *life*? What entails an *imminent threat*? Words can diminish or privilege.

So it is with EBPs. At first blush, there is universal agreement that we should use evidence as a guide in determining what works. It's like publicly prizing Mother and apple pie. Can anyone seriously advocate the reverse: nonevidence-based practice?

But it is neither as simple nor as consensual as that. Defining evidence, deciding what qualifies as evidence, and applying what is privileged as evidence are complicated matters with deep philosophical and huge practical consequences. For example, 60% to 90% of ESTs identified to date according to the Division 12 decision rules are cognitive–behavioral treatments (CBTs). The ESTs typically involve skill building, have a specific focus, involve relatively brief treatment, and rarely use traditional assessment measures (O'Donohue, Buchanan, & Fisher, 2000). The decision rules to require treatment manuals, rely on controlled research, focus on specific disorders, and validate specific treatment methods have all come under attack. In particular, EST lists do little for those psychotherapists whose patients and theoretical conceptualizations do not fall into discrete disorders (Messer, 2001). Consider the client who seeks more joy in his or her life, but who does not meet diagnostic criteria for any disorder, whose psychotherapy stretches beyond 20 sessions, and whose treatment objectives are not easily specified in measurable, symptom-based outcomes. Current evidence-based compilations have little to contribute to his or her therapist and his or her treatment. Not all psychotherapies or practitioners embrace an action-oriented, symptom-focused model.

Mental health professionals have become polarized on EBPs and separated into rival camps, with differing language systems and conflicting values. The controversy has spread into the professional literature and onto the floor of the APA Council of Representatives. EBPs have become the latest and most visible conflict in psychology's culture wars (Messer, 2004).

Part of these culture wars involves theoretical orientation, practice setting, and even professional associations. APA Division 12 and scientist–practitioners in the cognitive–behavioral tradition are, as a group, favorably disposed toward EBPs; APA Division 42 (Psychologists in Independent Practice) and full-time practitioners in the psychodynamic and humanistic traditions are, as a group, vigorously opposed. Tavris (2003), writing on this widening scientist–practitioner gap, opines that, today,

> calling it a "gap" is like saying there is an Israeli–Arab "gap" in the Middle East. It is a war, involving deeply held beliefs, political passions, views of human nature and the nature of knowledge, and—as all wars ultimately involve—money, territory, and livelihoods. (p. xiv)

And what of our (the editors') respective positions on EBP in mental health? Are not the editors' orientations and values potentially in play? Indeed they are.

The three of us are clinical psychologists, trained to value both practice and science. We have all taught at universities, all directed psychology departments or professional schools, all edited journals, all conducted private practices, all produced research, and all participated in the governance of the APA and its practice divisions. We are, at once, practitioners, researchers, teachers, and administrators of psychology.

Our bias is toward informed pluralism. We oppose zealots on both sides; we champion moderation in the middle. We value the integration of multiple perspectives and the mutual enrichment of practice and science. We are inveterate eclectics or integrationists, occupying the middle on many of these questions. Our most cherished value is to give full voice to the field's differences through respectful discourse.

Having said that and having emphasized our commonalities, those who know us and our professional contributions would probably align us slightly differently on many of the evidence-based questions. One of us (Ronald F. Levant) is perceived as more sympathetic to practitioners, one of us (Larry E. Beutler) is more inclined to scientists, and one of us (John C. Norcross) is a hopeless eclectic straddling the middle line. These differences, though small, have been exaggerated in political and professional circles. To the extent that these differences are real and meaningful, we are reasonably certain that they have helped us maintain a balance of perspectives in this volume.

Take the definition of evidence, for a prominent example. One of us (RFL) endorses the inclusive definition of EBP (Institute of Medicine, 2001, p. 147) as the integration of the best research evidence with clinical expertise and patient values. Levant does not privilege one component over another; he believes that a definition of practice based on evidence that equally values all three components will advance our knowledge and provide better accountability. Another one of us (JCN) embraces the same three components of best available research, clinical expertise, and patient values.

At the same time, Norcross would privilege best research and elevate it above the others in the hierarchy of evidence. The third one of us (LEB) is concerned about the movement in some quarters to include, within the definition of evidence, clinician expertise on the basis of personal beliefs, clinical experiences, and individual values. Beutler believes that, if unchecked against objective validity criteria, these are potential sources of bias in judgment and are the very sources of error that controlled research was designed to overcome.

Our relative differences on this and other EBP questions led us to invite contributions from champions of diverse perspectives for this book. More important, our own differences help to transcend polarizing characterizations on simplistic questions of evidence-based treatment to consider relative positions on the multiple, layered questions of EBP. Our hope is that the book will illuminate multiple horizons and perhaps a fusion of horizons.

NINE FUNDAMENTAL QUESTIONS

One of the immediate and overarching questions concerning evidence-based practice in mental health is what, exactly, qualifies as evidence. Must EBP be based on research (of some form)? Should the evidence include practitioner experience and expertise? And what about the consumer? Should the evidence include what patients value and prefer in their treatment? Put bluntly: What counts as evidence? Chapter 1 addresses this sticky wicket.

Definitions of EBP always embrace research as one of the sources of evidence and frequently privilege research findings as the most important guide to treatment selection. The "gold standard," particularly in the biomedical fields, has been the randomized clinical (or controlled) trial (RCT). However, in mental health fields, a spirited debate concerns the privileged status accorded to RCTs. Chapter 2 features five position papers on the question of what qualifies as research to judge effective practice in mental health.

Whatever form it may take, research on the effectiveness of mental health practices requires that patients receive similar, if not identically standardized, medication, treatment, or testing. In medication trials, this standardization involves administering the same medication at the same dose or following a standard protocol to determine dosage. In mental health research, this standardization has frequently involved the use of treatment manuals. Practitioners are asked to adhere to a psychotherapy manual, and subsequent fidelity or adherence checks are taken to ensure that the treatment is being implemented as specified in the manual. In fact, manualization has been deemed a prerequisite for inclusion in some compilations of ESTs or EBPs. The position papers in chapter 3 tackle the advantages and disadvantages of manualization in psychotherapy, particularly whether the use of manuals improves treatment outcomes.

EBPs seek to identify the most effective and efficient treatments in research studies so that those same treatments can be widely implemented in practice. However, such generalizations of research findings are not automatic or inevitable. Many hitches occur in generalizing and in transporting treatments from the lab to the clinic, and here we address two of these hitches. In chapter 4, we consider the pressing question of whether research patients and clinical trials are representative of clinical practice. Later, in chapter 9, we consider the related concern of whether efficacious laboratory-validated treatments readily transport to clinical practice.

Apart from the debate on the generalization and transportability of laboratory treatments is the broader question of what should be validated. What accounts for effective treatment? In biomedical research, it is traditionally the specific treatment method—the medication, the surgery, the discrete method applied to the patient—that is credited for effectiveness. In mental health research, however, there are diverse conceptual perspectives and conflicting research results. Some argue that the treatment method is the natural and inclusive target for research validation, whereas others argue that the psychotherapist, the therapy relationship, the patient, or the principles of change actually account for more of the success of psychotherapy and thus should be targets for research validation and EBPs. These arguments are presented in chapter 5.

The research enterprise itself—securing funding, selecting measures, collecting the data, interpreting the results, and then publishing the findings —is a complicated human task. As mental health professionals, we know that human behavior is materially influenced by a multiplicity of factors, some beyond our immediate awareness, and research is no exception. What is represented and published as evidence can be influenced by the funding sources, the researcher's theoretical allegiance, and conventional wisdom. These potential biases are considered in chapter 6.

In chapter 7, we tackle the bottom-line issue of effectiveness. Do therapies designated as ESTs for specific disorders produce outcomes superior to non-EST therapies? By definition, ESTs have outperformed no treatment, placebo, or treatment as usual (TAU). But do they outperform bona fide treatments that have not met the criteria for designation as ESTs? Two position papers provide contrasting answers.

In addition to their global effectiveness, we should also critically inquire if EBPs are effective for the historically marginalized segments of our population. Alas, insufficient research attention has been devoted in EBPs and TAUs to race–ethnicity, gender, sexual orientation, and disability status. Chapter 8 is the only chapter in which there was such unanimity that we could not locate an alternative position; all agree that EBPs to date have not satisfactorily addressed the various dimensions of diversity. The position papers in that chapter review the extant evidence and recommend directions that can make EBPs more applicable and effective in the future.

These nine questions, then, traverse the elemental controversies and real-life applications of evidence-based practices in mental health. Starting from the definition of evidence and ending at the transportability of laboratory-validated treatments to practice settings, these questions canvass the central territory of EBPs.

TOWARD PLURALISM AND HUMILITY

In the end, we hope that *Evidence-Based Practices in Mental Health* will present the fundamental questions in this fiercely contested debate and will provide balanced, informed positions on the salient questions. Proximity and dialogue help establish consensus and clarify disagreements; for this book, distinguished champions of particular positions came together and spoke directly to each other. Reading this book will certainly not solve the value problem or tell you what is the most effective practice, but it will assuredly enhance informed pluralism about EBPs.

In concluding his monumental *Principles of Psychology*, William James (1892/1985) tried desperately to resolve the conflicts between his hard head and his soft heart, his intuitive inclinations and his experimental aspirations. James offered two closing injunctions on the best ways we can facilitate progress in psychology. First, he tells us, we must understand how great the darkness is in which we grope. Second, we must never forget that our assumptions are provisional and reversible things. We would do well to heed his final admonishments and remain optimistically humble on the matter of evidence-based practices in mental health.

REFERENCES

American Psychological Association. (2002). Criteria for evaluating treatment guidelines. *American Psychologist, 57*, 1052–1059.

American Psychological Association. (2002). Criteria for practice guideline development and evaluation. *American Psychologist, 57*, 1048–1051.

Barlow, D. H. (2000). Evidence-based practice: A world view. *Clinical Psychology: Science and Practice, 7*, 241–242.

Boring, E. G. (1950). *A history of experimental psychology* (2nd ed.). New York: Appleton-Century-Crofts.

Chambless, D. L., Baker, M. J. Baucom, D. H., Beutler, L., Calhoun, K. S., Crits-Christoph, P., et al. (1998). Update on empirically validated therapies, II. *The Clinical Psychologist, 51*, 3–16.

Chambless, D., Sanderson, W. C., Shoham, V., Johnson, S. B., Pope, K. S., Crits-Christoph, P., et al. (1996). An update on empirically validated therapies. *The Clinical Psychologist, 49*, 5–14.

Chambless, D. L., & Hollon, S. D. (1998). Defining empirically supported therapies. *Journal of Consulting and Clinical Psychology, 64*, 497–504.

Department of Health. (2001). *Treatment choice in psychological therapies and counseling: Evidence-based practice guidelines*. London: Department of Health Publications.

Institute of Medicine. (2001). *Crossing the quality chasm: A new health system for the 21st century*. Washington, DC: Institute of Medicine.

James, W. (1985). *Psychology: The briefer course*. Notre Dame, IN: University of Notre Dame Press. (Original work published 1892)

Leff, H. S. (2002). A brief history of evidence-based practice and a vision for the future. In R. W. Manderscheid & M. J. Henderson (Eds.), *Mental health, 2003* (pp. 224–241). Rockville, MD: U.S. Department of Health and Human Services.

Messer, S. B. (2001). Empirically supported treatments: What's a nonbehaviorist to do? In B. D. Slife, R. N. Williams, & S. H. Barlow (Eds.), *Critical issues in psychotherapy* (pp. 3–19). Thousand Oaks, CA: Sage.

Messer, S. B. (2004). Evidence-based practice: Beyond empirically supported treatments. *Professional Psychology: Research and Practice, 36*, 580–588.

Nathan, P. E., & Gorman, J. M. (Eds.). (1998). *A guide to treatments that work*. New York: Oxford University Press.

Norcross, J. C. (Ed.). (2002). *Psychotherapy relationships that work: Therapist contributions and responsiveness to patient needs*. New York: Oxford University Press.

O'Donohue, W., Buchanan, J. A., & Fisher, J. E. (2000). Characteristics of empirically supported treatments. *Journal of Psychotherapy Practice and Research, 9*, 69–74.

Reed, G. M., McLaughlin, C. J., & Newman, R. (2002). American Psychological Association policy in context: The development and evaluation of guidelines for professional practice. *American Psychologist, 57*, 1041–1047.

Strauss, B. M., & Kaechele, H. (1998). The writing on the wall: Comments on the current discussion about empirically validated treatments in Germany. *Psychotherapy Research, 8*, 158–170.

Task Force for the Development of Guidelines for the Provision of Humanistic Psychosocial Services. (1997). Guidelines for the provision of humanistic psychosocial services. *Humanistic Psychologist, 25*, 65–107.

Task Force on Promotion and Dissemination of Psychological Procedures. (1995). Training in and dissemination of empirically validated psychological treatments: Report and recommendations. *The Clinical Psychologist, 48*, 3–23.

Task Force on Psychological Intervention Guidelines. (1995). *Template for developing guidelines: Interventions for mental disorders and psychosocial aspects of physical disorders*. Washington, DC: American Psychological Association.

Tavris, C. (2003). Foreword. In Lilienfeld, S. O., Lynn, S. J., & Lohr, J. M. (Eds.), *Science and pseudoscience in clinical psychology*. New York: Guilford Press.

Wampold, B. E., Lichtenberg, J. W., & Waehler, C. A. (2002). Principles of empirically-supported interventions in counseling psychology. *The Counseling Psychologist, 30*, 197–217.

1

WHAT QUALIFIES AS EVIDENCE OF EFFECTIVE PRACTICE?

Clinical Expertise

Geoffrey M. Reed

The most widely cited definition of evidence-based practice (EBP) is one adapted from Sackett and colleagues (2000) by the Institute of Medicine (2001):

> *Evidence-based practice* is the integration of best research evidence with clinical expertise and patient values. *Best research evidence* refers to clinically relevant research, often from the basic health and medical sciences, but especially from patient centered clinical research . . . . *Clinical expertise* means the ability to use clinical skills and past experience to rapidly identify each patient's unique health state and diagnosis, individual risks and benefits of potential interventions, and personal values and expectations. *Patient values* refers to the unique preferences, concerns and expectations that each patient brings to a clinical encounter and that must be integrated into clinical decisions if they are to serve the patient. (p. 147)

This definition speaks to an integration of three components, without implying that one is privileged over another, and is one that few practicing psychologists would disagree with as a model for practice. Yet practitioners who have been following the discussion on EBP are chagrined to find themselves regularly portrayed as either idiots or charlatans. A relatively typical statement is "that most of the theories and approaches that are used within the community of practitioners are unsupported by empirical evidence" (Beutler, 2000, ¶ 2). Although such statements may not be untrue according to the narrowest definition of evidence, they are generally offered without additional context and therefore as having much broader implications. Psychological treatments as they are routinely practiced in the community are characterized as being on the basis of beliefs, preferences, and unvalidated theories, as were "such widely varied practices as blood-letting, demonology, the inquisition, the holocaust, and the crusades as well as every other destructive political and religious philosophy" (Beutler, 2000, ¶ 3).

Carter (2002) characterized her experience of the discussion in this way:

> I keep waiting to meet the practitioners described by our scientist–academic colleagues . . . . Those practitioners are thoughtless, reckless, cavalier, and do not learn from experience. Since they follow charismatic-leader-driven treatment approaches without thought, they really need to be provided with manuals to tell them exactly what to do when . . . . They do not read, they do not think; and, above all, they have lost all capacity and interest in learning. (p. 1286)

How have we reached the point that intelligent people who are accepted into some of the most competitive doctoral programs in higher education, who complete what is generally a research-based doctoral degree, who undergo a minimum of two years of supervised clinical training, and who are able to pass national and state licensing exams are routinely discussed as though none of their knowledge is legitimate and their practice is no different from voodoo? And how has this come to be a core premise of the most widely touted initiatives in mental health?

This position paper explores some of the health system forces that have been fueling the deprofessionalization of health professionals and how these dynamics have interacted with the EBP movement. I conclude that reasserting and better defining clinical expertise is the key to helping psychology preserve its fundamentally human nature and, at the same time, meet the evidentiary standards necessary to advance health care policies that support our work.

EBP AS A PUBLIC IDEA

During the 1990s, EBP gained currency as a public idea (Tanenbaum, 2003). By this is meant an idea that both describes a public problem and suggests the wisdom of a particular response. The drunk driver, for example, became the focus of transportation safety efforts when a public idea cast him as the essential menace on American highways (Gusfield, 1981). The idea that drunk drivers cause accidents is not untrue, but accidents also have many other causes. A public idea focuses attention on one aspect of a complex problem and calls for the logical solutions to it.

In the health care arena, policy makers are indeed faced with a complex problem. Approximately 15% of the U.S. population is uninsured (Cohen & Ni, 2004; U.S. Census Bureau News, 2004). An even higher percentage (24%) has no mental health benefits, and only about half of those have coverage that could be considered reasonable (Maxfield, Achman, & Cook, 2004). We spend more per capita on health care than any other industrialized nation, yet we do not provide demonstrably better care (World Health Organization, 2001). Care is fragmented, with little coordination horizontally across systems or vertically among levels of care (Institute of Medicine, 2001). Health care costs also continue to rise. The future costs of entitlement programs, including Medicare, promise to create unacceptable burdens for the next generation. These problems seem intractable in the face of vested interests that oppose particular solutions.

Instead, Americans have been offered the public idea that the essential problem with the U.S. health care system is uninformed practice, which would be resolved if health care professionals practiced in ways that are consistent with research findings. This is the basic premise of EBP. Tanenbaum (2003) pointed out that EBP's potency as a public idea is based in part on its powerful rhetoric:

> It is, in fact, a rhetorical triumph, for who can argue with evidence? Critics of EBP literally have nothing to call themselves or their position; it is not evidence, but the limitations of certain evidence hierarchies they oppose . . . . Moreover, the rhetoric of EBP raises an important question in the listener's mind: if EBP is the introduction of evidence into practice, how have clinicians been practicing all along? What is there besides evidence? . . . Even if the public never gets specifics, however, it should be clear to them that clinicians are in the wrong. (p. 294)

EBP offers a further justification for the lay management of professional behavior that has been an operating principle of managed care. The way in which EBP as a public idea links problem and solution is not questioned. In a report of a national program to assess the applications of EBP to managed care, Keckley (2003) is typical in his assertion that the impact of clinicians not following evidence-based guidelines results in suboptimal care for patients and avoidable costs due to high levels of inappropriate variability in treatment patterns. Also typically, he provides no evidence that this is the case. He proposes that EBP can be a mechanism for managed care to improve its image among stakeholders and members. EBP can be "the fundamental basis for managing cost as well as quality" (p. 3) by providing a basis for coverage limitations and denials. This time the justification is framed in the language of science: the results of empirical research—especially randomized controlled trials—should override the judgment of the health professional in the treatment of any particular individual.

This perspective has been given legitimacy by clinical researchers eager to define the essential problem in health care services as the inadequate consumption and application of the research literature by clinicians. They argue that practice outcomes would be enhanced if psychotherapists limited their practice to the use of treatments that have substantial evidence of efficacy (e.g., Carpinello, Rosenberg, Stone, Schwager, & Felton, 2002; Chambless et al., 1996; Chorpita et al., 2002; Lampropoulos & Spengler, 2002; Nathan & Gorman, 1998). This chorus has been joined by federal research agencies eager to claim that their portfolios offer substantial public benefit and by service agencies that claim they hold the key to a system that works.

Health professionals' resistance is generally described as the major barrier to implementing EBP (e.g., Keckley, 2003). As a result, substantial resources are being devoted to programs aimed at increasing practitioner uptake of research-based services, in spite of the fact that virtually no evidence supports the underlying assumption that their implementation will improve health care outcomes. One example is a major joint initiative of the National Institute of Mental Health (NIMH) and the Department of Health and Human Services (DHHS) Substance Abuse and Mental Health Services Administration (SAMHSA) focusing on promoting and supporting the implementation of evidence-based mental health treatment practices into state mental health systems (e.g., National Institutes of Health, 2004). This initiative focuses on identifying the most effective and feasible methods for implementing EBP in state clinical practice settings and it also provides direct support to states and localities that are ready and committed to adopting EBP.

ARE RESEARCHERS A PART OF THE PROBLEM?

One question that may be asked is the extent to which clinical researchers have collaborated with or been used by managed care in its effort to deprofessionalize clinicians by removing their authority over treatment. Clearly, certain individuals denigrate practicing psychologists and discredit their treatments to practically anyone else who will listen. However, I believe they are a tiny (though vocal) minority and extremist subgroup that receives attention out of proportion with its number, often because its accusations make good media copy.

The best clinical scientists, however, have been engaged in different projects. For them, the central goal of the EBP movement is to demonstrate to external decision makers and stakeholders that psychological interventions have a scientific base and finally to put psychology on a par with medicine (see Tanenbaum, 2003, 2005). These researchers have been particularly concerned about widely disseminated practice guidelines that recommend the use of medications over psychological interventions in the absence of data supporting such recommendations (Barlow, 1996; Beutler, 1998; Muñoz, Hollon, McGrath, Rehm, & VandenBos, 1994; Nathan, 1998). Barlow (in press), in a forward-looking article, makes the case for the implementation of psychological treatments as mainstream health interventions in health systems around the world. He reviews data for psychological treatments for depression and panic disorder, for example, that meet the most stringent evidentiary criteria and that have been published in the most prestigious medical journals (e.g., Barlow, Gorman, Shear, & Woods, 2000; Keller et al., 2000).

However, making the case successfully for psychological interventions within the broader medical system requires meeting evidentiary standards as they are viewed by medicine (Davidson et al., 2003). Both health care policy makers and physicians are almost universally unfriendly to the argument that the gold standard of randomized clinical trials (RCTs) is not always the best model for investigating psychological interventions. From their point of view, the general message that "psychotherapy works" is equivalent to saying that "medication works." The finding that only a small proportion of outcome is predicted by intervention techniques makes it sound as though clinicians are not doing anything specifically important, and therefore that anyone could do it. Data regarding the importance of the therapeutic alliance may be seen as interesting, but is uninformative about what treatment should be offered to whom.

Although psychologists often view the purpose of RCTs as establishing causality, medical researchers and health care policy makers view the purpose of RCTs as providing a basis for health policy. At what age should which groups of women begin routine mammograms for breast cancer? At what cholesterol levels do statin drugs reduce cardiac risk in men? For example, on the basis of recent RCTs, routine hormone replacement therapy—for many years the most recommended treatment in North America—is now known to cause substantial harm in women by significantly increasing breast cancer rates (Chlebowski et al., 2003) and elevating cardiac risk (Manson et al., 2003). As a result, rates of hormone replacement therapy have plummeted (Hersh, Stefanick, & Stafford, 2004).

Unfortunately, adopting this framework in psychology has also meant accepting the "hierarchy of evidence" that evidence-based medicine has taken as its foundation (Sackett et al., 2000). An unfortunate consequence has been an enormous devaluation of the body of professional knowledge in our field. Psychological treatment as it is generally practiced in the community is fluid, self-corrective, not of fixed duration, and individualized

(Seligman, 1995). By definition, such treatment is vastly more difficult or impossible to support using RCT designs. Whether a treatment is deemed effective, then, is largely based on its compatibility with particular research methods (Tanenbaum, 2005). Further, manualization and evidence are confounded by using manualization as a criterion for whether psychological treatments can be evidence based (Chambless et al., 1996).

Widespread confusion exists in the public discussion of treatments that have been empirically disconfirmed with those that have not been tested using the methods emphasized by EBP, and a lack of clarity on this point also characterizes much of the professional literature (Westen, Novotny, & Thompson-Brenner, 2004). In corollary fashion, confusion occurs between treatments that are the "best available" and those that are more compatible with RCTs. For example, we do not in fact know that cognitive—behavior therapy (CBT) and interpersonal therapy are the most effective psychological treatments for depression, but only that these manualized, brief treatments are easier to test using RCT methodologies than alternative approaches. This has also led to a view of manuals as prescriptive and constitutive rather than representative of treatment, and it also contributes to a view of "psychotherapy as the job of paraprofessionals who cannot—and should not—exercise clinical judgment in selecting interventions or interpreting the data of clinical observation" (Westen et al., 2004, p. 639).

The challenge will be for psychology to have it both ways: to preserve the essentially human and individual nature of psychological work and, at that same time, meet the evidentiary standards that will be required of us to flourish in the health care system. Tanenbaum (2005) framed the policy-relevant question as

> Can EBP in mental health commit itself to an inclusive enough evidence hierarchy not to privilege technique unfairly over relationship? Can it do so without further stigmatizing psychology vis-à-vis medicine (including psychopharmacology), thus undermining mental health care's claim to effectiveness worthy of funding? (p. 166)

CLINICAL EXPERTISE: BACK TO THE FUTURE?

I believe that psychology can best overcome this challenge through a data-based reassertion of the importance of clinical expertise. Psychology's authority as a health profession is based on a body of specialized professional knowledge, which, together with a practitioner's individual experiences, forms the basis of a practitioner's clinical expertise. In EBP's most literal interpretation, a clinician's experience contributes little to, and is likely to detract from, appropriate treatment. It is ridiculous to imagine, however, that, faced with choosing a course of treatment for his mother's life-threatening illness, even the most ardent advocate of EBP would follow the advice of an intern who quoted the results of a single RCT over that of a widely respected physician who has treated 100 similar cases with successful results. It is obvious and inevitable that clinical expertise is of paramount importance in any form of health care, including psychological care.

Clinical expertise is certainly informed by controlled research, but controlled research may be unavailable, inconclusive, conflicting in conclusions, or misleading. A relevant example in psychology is an earlier report (Dobson, 1989) of a meta-analysis of 28 studies that reported cognitive therapy for depression had a greater effect than other treatments, including pharmacotherapy, behavior therapy, and other forms of psychotherapy. Later, Luborsky and colleagues (1999) conducted a meta-analysis of 29 treatment comparison studies in depression, incorporating measures of researchers' theoretical allegiance. They found that researcher allegiance accounted for two thirds of the variance in reported treatment differences. Cognitive therapists tended to find superior results for cognitive therapy, whereas psychodynamic researchers found more impressive results for more dynamic treatments. Not surprisingly, this phenomenon also extends to those with allegiance to the biomedical viewpoint who insist that pharmacotherapy is superior to psychotherapy in treating depression, in spite of substantial evidence from psychological research to the contrary (e.g., DeRubeis et al., in press; Hollon et al., in press).

Efficacy research should not be the sole basis for setting policies about what types of services should be encouraged or restricted. The rapid implementation of health care policies discouraging other forms of treatment than cognitive therapy on the basis of Dobson's 1989 review would likely have deprived Luborsky and colleagues of the data necessary to come to a corrective conclusion 10 years later. More important, it would have inappropriately restricted access to effective psychological services among a population that constitutes a major portion of U.S. disease burden and is dramatically undertreated (Kessler et al., 2003; World Health Organization World Mental Health Survey Consortium, 2004). In the context of other populations such as children and the persistently mentally ill, a tremendous need for interventions exists, but relatively few treatments meet the most narrowly defined criteria of evidence because of the difficulties associated with such documentation. An overemphasis on RCTs as evidence is likely to support the application of treatments that are relatively easy to study using this method, in particular the use of medication, which may not be in the best interests of these vulnerable populations. In some cases, an overreliance on controlled research may actually limit the development of cutting-edge treatments that are demonstrably better in terms of individual outcomes but that have not yet been tested in larger controlled designs. Warwick, a pediatrician whose clinic has achieved huge gains in the life expectancy of individuals with cystic fibrosis (more than 47 years as compared to a national average at research-based centers of 33 years) says that national research-based guidelines are "a record of the past, and little more—they should have an expiration date" (Gawande, 2004, p. 82).

The appropriate application of research findings in real-world health care is a primary subject of clinical expertise. Goodheart (2004a) defined clinical expertise in psychology as the ability to integrate knowledge, experience, technical and relational skill, critical thinking, prediction, decision-making, and self-assessment within a fluid situation that often is uncertain and ambiguous. Clinical expertise is required to evaluate the client's clinical state, prioritize treatment needs, form a therapeutic alliance with the patient, select appropriate interventions and evaluate their potential risks and benefits for the individual patient, apply these interventions skillfully, monitor progress, and adjust treatment accordingly. Clinical expertise is also necessary for effective communication with the patient and relevant others to assess the patient and family's goals, values, choices, and desired role in treatment. Clinical expertise also entails considering an array of client factors, including age and developmental stage, culture, language, social class, personality (e.g., strengths and limitations, as well as coping style), behavioral factors (e.g., health risk behaviors and the ability to comply with complex treatments), and relevant systems factors (e.g., family and school).

It is impossible for research to direct clinical decision-making at this level of specificity. For example, research is largely unavailable regarding the impact of most psychological interventions on U.S. minority populations. The hard-line EBP stance would suggest that this makes no difference in treatment selection. I once heard a prominent researcher argue that the group psychological interventions for women with breast cancer that had been developed and tested primarily with a middle-class White population should initially be applied without modification by a community-based organization working with Spanish-speaking immigrant women because evidence exists for the intervention as previously applied and no evidence has been provided for a modification. Such a recommendation would strike most clinicians as bizarre and certainly not based on a consideration of the relevant evidence. It ignores the principles and research of community and multicultural psychology; evidence regarding the enormous impact of language, culture, and context on beliefs about illness and interactions with the health care system; and clinical knowledge regarding the importance of respect for culture and context.

The researcher's recommendation is a direct consequence of inappropriately emphasizing and overgeneralizing from RCTs. RCTs yield group-level probabilities, often on the basis of very narrowly defined groups. Available data indicate that substantial differences can be found between patient samples enrolled in clinical trials and those seen in clinical practice (Zarin, Young, & West, in press), but EBP has tended to assume away the inferential leap required to apply aggregate findings to individual cases (Tanenbaum, 1999). EBP suggests that treatment of the next individual patient can be directly determined by the calculated probability of an outcome associated with specific therapy techniques. Given that other factors are likely to be more important in determining outcome—that is, the patient, the clinician, the culture and context, the therapeutic relationship, and the match between patient and treatment—a practice that is truly evidence-based has to consider all of them.

Critics of clinical decision-making (e.g., Garb, 1998; Meehl, 1954) have tended to emphasize that clinicians are subject to information-processing biases and heuristics in aggregating data and making predictions on the basis of them, as, indeed, is everyone (Kahneman & Tversky, 1973; Nisbett & Ross, 1980). These critiques generally assume that the central goal of clinical decision-making is to predict behavior (Westen & Weinberger, in press). Indeed, statistical prediction generally outperforms clinical prediction in predicting relatively broad or distal behavioral outcomes, and clinical experience does not confer much benefit in such prediction. However, with the exception of specific legal situations, behavioral prediction is not the focus of clinical training or clinical work. Westen and Weinberger (in press) review data that make a strong argument for clinical expertise related to decisions that more closely approximate clinical training and clinical work, including judgments at moderate levels of inference, judgments in contexts in which clinicians are likely to develop expertise (e.g., diagnosis and intervention), and conditions that optimize the expression of expertise (e.g., psychometric instruments designed for expert observers).

Critiques of clinical decision-making also often focus on questions about the predictive validity of certain psychological tests (e.g., Garb, 1998). However, although a wide array of evidence indicates that psychological tests are at least as predictive of a variety of important outcomes as many medical tests (Meyer et al., 2001), this is a separate question from whether the decisions that clinicians make as a part of their assessments and treatments lead to maximally helpful results for their patients. With specific regard to diagnosis, much attention has been devoted to the lack of interrater reliability among clinicians in making a diagnosis on the basis of the *Diagnostic and Statistical Manual of Mental Disorders, Fourth Edition* (DSM–IV; American Psychiatric Association, 1994), particularly as compared to structured interviews (e.g., Basco et al., 2000; Ventura, Liberman, Green, Shaner, & Mintz, 1998). However, although the fine-grained distinctions of the *DSM–IV* may be important for the construction of homogenous patient groups for research, many are of little relevance to clinicians in making or implementing treatment recommendations. As Westen and Weinberger stated (in press, p. 7), "From a strictly empirical perspective, we are aware of no evidence that patients who fall just below or just above threshold for the categorical diagnosis of any *DSM–IV* diagnosis respond differently to any form of treatment, have different etiologies, or differ in any other important respect." A lack of diagnostic reliability may be more properly seen as a problem with the clinical validity of *DSM–IV* rather than with clinical judgment.

Perhaps more relevant to the question of clinical expertise are findings about differences in decision-making between novices and experts that have been tested across many content areas (see Bransford, Brown, & Cocking, 1999). Goodheart (2004a) summarized them as follows: First, experts have acquired extensive content knowledge, organize it in a way that reflects deep understanding, and are able to retrieve elements of this knowledge with little attentional effort. Experts are flexible in their approach to new situations and attend to features and patterns that are not noticed by novices, of whom rote rule-following is more characteristic (Klein, 1998). Expert knowledge cannot be reduced to a set of facts or propositions but is linked to contexts of applicability. Finally, in spite of their level of knowledge, experts may not be able to communicate that knowledge and how they use it clearly to others. This point has relevance for the present discussion.

Recent evidence from RCTs supports the importance of therapist experience and expertise in maximizing therapeutic outcomes (e.g., Huppert et al., 2001; Klein et al., 2003). For example, when Jacobson and Hollon (1996) examined the data from the only RCT that found medications to be more effective than cognitive therapy in treating depression, they found that the site with the most experienced cognitive therapists achieved outcomes that were equal to those of medication, whereas the sites with less experienced therapists did less well. Specific strategies that experienced therapists use in response to individual patients are important in determining outcomes (Anderson & Strupp, 1996; Beutler, Moleiro, & Talebi, 2002; Castonguay, Goldfried, Wiser, Raue, & Hayes, 1996). Available data suggest that rigid adherence to a treatment manual may detract from the therapeutic alliance by increasing the frequency and severity of therapeutic ruptures (Norcross & Hill, 2004), resulting in poorer therapy outcomes (Wampold, 2001).

In an editorial in the *Evidence-Based Medicine Notebook*, Haynes, Devereaux, and Gordon (2002) indicated that early conceptualizations of expertise focused on identifying the relevant research and applying it, deemphasizing other factors in clinical decision-making. They proposed a new model that locates clinical expertise at the intersection of the patient's clinical state and circumstances, the patient's preferences and actions, and the research evidence. In the psychotherapy arena, Beutler (2000) listed five therapeutic competencies: (a) communicating an attitude that is conducive to a therapeutic relationship; (b) therapeutic knowledge of principles of change; (c) therapeutic skill to implement effective techniques; (d) being sensitive to the demands and uses of time in selecting interventions; and (e) using creative imagination when established techniques are not available. Norcross and Hill (2004) similarly offered research-based descriptions and recommendations related to psychotherapy relationships.

EBPs require multiple streams of evidence, always including clinician expertise (Goodheart, 2004a). It is important to recognize that much contemporary clinical research, and the best discussions of EBP, do not support cookbook, one-size-fits-all models of treatment. More sophisticated and experientially accurate models of clinical expertise will shift our understanding of the uses of controlled research. Research is informative, but it can rarely be prescriptive in its application to an individual patient. For the most part, clinical research is most helpfully viewed as a way to assess interventions that may prove useful at particular junctures in work that is guided by clinical expertise. Framing good psychological practice, including a sophisticated understanding of clinician expertise, in terms that draw on the empirical literature will be important in reclaiming respect for the professional role and in advancing the profession in the current climate of health care.

Scientific Research

John F. Kihlstrom

Scientific research is the only process by which clinical psychologists and mental-health practitioners should determine what "evidence" guides EBPs.

THE BACKGROUND IN EVIDENCE-BASED MEDICINE

When the *New York Times* listed "evidence-based medicine" as one of the breakthrough ideas of 2001, many of its readers probably thought, "As opposed to *what*? Are there any medical treatments that are *not* evidence based?" (Hitt, 2001). The simple, straightforward answer to this question is "Yes." Although the medical profession has long cloaked itself with the mantle of science, the fact is that until surprisingly recently physicians had relatively few effective treatments for disease. The available treatments were mostly palliative in nature, intended to ameliorate the patient's symptoms, and make the patient comfortable while nature took its course, or else physicians simply removed diseased organs and tissues through surgery. In a very real sense, scientific medicine really only began in the latter part of the 19th century (about the same time scientific psychology began) with the laboratory revolution of Claude Bernard, and the microbe-hunting of Louis

I thank Lucy Canter Kihlstrom for many stimulating discussions that have helped me clarify my ideas about the relations between science and practice.

Pasteur and Robert Koch, followed by successive phases of the pharmaceutical revolution of the 20th century (Magner, 1992; Porter, 1997).

Nevertheless, almost 150 years after Bernard, and more than a century after Pasteur and Koch, the *Times* article cited a recent estimate that only about 20% of common medical practices were "based on rigorous research evidence," as opposed to being "a kind of folklore" (Hitt, 2001, p. 68). It is only in the last few years that researchers have begun to systematically evaluate medical practices to determine whether they actually work, which ones work better than others, and which are cost effective (Davidoff, Haynes, Sackett, & Smith, 1995; Evidence-Based Medicine Working Group, 1992; Rosenberg & Donald, 1995; Sackett, Straus, Richardson, Rosenberg, & Haynes, 1997). But now evidence-based medicine—defined as "the conscientious, explicit and judicious use of current best evidence in making decisions about the care of individual patients" (Sackett, Rosenberg, Muir-Gray, Haynes, & Richardson, 1996, p. 71), and more broadly renamed as EBPs (Institute of Medicine, 2001)—is the way medicine increasingly does business.

SCIENCE, PSYCHOTHERAPY, AND MANAGED CARE

We can trace a parallel history in psychology. Clinical psychology owes its professional status, including its autonomy from psychiatry and its eligibility for third-party payments, to the assumption that its procedures for diagnosis, treatment, and prevention are based on a substantial body of scientific evidence. But for a long time after the invention of psychotherapy in the latter part of the 19th century, this assumption simply went unchecked. It must have been a shock when, reviewing the paltry literature then available, Eysenck cast doubt on the proposition that psychotherapy had any positive effect at all, over and above spontaneous remission (Eysenck, 1952). It was certainly not good news for a profession facing competition from the first generation of psychotropic drugs, including lithium (introduced in 1949), the phenothiazines, imipramine, Miltown, and other benzodiazepines. For an embarrassingly long time afterward, the chief counterweight to Eysenck's expose was the assertion that psychotherapy did have effects after all, but that the negative effects balanced the positive ones, creating an illusion of no change (Bergin, 1966). It took another 25 years and the development of new meta-analytic techniques, which not only provided quantitative summaries of data trends but also enabled investigators to aggregate weak effects into strong ones, for researchers to demonstrate that psychotherapy did, in fact, on average, have a greater positive effect than nothing at all (see also Lispey & Wilson, 1993; Smith & Glass, 1977; Smith, Glass, & Miller, 1980).

One positive legacy of Eysenck's expose, and Bergin's rejoinders to it, was research intended not only to demonstrate that psychotherapy did work after all but to identify conditions, and techniques, that would magnify the positive outcomes of psychotherapy and minimize the negative ones (Bergin & Strupp, 1970; Fiske et al., 1970; Garfield & Bergin, 1971; Strupp & Bergin, 1969). Following the rise of psychotropic drugs, the professional landscape within psychotherapy became even more competitive with the emergence of behavioral (Wolpe, 1958) and cognitive (Beck, 1970) therapies to rival more traditional psychodynamic and client-centered treatments. The first generation of behavioral and cognitive therapists took clinical psychology's scientific rhetoric seriously, and systematically set about to demonstrate the effectiveness of what they did (Yates, 1970). By the time that Smith and Glass did their meta-analysis, it did indeed seem that the CBTs were able to deliver the goods in a way that more traditional insight-oriented approaches did not. Although some observers concluded from the Smith and Glass that "everyone has won and so all must have prizes" (Luborsky, Singer, & Luborsky, 1975), this was not really the case. Even in the Smith and Glass study, the effect sizes associated with cognitive and behavioral therapies were larger than those associated with psychodynamic and humanistic ones (Smith & Glass, 1977; Smith et al., 1980). Over the succeeding years, the CBTs have gradually emerged as the standard of psychotherapeutic care.

Still, the analysis of Smith and Glass (Smith & Glass, 1977; Smith et al., 1980) suggested that there was enough success to go around, and that would probably have been enough to permit psychoanalysts, Rogerians, and behavior therapists alike to enjoy good professional livelihoods, except that the professional landscape changed once again, with the rise of health maintenance organizations and other forms of managed care. Patients and clients can pay for whatever treatment they want out of their own pockets, regardless of whether it works well or efficiently, so long as they believe they are getting some benefit—or are persuaded that some benefit will ultimately accrue to them. But when third parties foot the bill (patients and therapists are the first and second parties), strong demands for professional accountability come with the package, and this is no less true for mental health care than it is for the rest of the health care industry (Kihlstrom & Kihlstrom, 1998). As a result, the demands of managed care have combined with the rhetoric of science, and competition from both cognitive and behavioral therapy and psychotropic drugs is fostering the development of standards for ESTs (Chambless & Ollendick, 2001; Task Force, 1995) or, again, more broadly, EBP within clinical psychology.

"EFFICACY" AND "EFFECTIVENESS"

Viewed from a historical perspective, EBPs are something that clinical psychology should have been striving for, and promoting, all along, and they have a real flavor of historical inevitability to them. Remarkably, though, at least from the standpoint of a profession that takes pride in its scientific base, there has been considerable resistance to the demand for EBPs. As tempting as it might be to dismiss this resistance as coming from private-practice entrepreneurs who simply want to continue doing what they've always done and resent any infringements on their livelihoods, I suspect things are more complicated than that. Just as some well-intentioned physicians have bridled at having their clinical judgment checked by managed-care bureaucrats, some well-intentioned psychotherapists argue against any standards or guidelines at all, on the grounds that they should be free to pick whatever treatment they think will be best for the individual patient. But physicians don't have this freedom; they have to conform their practices to the available evidence, and where evidence is lacking, to the prevailing standard of care. Why should psychotherapists be any different?

Other resisters, including some clinical scientists, believe that the "efficacy" research that provides the basis for EBPs is inappropriate, or at least insufficient, because the studies are conducted under somewhat artificial conditions that do not represent the problems encountered in actual practice (e.g., Levant, 2004; Seligman, 1995; Seligman & Levant, 1998; Westen & Morrison, 2001; Westen, Novotny, & Thompson-Brenner, 2004). Instead, they propose that ESTs be based on "effectiveness" research, which, they argue, is more ecologically valid. But the distinction between efficacy research and effectiveness research seems strained. Research is research. Clinical drug trials are somewhat artificial too, but their artificiality does not prevent physicians from prescribing effective drugs in actual practice, based in large part on carefully controlled studies that show that the drugs in question really do improve the conditions being treated.

To the extent that effectiveness research attempts to extend the logic of efficacy research to more ecologically valid treatment settings—studying patients with comorbid conditions, for example, or with diagnoses on Axis II as well as Axis I, or more extended treatments—no essential difference exists between the two. But to the extent that effectiveness research loosens the standards for methodological rigor characteristic of efficacy research, then effectiveness research is a step backwards. In the *Consumer Reports* study, for example (*Consumer Reports*, 1995; Kotkin, Daviet, & Gurin, 1996; Seligman, 1995), the outcome of psychotherapy was measured by patients' self-reported satisfaction with their treatment, instead of objective evidence of actual improvement. There were no controls for a sampling bias, nor any untreated control group—a particularly egregious problem in the wake of Eysenck's (1952) analysis. It did not ask about the specificity of treatments, a question critical to distinguishing a genuine effect of psychotherapy from placebo, and for evaluating the differential effectiveness of various forms of therapy.

If the *Consumer Reports* study is an example of effectiveness research, then effectiveness research is a step backward, not a step forward, in the journey toward evidence-based treatments. Efficacy research, modeled on randomized clinical trials in drug research, is a good place to begin research on psychotherapy outcomes. Any deficiencies that efficacy studies might have with respect to ecological validity, deficiencies that might be remedied in the future by properly designed and controlled effectiveness studies, should not be taken as an excuse for discounting them in the meantime.

RATCHETING UP THE STANDARDS

At present, the standards for EBP in psychotherapy are roughly modeled on the clinical trials required before drugs are marketed (Chambless & Ollendick, 2001). To qualify as "empirically supported" on the list maintained by the Society of Clinical Psychology (Division 12, Section III, of the APA), a treatment must yield outcomes significantly better than those associated with an adequate control (typically, patients who receive no treatment at all) in at least two studies, preferably conducted by independent research groups. These standards are a good start for putting psychotherapy, at long last, on a firm scientific base, but they are also somewhat minimal, and over time they should be progressively ratcheted up (the opposite of defining them down; Moynihan, 1993) to improve the quality of psychotherapeutic practice.

For example, two studies out of how many? The current EST standard is modeled on current Food and Drug Administration (FDA) standards, which require only two positive trials, regardless of how many negative or inconclusive trials there are, raising the file-drawer problem and the issue of selective publication of positive results. Just as the medical community is ratcheting up this requirement by requiring drug companies to preregister all drug trials as a condition of accepting reports of them for publication (Vedantam, 2004), so we might find a way to register ongoing psychotherapy outcome studies before their results are in. Certainly, this is possible for major, collaborative studies supported by federal funds.

More substantively, we might wish to drop the no-treatment control as an appropriate comparison group in favor of either an appropriate placebo or some alternative treatment. It is something to prove that psychotherapy is better than nothing, but surely it is not much. Placebo controls are not easy to implement in psychotherapy research, because it is difficult to keep psychotherapists blind to the treatment they are delivering. In drug research, especially when ethical concerns have arisen about the use of placebo controls, new medications may be evaluated against the current standard of care instead. If a new drug is not discriminably better than what is already available, and certainly if it is discriminably worse, then it is incumbent on its proponents to show that it is a reasonable alternative treatment for some individuals, for whom the currently available medications are ineffective or inappropriate. An example of such a comparison might be the NIMH Treatment of Depression Collaborative Research Program (TDCRP), where the antidepressant drug imipramine might be construed as the established standard of (medical) care, and psychotherapy as the alternative, as well as, for that matter, CBT as the alternative to the more established interpersonal therapy (Elkin et al., 1989).

Next is the matter of how to evaluate the significance of outcomes. Long ago, Jacobson and his colleagues pointed out that a statistically significant change in some criterion measure may not reflect a clinically significant change in terms of the patient's status (Jacobson, Follette, & Revenstorf, 1984; Jacobson & Revenstorf, 1988). The question is, what are the standards for clinical significance? Although I continue to believe (Kihlstrom, 1998) that the null-hypothesis statistical test is the foundation of principled argument in psychology (Abelson, 1995), psychotherapy outcome is one case where effect sizes really *are* preferable to tests of statistical significance (Cohen, 1990, 1994). Although even small effects can be practically significant (Rosenthal, 1990), there is no question that big effects are better, and probably more significant clinically as well.

One reasonable standard for clinical significance is that a patient who enters psychotherapy by virtue of receiving a diagnosis of mental disorder should no longer qualify for that diagnosis at the end of treatment. Accordingly, Jacobson and his colleagues suggested that the outcome of psychotherapy be deemed successful if the treated patient's scores on some criterion measure fall within normal limits (e.g., within 2 SD of the population mean), more than 2 SD of the untreated patient mean, or preferably both (Jacobson et al., 1984; Jacobson & Revenstorf, 1988). Such standards are occasionally applied to the evaluation of therapeutic outcomes, including the TDCRP (Ogles, Lambert, & Sawyer, 1995). Of course, it might turn out that some mental disorders are chronic in nature, meaning that a cure, so defined, is impossible. Even so, clinically relevant standards for evaluating outcome in the treatment of chronic mental disorders might be modeled on evolving procedures for evaluating the management of chronic physical illnesses such as asthma or diabetes (Fox & Fama, 1996).

Again, this is a start, but one can imagine at least two improvements. One is to assess outcomes in terms of laboratory measures of mental and behavioral functioning, instead of symptoms, especially self-reported symptoms. In the TDCRP, for example, outcomes were measured by patients' scores on the Beck Depression Inventory (BDI), the Hamilton Rating Scale of Depression (HRSD), and the Hopkins Symptom Checklist. But although the diagnosis of mental disorder (as represented by *DSM–IV*) is based on signs and symptoms, just as it was in the 19th century, in the rest of health care the diagnosis of illness and the evaluation of treatment outcome are increasingly based on the results of objective laboratory tests, such as blood tests and radiological scans, interpreted in light of an increasingly sophisticated understanding of normal structure and function. It is long past time (Kihlstrom & Nasby, 1981; Nasby & Kihlstrom, 1986) that psychology began to move away from questionnaires and rating scales, and toward a new generation of assessment procedures on objective laboratory tests of psychopathology (Kihlstrom, 2002b).

The interest of third-party payers in the outcome of both treatment and disease management suggests yet another more macroscopic approach to the evaluation of outcomes, which is to assess how the treated patient fares in the ordinary course of everyday living. Couples who go through marital therapy might reasonably expect to have happier children than they did before, and employers who pay for their employees to participate in alcohol or drug-abuse treatment programs might reasonably ask if their employees do, in fact, become more productive after treatment. These examples remind us that other stakeholders are involved in the treatment process than just the patients themselves, and that their evaluation of treatment outcome also counts.

As an example of what might be done, Rosenblatt and Attkisson have proposed a conceptual framework in which outcome evaluation proceeds along three dimensions (Rosenblatt & Attkisson, 1993): the respondent (the patient, family members, social acquaintances, the therapist, or an independent evaluator), the social context (personal, family, work or school, and community), and domain (clinical status, functional status, life satisfaction and fulfillment, and safety and welfare). So, for example, in addition to measuring clinical status with scales such as the BDI or HRSD, we could evaluate the degree to which the patients' families and coworkers notice a difference (Sechrest, McKnight, & McKnight, 1996) after treatment, or the degree to which these "third parties" feel that their own life satisfaction has improved. Such a proposal transcends quibbles about the quantitative threshold for clinical significance and brings qualitative considerations of ecological validity into the measure of treatment outcome.

Finally, it should be understood that EBPs include more than *treatments*; they also include the procedures by which patients are diagnosed and treatment outcomes are assessed. Many of the assessment techniques traditionally used by clinical psychologists (Rapaport, Gill, & Schafer, 1968) appear to rest on a surprisingly weak evidentiary base (Wood, Nezworski, Lilienfeld, & Garb, 2003). We need to extend the logic of EBPs to assessment as well as treatment, establishing and improving the validity of our current techniques, and abandoning those that do not pass muster. Moreover, it should go without saying that the logic of EBPs extends beyond clinical psychology to the broader range of professional psychology, including counseling, educational, and industrial/organizational psychology, as well as other domains where scientific knowledge is put into practice.

THE THEORY BEHIND THE THERAPY

Documenting treatment efficacy is not just a purely empirical matter; theoretical considerations also play a part in the evaluation of any form of treatment. As my spouse once put it in a conversation about an innovative treatment, "What made them think that would work?" It is not enough that a treatment proves empirically to be efficacious. Just as sound medical treatment is based on a scientific understanding of anatomy and physiology, so sound psychotherapy must be based on a scientifically valid understanding of mental and behavioral processes. Here is where placebos and other controls may have their real value—not merely in going one step further than showing that psychotherapy is better than nothing but in evaluating claims concerning the mechanism by which a treatment achieves its effects. If some form of psychotherapy does no better than an appropriate placebo, we can begin to doubt whether that treatment has any specific effects at all. Of course, this assumes that psychotherapy is more than a placebo treatment to begin with (Frank, 1961; Rosenthal & Frank, 1956), which, in fact, is my assumption.

Other kinds of controlled therapy outcome research can also evaluate the scientific validity of certain psychotherapeutic practices. For example, Wolpe's (1958) invention of systematic desensitization was predicated on Hullian learning theory. The only problem was that psychology already had grounds to suspect that Hullian learning theory was not correct (Gleitman, Nachmias, & Neisser, 1954). Fortunately, later research (e.g., Wilson & Davison, 1971) showed that exposure was the active ingredient in systematic desensitization, a conclusion that was consistent with the new, improved, cognitive view of learning that emerged in the 1960s. Along similar lines, a more recent spate of dismantling studies indicates that exposure, not eye movement, is also responsible for the effectiveness of eye-movement desensitization and reprocessing (EMDR; e.g., Lohr, Lilienfeld, Tolin, & Herbert, 1999). Although EMDR may pass the narrowly empirical test for efficacy, claims in its behalf may be undercut by the lack of evidence for its underlying theory.

The point here is that sound treatments are not just those that are empirically supported. Sound treatments are based on scientifically valid theories of mind and behavior. Whenever an innovative therapy is accompanied by a theoretical statement of its underlying mechanism, the therapy should be evaluated not just in terms of whether it works but in terms of its proponents' theory of *why* it works. In this way, we validate the general principles that the treatment is based on and that can form the basis for other therapeutic innovations as well (Rosen & Davison, 2003). We also avoid the trap of using efficacy research to legitimize proprietary, even trademarked, therapies.

To take an example from the history of hypnosis, Mesmer's animal magnetism was not rejected by the Franklin Commission because it did not work (Kihlstrom, 2002a). Everyone agreed that it did work, and, in fact, Mesmer had previously scored a win for scientific medicine by showing he could duplicate the effectiveness of exorcisms with a technique that was materialist, rather than supernatural, in nature. Animal magnetism was rejected solely because Mesmer's theory was wrong, and nobody had a good theory to replace it (scientific psychology not having been invented yet). Exorcism might work empirically, but even if it did, medicine would reject it as a legitimate treatment because its underlying theory—that disease is caused by demon possession—is inconsistent with everything we know about how the body works.

SCIENCE AS THE BASIS OF PRACTICE

The examples of Mesmer and hypnosis make it clear that the relation between science and practice is not unidirectional. Studies of psychopathology and psychotherapy can alter our understandings of normal mental and behavioral functions (Kihlstrom, 1979; Kihlstrom & McGlynn, 1991), but they also underscore the point that we want our EBPs not only to be empirically valid but based on valid scientific principles as well. The scientific method is the best way we have of understanding how the world works and why. Therefore, it is also the best way we have of knowing which of our practices work (and why). In establishing the validity of our theories and practices, anecdotal evidence, impressionistic clinical observations, and customer-satisfaction ratings simply will not suffice. Enhancing the scientific basis for clinical practice by determining which practices are scientifically valid and promoting, and letting the others wither away, is the best way that clinical psychology can meet the competition from psychiatry and drugs, and meet the demands for managed care. It is the best way for clinical psychology to promote public welfare. And it is the only way for clinical psychology to achieve its aspirations.

Patient Values and Preferences

Stanley B. Messer

According to the Institute of Medicine's definition of quality health care for the 21st century (2001, p. 147), "Evidence-based practice is the integration of best research evidence with clinical expertise and patient values . . . . Patient values refers to the unique preferences, concerns and expectations that each patient brings to a clinical encounter and that must be integrated into clinical decisions if they are to serve the patient." Along with clinical expertise, taking account of patients' concerns and satisfaction is the nonevidence-based part of the Institute's definition. The need for research evidence notwithstanding, the framers of this statement recognized that without paying attention to patients' preferences and what they expect from the practitioner, they are served neither fully nor well.

In agreement with this viewpoint, this position paper argues that, despite their utility for some purposes, neither an evidence-based *DSM* diagnosis nor a manual-based EST is sufficient to treat psychotherapy patients. Diagnoses cannot capture the unique qualities and concerns that patients bring to the clinician nor the specifics of the context in which their problems emerged in the past and are taking place in the present. For that matter, many patients seeking psychotherapy do not carry a formal diagnosis at all, which means that one has to look beyond ESTs for guidance—to empirically supported relationships (ESRs), for example (Norcross, 2002). The strength of ESTs, which are based on randomized clinical trials, or ESRs, which typically rely on correlational data, is their application to patients in general. The clinician, although needing to attend to such empirical findings, must go beyond them to take cognizance of patients' unique qualities, circumstances, and wishes (cf. Goodheart, 2004b). In Beutler's (2004, p. 228) pithy statement, the clinician wants to know, "What can I do, given my own particular strengths and weaknesses, to help this patient, with this problem, at this time?" In other words, nomothetic and idiographic information each have a role to play in clinical practice.

The problems that patients present when first encountering a helping professional may be simply a "calling card." As patients' relationship to the therapist deepens and comfort and trust are more firmly established, the complexity of their lives becomes apparent. The nature of their problems and the specifics for which they are seeking help seem less straightforward. In other words, unless a patient and clinician are intent on treating only the *DSM* disorder as such, for which there may or may not be a prescribed EST, it is necessary to take a broader view of what troubles the patient. Issues are often subtle or may be unconscious, and patients are frequently conflicted and ambivalent about how to proceed with their lives. Although it has been argued that *DSM* disorders can be treated sequentially, say, with one EST followed by another (e.g., Wilson, 1998), patient problems, as I will demonstrate, are typically so intertwined as to preclude entirely separate treatments for each problem area.

This chapter portion presents two cases that illustrate the context-specific and complex nature of what clinicians face daily. In these presentations, I underscore the value of attending to unique patient preferences and satisfactions in effective practice. Certainly, clinicians should draw upon their clinical expertise and be knowledgeable about whatever research evidence exists as it applies to the practice of psychotherapy in general. At the same time, they must be open to patients' special concerns, expectancies, and preferences.

Both of the following two patients presented with symptoms of post-traumatic stress disorder (PTSD). In each case, I drew upon empirical findings and theoretical principles to help treat the PTSD. Nevertheless, as is usually the case, therapy was not straightforward. The nature of the PTSD did not readily fit the ESTs available, the patients wanted more than help with the PTSD despite its initially appearing otherwise, and the specific features and comorbidities of the two patients carrying the same diagnosis were very different. All these features underscore the Institute of Medicine's call for clinicians to take account of patients' unique concerns.

PTSD IN AN ARMY VETERAN: THE CASE OF TOM

Tom is a 26-year-old, single office worker who recently returned from a 1-year tour of army duty in a country where he subsequently spent an additional two years as a civilian worker.

Presenting Problems

Tom came in complaining that since he returned from abroad 3 months ago he has been experiencing disturbing symptoms related to a combat event. He was with soldiers from his unit in an exposed situation where grenades were going off and shots were being fired. He suffered injury to his hand, which had to be bandaged to stop the bleeding, but Tom continued to fight on during the battle. Some scars remain on his hand from the incident, but no physical impairment occurred.

Tom reported that he was emotionally numb at the time and in fact only started thinking about the event when he returned stateside. On the anniversary of the battle, he had a distressing recollection of the battle, which led to heart pounding and labored breathing. At times, he feels the incident was not real, comparing his recollection to looking at a photo. He has been having recurring dreams in which he hears the loud noise of an exploding grenade, sees a flash of light, and looks at his hands to see if they are bloody. He wakes up in a sweat, feeling very anxious, and is disoriented as to his location. He is fearful now in a way that he was not at the time of the incident.

Tom tries to avoid conversations about the trauma, which is why, he said, he delayed coming to see me for three months. He cried when he told his girlfriend about it and has mentioned it to no one but her and me. He has had trouble sleeping, is hyper-vigilant, and experiences a startle response; for example, when a friend tried to hug him from behind, "I put him on the floor." When he walks down the street, he looks over his shoulder, believing that someone may be on a roof about to shoot him. He will look at a stranger and wonder if he has a bomb, although he acknowledges that the thought is ridiculous. He was seeking help overcoming his readily diagnosable PTSD.

In our third session, Tom let me know he has suffered from Tourette's syndrome (TS) since he was a child. In Tom's case, he has mild facial tics around his nose and cheek, drums his fingers on his leg, and occasionally makes soft clicking noises with his throat. He suppressed the symptoms in our first two meetings and perhaps only after feeling a little more comfortable with me did he reveal his condition and manifest the behaviors, which are relatively mild. He wanted help with this problem as well, because he found it had worsened in recent months. Interestingly, it was not only that Tom wished for a decrease in symptoms, but, more important to him, he hoped to become comfortable with himself as a person who has TS. He wanted to be able to manifest the behaviors in public without feeling so self-conscious. In addition to the PTSD and TS, the client suffered from attention-deficit/hyperactivity disorder (ADHD) since childhood. He cannot sit still for too long and has trouble with written expression (dysgraphia).

Tom has very recently met the woman he plans to marry. As the two of them have gotten to know each other better, inevitable differences have surfaced, which he wanted help to understand and negotiate. For example, he finds himself annoyed and upset when his girlfriend spends time with her friends. In addition, as the wedding day approaches, he feels increasingly nervous about taking on new responsibilities and losing his freedom as a single man.

Yet one more issue troubled Tom. While in the military, he felt a great sense of purpose in his life. He garnered respect from others, which raised his self-respect. He also developed close friendships, which have been hard to sustain over time and distance, and which enhances his need for companionship with his girlfriend. He would like to find the kind of part-time work that would improve his self-esteem.

Therapy Choice and Process

Are there evidence-based treatments, pharmacological or psychological, that would be suitable for treating Tom's PTSD? To start with the medication option, some studies support the use of Selective Serotonin Reuptake Inhibitors (SSRIs) in the treatment of PTSD, but more confirmation is needed (Yehuda, Marshall, Penkower, & Wong, 2002). Are the empirical findings particular to combat-induced trauma? There have been four published clinical trials on the use of SSRIs specifically with U.S. war veterans, three of which showed no improvement over placebo, which gave me pause about referring Tom for medication. On the other hand, many of the subjects in these trials had been refractory to other treatments attempted, which was not true of Tom. Of most relevance to our present focus on considering patient preferences, however, was Tom's stance that he would only consider medication as a last resort.

Turning to psychological treatments, is there an EST that fits the case at hand? The answer is "not too well." Therapies for PTSD that are considered efficacious do not pertain to combat but to rape, genocide, and natural disasters (Keane & Barlow, 2002). Furthermore, many PTSD studies apply only to treatment that takes place soon after the trauma (Litz, Gray, Bryant, & Adler, 2002), which was not Tom's situation. Nevertheless, a substantial amount of empirical research on PTSD and other anxiety disorders points to two important treatment factors: anxiety management and exposure, whether *in vivo* or imaginal (Keane & Barlow, 2002). I drew upon these principles in helping Tom talk about the details of the event with the accompanying emotion to help him gain a greater mastery over memories of it. Incidentally, as Keane and Barlow pointed out, it was Janet and Freud who most influenced these CBT approaches to PTSD, so that it was not difficult for me as an "assimilative" psychodynamic therapist to adapt them to the therapy. (Assimilative integration refers to the incorporation of techniques or perspectives from one theoretical orientation into one's preferred, theoretically based therapy; Messer, 2001.)

To view Tom's problems more broadly, a central dynamic ran through the three diagnoses: control. He had always connected the ADHD and TS in his mind, feeling that, because he had some measure of control over the ADHD symptoms, he should be able to do so with the TS symptoms as well, which was not the case. As a child, he was frequently out of control and feared adult situations in which this might occur as well. Tom's way of coping with these fears was taking on heroic tasks such as dangerous army duty. The traumatic combat event he experienced was especially troubling in that he felt not in control. In fact, when recounting the combat event during therapy, he reported that because civilians were close to the action he was not able to shoot back, leaving him feeling particularly helpless.

Regarding his TS, I referred him to a specialty clinic in the area where a therapist helped him learn how to focus less on the tics and "to let go," so that he could concentrate on the matter at hand. The therapist also taught him to meditate. All the while, and in accordance with his request, I worked with him to bolster his self-acceptance as a person with TS. It should be noted that no EST has been established for TS (which is sometimes considered a form of obsessive–compulsive disorder [OCD] or is comorbid with it) and no cure has been found. However, medication (albeit with side effects; Erenberg, 1999) and behavioral techniques, such as habit reversal along with parental support, have been shown to be helpful to children and younger adolescents (e.g., Azrin & Peterson, 1990).

In Tom's therapy, I also paid attention to his current dependency on his girlfriend, which was due to the fact that he no longer had the companionship of his army buddies available, and which created tension between them. He became aware that his dependency was not the result of any purposeful deprivation on her part but rather was because of his own neediness in the current circumstances, which he subsequently took steps to change. Similarly, he found part-time work at a hospital that helped satisfy his need to be helpful to others and which augmented his sense of self-respect.

After 8 months of therapy, the PTSD was very much improved and his concern with the TS lessened. He is in the process of working out his conflicts with his girlfriend. A recent incident, however, indicated that the PTSD still lurks in the background. When firecrackers went off unexpectedly on July 4, he was very startled, his heart raced, and he broke into a cold sweat. However, he calmed down quickly, drew on his girlfriend's soothing support and now feels confident that he will be better able to handle loud noises in the future.

The Take-Home Point in the Case of Tom

The therapy was guided by the client's wishes, expectancies, and concerns about his psychological and neurological problems in conjunction with my knowledge of empirical research, theoretical predilection, and clinical expertise. I did not impose a set treatment on Tom nor did I narrow my focus to the specific diagnosis he initially presented. I followed the patient's wishes to avoid medication if possible and treated issues outside the triple diagnosis he carried. These included his relationship with his girlfriend and his sense of lost purpose in life. Had I not done so, I am quite sure that he would not have been helped as much and would have been much less satisfied with the therapy I offered. Together, we also came to understand the common dynamic thread around his concern with control, which he found enlightening and helpful in becoming less preoccupied with and ruled by it.

I turn now to a second case of PTSD in an effort to demonstrate the variety typically encompassed by any single diagnosis, and the necessity for clinical sensitivity to patients' individual concerns and satisfaction.

PTSD IN A BUSINESS MANAGER: THE CASE OF MRS. T

Mrs. T is a 42-year-old woman who is married with two teenage sons and one preteen daughter. She is of European background and grew up abroad. On September 11, 2001, Mrs. T witnessed the second plane crash into the World Trade Center while knowing that several of her close associates were in that building for a meeting. At the time, she had a very responsible, human relations position at a corporation where she did the hiring. In this role, she arranged the funeral services for two of the employees and served as the liaison for their families, taking care of matters such as insurance and death certificates. She was also an emotional support for the bereaved families.

Presenting Problems

Since a few months after that time and the subsequent loss of her managerial job, she has suffered from frequent crying spells, anxiety attacks, and a sense of despondency. She finds that her thoughts are disconnected, making her unable to focus on any task. Beset by physical problems, such as high blood pressure and a severe facial rash, Mrs. T has also experienced chest pains and heart palpitations, making her feel as if she were having a heart attack. Complaining of diminished libido, the client has less interest in being intimate with her husband, with whom there have been increased marital tensions. Not long after 9/11, Mrs. T withdrew from social activities, preferring to be by herself. Her feelings, except for grief, sadness, and irritability, have been numbed.

Mrs. T came to see me in a very distraught, tearful state despite a year having elapsed since 9/11. Referring to her experience at that time, Mrs. T told me she had learned that one of her female associates left the building with her body on fire and succumbed shortly afterwards. Mrs. T still imagines herself in conversation with the deceased employees who were also her friends. The 9/11 events are replayed in her mind both in the waking state and in her disturbing nightmares. Mrs. T believes she was indirectly responsible for her associates' deaths, which has been one important focus of therapy.

Due to the business downturn in New York City after 9/11, her firm decided not to do any more hiring and Mrs. T was let go. (Job loss is a frequent complication in people with PTSD; Levant, Barbanel, & DeLeon, 2003.) The termination of her high-paying, challenging position was a big blow to her self-esteem. Although she made an effort to find other employment, she was not successful and soon became unable to pursue it further because of her increasingly debilitating symptoms. Her financial situation deteriorated, made worse by her husband losing his job as well. She first sought treatment with a psychologist a few months after 9/11, which was helpful but which she had to terminate when she no longer had insurance coverage. A psychiatrist who prescribed antidepressant and antianxiety medications has also seen her.

Therapy Choice and Process

Is there an EST suitable for Mrs. T? Regarding medication, Mrs. T had already been taking an antidepressant SSRI and a mood stabilizer for a year, which, although helpful, were not sufficient to restore her mental stability and life functioning. With reference to psychological treatments, just as no obvious EST was available for treating Tom, the same was true of Mrs. T. (The jury is still out on the use of eye-movement desensitization and reprocessing [EMDR] for civilian PTSD; Resick & Calhoun, 2001). As in Tom's case, I drew upon the principles of anxiety management and exposure, as recommended by Keane and Barlow (2002), to help Mrs. T face up to and start to master the 9/11 trauma, as well as to reduce her avoidance of social interactions and vocational pursuits.

In both cases, I called upon therapist factors that have been shown to correlate with therapy outcomes. For example, strong empirical evidence shows that therapeutic alliance has a significant and reliable relationship to outcome (Martin, Garske, & Davis, 2000). In a recent review of therapist characteristics and techniques that enhance the therapeutic alliance, Ackerman and Hilsenroth (2003) found the following personal attributes of the therapist to be important: being flexible, honest, respectful, trustworthy, confident, warm, interested, and open. Apropos of techniques, they found the following kinds of interventions to contribute positively to the alliance: exploration, reflection, noting past therapy success, accurate interpretation, facilitating the expression of affect, and attending to the patient's experience.

Although these personal characteristics and technical approaches were of some help in Mrs. T's therapy, they were only partially successful in restoring her mental health. A primary question that arose in my mind was why her symptoms had persisted so long and with such virulence. Was there something more to it than a natural, human response to disaster? Why did she feel so responsible for the fate of her employees who were simply going about their business in a usual way? After all, she did not deliberately send them to their death and was only "responsible" to the extent that she had hired them and made the case for keeping on one of them when the boss wanted to let her go. What individual characteristics and expectancies might be maintaining the symptoms?

When I asked Mrs. T to tell me what came to mind about her feeling responsible for the employees' demise, she informed me that she had long believed that she possessed magical powers, that she was, in her words, "a small deity." I asked her for examples of what she meant. In response, she told me how she is able to locate objects even years after others have lost them simply by holding something of theirs in her hand. As another example, on three separate occasions she had heard a knock on the door although no one was there, and knew instantly that someone in the family had died.

It became clear to both of us that her sense of specialness had played an important role in her slow recovery from the trauma. If she could foresee the future, she posited, why had she not prevented her associates from going into the World Trade Center on that fateful day? When I pointed out that her excessive guilt over their deaths was closely linked to her belief in her special powers, she responded ruefully that if she were more humble she might not be suffering so much. This dynamic also helped her to understand that her sadness was not related only to the 9/11 losses but also to the diminution of her secret sense of being powerful and special. At first, she experienced this revelation as a considerable narcissistic blow (to use the language of self-psychology). With further exploration and reflection about this unusual feature of her personality, her narcissism diminished to some degree as she became more accepting of herself as an ordinary mortal. These reflections also helped her to recognize her own role in her strong reaction to 9/11. Although the insight caused her grief, it also produced relief at its exposure in a safe therapeutic setting.

Very briefly, other features of the therapy included my encouraging Mrs. T to express her mixed feelings about her marriage and her coming to the realization that she no longer wanted the kind of high-powered job she once enjoyed. That job had meant giving up what she now saw as precious time with her growing children and having too little time for herself and her husband. Although Mrs. T is not yet fully recovered after one and a half years of therapy, she is much less subject to anxiety and mood swings, is working part time, and is functioning better on a day-to-day basis. Her medications have also been substantially reduced.

The Take-Home Point in the Case of Mrs. T

An EST, although of some help in this case, could not by itself cover other ground that truly mattered to this woman. Hers was not a case of pure or even typical PTSD, as is also true of many cases that are triply diagnosed or multifaceted. In fact, the complexity of peoples' lives is not readily captured by diagnosis, which is why individual client expectancies, preferences, and concerns need to be addressed. For example, after reviewing the influence of client variables on psychotherapy, Clarkin and Levy (2004, p. 214) concluded that "Nondiagnostic client characteristics may be more useful predictors of psychotherapy outcome than DSM-based diagnoses. The diagnostic categories allow for too much heterogeneity in personality traits to serve as useful predictors or matching variables." Similarly, Beutler et al.'s (2004, p. 291) review of therapist variables led them to state that "evidence is accumulating on the role of patient moderators in determining the effectiveness of interventions." The client's functional impairment, resistance level, coping style, and stage of change and expectations, among other features, are all evidence-based, transdiagnostic means of customizing therapy to improve outcomes (Norcross, 2002). In other words, it is frequently more important to know what kind of patient has the disorder than what kind of disorder the patient has.

CONCLUDING COMMENTS

Many psychological complexities characterize these two cases that, to be treated optimally, call for a knowledge of ESTs, ESRs, therapist variables, client factors, and their interaction; the recognition of intrapsychic and interpersonal themes; a degree of psychotherapy integration; and an appreciation of unique patient needs (Messer, 2004). Both patients suffered from the same condition, PTSD, yet the nature of the trauma, its severity, and effect were very different, similarities notwithstanding. Tom's PTSD is combat related, whereas Mrs. T's is a vicarious response to witnessing the attack on the twin towers and a result of losing friends there. Tom wants medication only as a last resort, whereas Mrs. T is already on medication. Tom is multiply comorbid on *DSM* Axis I, whereas Mrs. T has Axis II traits that complicate the PTSD. One could not simply apply a packaged EST to them even for a diagnosis where such treatments do exist. In both cases, one would be hard pressed to limit the therapy to symptom alleviation without leaving the client dissatisfied.

In this connection, it is difficult to establish a single, consensual definition of success in psychotherapy. To be considered are the perspectives of at least four parties—client, therapist, independent judge, and society—and these are only moderately correlated (Luborsky, 1971). Although I do not advocate ignoring the other perspectives, I have emphasized the necessity of taking into account the patient's viewpoint on what matters regarding choice of treatment, its content, and its effectiveness. The patient's evaluation is a critical component of effective practice. To achieve patient satisfaction with any psychological treatment, the therapist must be flexibly attuned to the vicissitudes of patients' needs and pay careful attention to their unique characteristics, concerns, and preferences.

Dialogue: Convergence and Contention

Geoffrey M. Reed

In their position papers, Kihlstrom and Messer cover much of the ground that I might have in a more complete discussion of my own point of view, as compared to my assigned focus on clinical expertise. In fact, Messer makes the case for clinical expertise more compellingly through his description of two cases, and his conclusions about the necessary ingredients of appropriate treatment are similar to my own. I agree generally with Kihlstrom about the importance of research as a foundation for practice. I concur particularly with his emphasis on psychotherapy outcomes and share the perspective that psychologists will soon be required to document the outcomes of the treatment they provide. There are serious issues about the selection of measures and the funding and infrastructure for outcomes assessment, and we should be placing substantial energy as a field in addressing them.

However, I struggle with Kihlstrom's argument for the same reasons that professional psychologists struggle with the current discussion of EBP: its narrowness and the major implications of what it leaves out. The meaning of his opening assertion that "scientific research is the only process by which ... practitioners should determine what 'evidence' guides EBPs" (p. 23) is unclear. Does this imply that Messer's use of the patient's wishes and goals for treatment, the developing therapy alliance, and his formulation of the deeper themes of control and narcissism does not constitute EBP? Should Messer have instead identified the treatment manual that most closely corresponded to the characteristics of these patients and implemented that treatment as described? Or, given the lack of efficacy trials of PTSD treatments with patients whose clinical characteristics matched those of Messer's patients, should no treatment have been offered at all?

Kihlstrom frames his argument around a dichotomous distinction: Either a practice is "based on rigorous research evidence" or "a kind of folklore" (p. 24, citing Hitt, 2001). However, this claim assumes that knowledge on the basis of evidence other than specific experimental manipulations either cannot be rigorous or cannot be research. Therefore, health services on the basis of such evidence are the modern equivalent of bloodletting. Such dichotomies are polemic and specious. The assertion that there is a lack of evidence supporting psychological practice is based on a highly selective and narrow reading of the literature, the result of filtering the knowledge base of professional psychology through the Division 12 evidentiary criteria to which Kihlstrom refers. By their very nature, these criteria legitimate some approaches to psychotherapy and delegitimate others (Tanenbaum, 2003), one reason that the emotional pitch of the EBP discussion within psychology is so high. A glance at the lists of evidence-based psychological treatments indicates that these are overwhelmingly behavioral or cognitive–behavioral, supporting Kihlstrom's assertion that such treatments are the standard of care. However, this conclusion arises from a confounding of the criteria with the characteristics of the treatments they are used to assess (Tanenbaum, 2005; Westen, Novotny, & Thompson-Brenner, 2004).

Kihlstrom's call for randomized comparisons of one specific treatment or modality to another as the most authoritative source of knowledge can be linked directly to the criteria. This emphasis ignores the two most robust findings in the psychotherapy literature: (a) specific treatment techniques account for little variance in psychotherapy outcomes and (b) the strongest and most consistent predictors of psychotherapy outcomes are the characteristics of the therapist and the nature of the treatment relationship. In this regard, the EBP movement has been remarkably impervious to much of the evidence.

Kihlstrom describes the confluence of the demands of managed care and the rhetoric of science as a positive development that fosters professional accountability. Indeed, organized health care systems are moving to formulate lists of evidence-based treatments with the goal of making these the basis for reimbursement policies, and they are soon likely to attempt to proscribe treatment on this basis. EBP proponents argue that the "tested" treatments that appear on the lists of ESTs, in contrast to the "untested" treatments practiced widely in the community, are what should be offered and reimbursed until equivalent evidence is available for other forms of treatment (an eventuality that the nature of the criteria effectively prevents).

I concur that we have passed the point when it is acceptable to compare psychological treatments to no treatment. But if we propose to use these comparisons as a basis for restricting patient choice, directing reimbursement, or compelling practitioners to use particular approaches, I contend that the required comparison should be between the outcomes of the treatment being tested and those achieved by respected therapists in the community. Such comparisons have virtually never been undertaken (cf., Westen et al., 2004).

Kihlstrom is silent on the commercial interests of the managed care organizations he portrays as allies for accountability. The EBP discussion within managed care focuses clearly on limiting utilization, in spite of compelling evidence that a much higher rate of mental health services should be provided than is currently the case. The great majority of people with mental health problems delay or avoid seeking help, and, when they do, their care is dispersed through a fragmented service delivery system (Narrow, Regier, Rae, Manderscheid, & Locke, 1993; Regier et al., 1993). Many mental health disorders are chronic in nature, contributing heavily to worldwide disability and associated costs (World Health Organization, 2001). Their onset is typically early in life, and the costs and consequences of failing to treat them are cumulative across the lifespan (Kessler et al., 2003). Barely half of those in the U.S. with severe mental heath problems and a minority of those with moderate problems receive any treatment at all (World Health Organization World Mental Health Survey Consortium, 2004), and treatment is often inadequate. If the goal of EBP is to improve U.S. health care, we must replace the pursuit of "psychotherapy tinkering" studies (Humphreys & Tucker, 2002, p. 130) with a focus on how we can best deliver treatment to the population in need and thereby increase the population impact of services for mental health disorders.

In medicine, EBP has three components: The "best research evidence" is integrated with "clinical expertise" and "patient values" in an effort to optimize treatment outcome and patient satisfaction (Institute of Medicine, 2001, p. 147). So far as psychotherapy is concerned, the three contributors to this chapter are all agreed on this general formula, in principle, but disagree about the place that controlled research occupies in the hierarchy of practice-relevant evidence. Geoffrey Reed laments the "deprofessionalization of health professionals" (p. 14) and reasserts the "paramount importance" (p. 19) of clinical expertise, by which he means the combination of "a body of specialized professional knowledge" with the clinician's "individual experiences" (p. 18). Stanley Messer, for his part, argues that research evidence about "patients in general" is insufficient when it comes to "patients' unique qualities, circumstances, and wishes" (p. 32). Both arguments make good points but do not contradict the fundamental proposition that good treatment relies, first and foremost, on good research.

To see why this is so, let us return to the definition of EBP given previously, and cited by both Reed and Messer. When diagnosing and treating illness, physicians apply the best medical knowledge to the individual case. When a patient presents with a fever, for example, they understand, from medical science, that fevers are symptoms of underlying infections. They then use scientifically validated laboratory tests to determine the nature of that infection and prescribe a particular antibiotic that scientific evidence, summarized by practice guidelines, suggests will be most effective in treating that particular infection. If several appropriate treatments are available, the physician may prescribe the one that is older, and thus whose side effects and risks are better known. Or perhaps he or she will prescribe a generic drug that is cheaper than a proprietary product. If this does not work, the physician may try another antibiotic or order another panel of tests. But in any event, scientific evidence informs the entire process from beginning to end. Why should psychotherapy be any different?

Of course, practitioner expertise is important. But expertise in what? In medicine, the physician's expertise consists largely in applying scientific evidence, and scientifically based techniques, to the diagnosis and treatment of the individual case. Like psychotherapists, physicians treat individual patients, but this offers no dispensation from the obligation to base treatments on the best scientific evidence. To continue the fever example: If the patient presents some contraindication to the treatment of first choice, then the physician will select an alternative that has also been proven effective, but which bypasses the relevant contraindications. The physician may also have expertise in building rapport with patients, taking a history, performing a physical examination, finding a vein, and delivering bad news. But these practical skills mean nothing unless the physician is making decisions on the basis of the best evidence available. Why should psychotherapy be any different?

And besides, how do we know that a clinician is an expert? We know that someone is an expert because we have empirical evidence concerning the outcomes of his or her encounters with patients. That evidence comes from research. In the classic scientist–practitioner model, the practitioner's scientific credentials come in two forms. First and foremost is the assumption that psychotherapy would be based on the best available knowledge about mind and behavior, and the best available evidence as to what specific treatments work best for specific conditions. These results of nomothetic research are to be complemented by idiographic research in which practitioners study their own outcomes. Physicians acquire reputations as experts, and hospitals acquire reputations as collections of experts, because empirical evidence shows that their patients get better. The collection of such data is simply another form of research. Why should psychotherapy be any different?

And, of course, patient values are important too, but they do not trump scientific evidence. With few exceptions, mostly in the domain of public health, a patient is free to reject a physician's treatment plan, but the plan itself must be based on the best available scientific evidence. A patient may appear for a diagnosis to find out what is wrong with him or her but ultimately decline treatment for religious or financial reasons. Or the patient may prefer palliative care to active treatment that is too risky or has undesirable side effects. A patient may prefer to be treated by someone of the same gender. All these patient values, and others like them, can be accommodated within the framework of EBP by allowing patients to select, among scientifically validated practices, those that are most compatible with their values. Why should psychotherapy be any different?

Even though the presenting case may be complex, there is no reason to think that EBPs do not provide the best approaches to treatment. Arguably, the most important "therapist factor" is the wisdom to be guided by available research evidence, even if the research base does not precisely match the features of the case at hand. And the most important feature of the relationship between the patient and the therapist is the patient's confidence that what the therapist does is based on the best available scientific evidence.

The constraints of EBP, including the placement of scientific research at the top of the hierarchy of evidence, over and above expertise and patient values, do not in any respect "deprofessionalize" health care. The professional status of psychotherapy and the professional autonomy of clinical psychology from psychiatry depend critically on the assumption that therapeutic practices are grounded in a firm base of scientific evidence. Professions are defined precisely by practices on the basis of specialized bodies of knowledge (Abbott,

1988; Friedson, 1970; Starr, 1982). That is what it means to be a professional, as opposed to an amateur or a dilettante. If clinical psychology is to retain its status as a profession, it needs more research, not less; the best research, not excuses; and sooner, rather than later.

Stanley B. Messer

A fundamental difference in outlook exists between the point of view presented by Reed and me, on the one hand, and by Kihlstrom, on the other. Reed and I emphasize the importance of taking full account of the nature of the players involved in EBP, whether it is the clinician (Reed) or the client (Messer). I would characterize our stance as falling within the romantic vision, which prizes individuality, subjectivity, and the unique qualities of every human being. By contrast, Kihlstrom's approach views individuals as interchangeable and their subjectivity an unfortunate impediment, particularly in the assessment of psychotherapy outcomes. Closely tied to this outlook is his strong reliance on the medical metaphor for describing psychological problems in which one diagnoses and treats psychopathology much like one diagnoses and treats cancer. In this view, psychotherapy is equivalent to a drug, a control condition is akin to a placebo, techniques are administered via manualized instructions, and outcomes are measured in labs through the analog of blood tests. The approach valorizes mechanism, objectivity, and technical aspects of therapy over artistry, client subjectivity, and quality of the therapeutic relationship. In this brief commentary, I will stress the importance of attending to the patient's needs and preferences and will point to some drawbacks of Kihlstrom's more objective and externally oriented position.

Regarding psychotherapy outcome measurement, Kihlstrom criticizes the *Consumer Reports* study, which used patients' self-reported satisfaction with their treatment "instead of objective evidence of actual improvement" (p. 26). Within an epistemological stance that takes patients' subjectivity seriously, their own evaluation of outcome is as "actual" as any other form of outcome assessment. Although it is different than an objective assessment, this does not make it any less real or less important, especially in the context of the highly personal realm of psychotherapy. In the same vein, Kihlstrom argues that "it is long past time that psychology began to move away from questionnaires and rating scales, and toward a new generation of assessment procedures on objective laboratory tests of psychopathology" (p. 29). If we were to do so, however, how would we judge results that showed a lessening of psychopathology on a physiological measure, alongside a patient's continuing unhappiness with the therapy or him- or herself? For example, what if the patient's anxiety subsided after treatment, but she was still unable to achieve the intimacy she craves and continued to feel lonely and isolated? Her subjectively experienced life satisfaction, it can be argued, is every bit as important as the decrease of pathology as gauged by objective instruments.

Along similar lines, Kihlstrom is more interested in how third parties view the results of therapy than he is in the participants' satisfaction, giving as one example that couples who go through therapy "might reasonably expect to have happier children than they did before" (p. 29). What if, as a result of therapy, the couple decides to divorce, which leads to greater ultimate happiness for them but less immediate happiness for their children? In other words, can we judge the outcome of the therapy only or primarily by the children's assessment or should we not consider the major participants' desires as well? Further regarding the role of third parties, Kihlstrom states, "employers who pay for their employees to participate in alcohol or drug abuse treatment might reasonably ask if their employees do, in fact, become more productive after treatment" (p. 29). What if the client comes to realize after therapy that she is in the wrong job or even the wrong career, which has contributed to her alcohol or drug abuse? She then stops drinking or taking other drugs, leaves the company, goes back to school, and eventually becomes both happier and more productive elsewhere. Should the company be paying only for an improvement in its bottom line? Is this the kind of corporate outlook that we, as mental health practitioners, wish to promote?

Finally, Kihlstrom also proposes that we assess psychotherapy outcomes according to whether third parties "feel that their own life satisfaction has improved" (p. 29) because of the client's therapy. He refers, in this connection, to the client's family and coworkers. (It should be noted here that Kihlstrom is unwilling to grant epistemological legitimacy to the client's felt improvement in his or her life satisfaction but is prepared to do so for a third party.) But imagine, for the moment, a timid woman who becomes more self-confident, assertive, and challenging of her domineering husband because of therapy. In addition, she begins to stand up for herself at work, where her boss has quite regularly taken advantage of her timidity. Should we consider her husband's or boss's decreased satisfaction as an indicator of a failed therapy? Coming to such a conclusion is one of the risks of relying on outside parties in the service of objectivity.

To reiterate my main point, there is no escape from the subjectivity of the patient whose preferences, values, and expectations the clinician must always keep firmly in mind. Nor is there any escape from the valuative dimension of therapy, which reminds us that decisions about the way we characterize peoples' problems, conduct therapy, and assess outcomes are not determined by scientific criteria alone (Messer & Woolfolk, 1998).

REFERENCES

Abbott, A. (1988). *The system of professions: An essay on the division of expert labor.* Chicago: University of Chicago Press.

Abelson, R. P. (1995). *Statistics as principled argument.* Hillsdale, NJ: Erlbaum.

Ackerman, S. J., & Hilsenroth, M. J. (2003). A review of therapist characteristics and techniques positively impacting the therapeutic alliance. *Clinical Psychology Review, 23,* 1–33.

American Psychiatric Association. (1994). *Diagnostic and statistical manual of mental disorders* (4th ed.). Washington, DC: Author.

Anderson, T., & Strupp, H. H. (1996). The ecology of psychotherapy research. *Journal of Consulting and Clinical Psychology, 64,* 776–782.

Azrin, N. H., & Peterson, A. L. (1990). Treatment of Tourette syndrome by habit reversal: A waiting-list control group comparison. *Behavior Therapy, 21,* 305–318.

Barlow, D. (1996). The effectiveness of psychotherapy: Science and policy. *Clinical Psychology: Science and Practice, 1,* 109–122.

Barlow, D. H. (in press). Psychological treatments. *American Psychologist.*

Barlow, D. H., Gorman, J. M., Shear, M. K., & Woods, S. W. (2000). Cognitive-behavior therapy, imipramine, or their combination for panic disorder: A randomized controlled trial. *Journal of the American Medical Association, 283,* 2529–2536.

Basco, M. R., Bostic, J. Q., Davies, D., Rush, A. J., Witte, B., Hendrickse, W., et al. (2000). Methods to improve diagnostic accuracy in a community mental health setting. *American Journal of Psychiatry, 157,* 1599–1605.

Beck, A. T. (1970). Cognitive therapy: Nature and relation to behavior therapy. *Behavior Therapy, 1,* 184–200.

Bergin, A. E. (1966). Some implications of psychotherapy research for therapeutic practice. *Journal of Abnormal Psychology, 71,* 235–246.

Bergin, A. E., & Strupp, H. H. (1970). New directions in psychotherapy research. *Journal of Abnormal Psychology, 76*(1), 13–26.

Beutler, L. E. (1998). Identifying empirically supported treatments: What if we didn't? *Journal of Consulting and Clinical Psychology, 66,* 113–120.

Beutler, L. E. (2000). Empirically based decision making in clinical practice. *Prevention and Treatment, 3*(27). Retrieved November 29, 2004, from http://journals.apa.org/prevention/volume3/pre0030027a.html

Beutler, L. E. (2004). The empirically supported treatments movement: A scientist–practitioner's response. *Clinical Psychology: Science and Practice, 11,* 225–229.

Beutler, L. E., Malik, M., Alimohamed, S., Harwood, M. T., Talebi, H., Noble, S., et al. (2004). Therapist variables. In M. J. Lambert (Ed.), *Bergin and Garfield's handbook of psychotherapy and behavior change* (5th ed., pp. 227–306). New York: Wiley.

Beutler, L. E., Moleiro, C., & Talebi, H. (2002). How practitioners can systematically use empirical evidence in treatment selection. *Journal of Clinical Psychology, 58,* 1199–1212.

Bransford, D., Brown, A. L., & Cocking, R. R. (Eds.). (1999). *How people learn: Brain, mind, experience, and school.* Washington, DC: National Academy of Sciences.

Carpinello, S. E., Rosenberg, L., Stone, J., Schwager, M., & Felton, C. J. (2002). New York State's campaign to implement evidence-based practices for people with serious mental disorders. *Psychiatric Services, 53*(2), 153–155.

Carter, J. A. (2002). Integrating science and practice: Reclaiming the science in practice. *Journal of Clinical Psychology, 58,* 1285–1290.

Castonguay, L. G., Goldfried, M. R., Wiser, S., Raue, P. J., & Hayes, A. M. (1996). Predicting the effect of cognitive therapy for depression: A study of unique and common factors. *Journal of Consulting and Clinical Psychology 64,* 497–504.

Chambless, D. L., & Ollendick, T. H. (2001). Empirically supported psychological interventions: Controversies and evidence. *Annual Review of Psychology, 52,* 685–716.

Chambless, D. L., Sanderson, W. C., Shoham, V., Johnson, S. B., Pope, K. S., Crits-Christoph, P., et al. (1996). An update on empirically validated therapies. *The Clinical Psychologist, 49*(2), 5–18.

Chlebowski, R. T., Hendrix, S. L., Langer, R. D., Stefanick, M. L., Gass, M., Lane, D., et al. (2003). Influence of estrogen plus progestin on breast cancer and mammography in healthy postmenopausal women. *Journal of the American Medical Association, 289,* 3243–3253.

Chorpita, B. F., Yim, L. M., Donkervoet, J. C., Arensdorf, A., Amundsen, M. J., McGee, C., et al. (2002). Toward large-scale implementation of empirically supported treatments for children: A review and observations by the Hawaii empirical basis to services task force. *Clinical Psychology: Science and Practice, 9,* 165–190.

Clarkin, J. F., & Levy, K. N. (2004). The influence of client variables on psychotherapy. In M. J. Lambert (Ed.), *Bergin and Garfield's handbook of psychotherapy and behavior change* (5th ed., pp.194–226). New York: Wiley.

Cohen, J. (1990). Things I have learned (so far). *American Psychologist, 45,* 1304–1312.

Cohen, J. (1994). The earth is round (p < .05). *American Psychologist, 49,* 997–1003.

Cohen, R. A., & Ni, H. (2004). *Health insurance coverage for the civilian noninstitutionalized population: Early release estimates from the National Health Interview Survey, January–June 2003.* Retrieved November 19, 2004, from www.cdc.gov/nchs/nhis.htm

Davidoff, F., Haynes, B., Sackett, D. L., & Smith, R. (1995). Evidence based medicine. *British Medical Journal, 310,* 1085–1086.

Davidson, K. W., Goldstein, M., Kaplan, R. M., Kaufmann, P. G., Knatterud, G. L., Orleans, C. T., et al. (2003). Evidence-based behavioral medicine: What is it, and how do we achieve it? *Annals of Behavioral Medicine, 26,* 161–171.

DeRubeis, R. J., Hollon, S. D., Amsterdam, J. D., Shelton, R. C., Young, P. R., Salomon, R. M., et al. (in press). Cognitive therapy vs. medications in the treatment of moderate to severe depression. *Archives of General Psychiatry.*

Dobson, K. S. (1989). A meta-analysis of the efficacy of cognitive therapy for depression. *Journal of Consulting and Clinical Psychology, 57,* 414–419.

Elkin, I., Shea, M. T., Watkins, J. T., Imber, S. D., Sotsky, S. M., Collins, J. F., et al. (1989). National Institute of Mental Health Treatment of Depression Collaborative Research Program: General effectiveness of treatments. *Archives of General Psychiatry, 46,* 971–982.

Erenberg, G. (1999). Tics. In R. A. Dershewitz (Ed.), *Ambulatory pediatric care* (3rd ed., pp. 806–809). Philadelphia: Lippincott–Raven.

Evidence-Based Medicine Working Group. (1992). Evidence-based medicine: A new approach to the teaching of medicine. *Journal of the American Medical Association, 268,* 2420–2425.

Eysenck, H. J. (1952). The effects of psychotherapy: An evaluation. *Journal of Consulting Psychology, 16,* 319–324.

Fiske, D. W., Hunt, H. F., Luborsky, L., Orne, M. T., Parloff, M. B., Reiser, M. F., et al. (1970). Planning of research on effectiveness of psychotherapy. *Archives of General Psychiatry, 22,* 22–32.

Fox, P. D., & Fama, T. (Eds.). (1996). *Managed care and chronic illness: Challenges and opportunities.* Gaithersburg, MD: Aspen Publishers.

Frank, J. D. (1961). *Persuasion and healing.* Baltimore: Johns Hopkins University Press.

Friedson, E. (1970). *Profession of medicine: A study of the sociology of applied knowledge.* Chicago: University of Chicago Press.

Garb, H. N. (1998). *Studying the clinician: Judgment research and psychological assessment.* Washington, DC: American Psychological Association.

Garfield, S. L., & Bergin, A. E. (1971). Therapeutic conditions and outcome. *Journal of Abnormal Psychology, 77,* 108–114.

Gawande, A. (2004, December 6). The bell curve: What happens when patients find out how good their doctors really are? *The New Yorker,* 82–91.

Gleitman, H., Nachmias, J., & Neisser, U. (1954). The S-R reinforcement theory of extinction. *Psychological Review, 61,* 23–33.

Goodheart, C. D. (2004a). Multiple streams of evidence for psychotherapy practice. In C. D. Goodheart & R. F. Levant (Co-chairs), *Best psychotherapy based on the integration of research evidence, clinical judgment, and patient values.* Symposium presented at the 112th Annual Convention of the American Psychological Association, Honolulu, HI.

Goodheart, C. D. (2004b). Evidence-based practice and the endeavor of psychotherapy. *The Independent Practitioner, 24,* 6–10.

Gusfield, J. R. (1981). *The culture of public problems: Drinking-driving and the symbolic order.* Chicago: University of Chicago Press.

Haynes, B. P., Devereaux, P. J., & Gordon, H. G. (2002). Clinical expertise in the era of evidence-based medicine and patient choice. *Evidence-Based Medicine Notebook, 7,* 1–3.

Hersh, A. L., Stefanick, M. L., & Stafford, R. S. (2004). National use of postmenopausal hormone therapy: Annual trends and response to recent evidence. *Journal of the American Medical Association, 291,* 47–53.

Hitt, J. (2001, December 9). Evidence-based medicine. *New York Times Magazine*, p. 68.

Hollon, S. D., DeRubeis, R. J., Shelton, R. C., Amsterdam, J. D., Salomon, R. M., O'Reardon, J. P., et al. (in press). Prevention of relapse following cognitive therapy versus medications in moderate to severe depression. *Archives of General Psychiatry*.

Humphreys, K., & Tucker, J. A. (2002). Toward more responsive and effective intervention systems for alcohol-related problems. *Addiction, 97*, 126–132.

Huppert, J. D., Bufka, L. F., Barlow, D. H., Gorman, J. M., Shear, M. K., & Woods, S. W. (2001). Therapists, therapist variables, and cognitive–behavioral therapy outcome in a multicenter trial for panic disorder. *Journal of Consulting and Clinical Psychology, 69*, 747–755.

Institute of Medicine. (2001). *Crossing the quality chasm: A new health system for the 21st century*. Washington, DC: National Academy Press.

Jacobson, N. S., Follette, W. C., & Revenstorf, D. (1984). Psychotherapy outcome research: Methods for reporting variability and evaluating clinical significance. *Behavior Therapy, 15*, 336–352.

Jacobson, N. S., & Hollon, S. D. (1996). Prospects for future comparisons between drugs and psychotherapy. *Journal of Consulting and Clinical Psychology, 64*, 104–108.

Jacobson, N. S., & Revenstorf, D. (1988). Statistics for assessing the clinical significance of psychotherapy techniques: Issues, problems, and new developments. *Behavioral Assessment, 10*, 133–145.

Kahneman, D., & Tversky, A. (1973). On the psychology of prediction. *Psychological Review, 80*, 237–251.

Keane, T. M., & Barlow, D. H. (2002). Posttraumatic stress disorder. In D. H. Barlow (Ed.), *Anxiety and its disorders* (2nd ed.). New York: Guilford Press.

Keckley, P. H. (2003). *Evidence-based medicine and managed care: Applications, challenges, opportunities—Results of a national program to assess emerging applications of evidence-based medicine to medical management strategies in managed care*. Nashville, TN: Vanderbilt University Center for Evidence-based Medicine.

Keller, M. B., McCullough, J. P., Klein, D. N., Arnow, B., Dunner, D. L., Gelenberg, A. J., et al (2000). A comparison of nefazodone, the cognitive behavioral-analysis system of psychotherapy, and their combination for the treatment of chronic depression. *New England Journal of Medicine, 342*, 1462–1470.

Kessler, R. C., Berglund, P., Demler, O., Jin, R., Koretz, D., Merikangas, K. R., et al. (2003). The epidemiology of major depressive disorder: Results from the National Comorbidity Survey Replication (NCS-R). *Journal of the American Medical Association, 289*, 3095–3105.

Kihlstrom, J. F. (1979). Hypnosis and psychopathology: Retrospect and prospect. *Journal of Abnormal Psychology, 88*(5), 459–473.

Kihlstrom, J. F. (1998). If you've got an effect, test its significance: If you've got a weak effect, do a meta-analysis [Commentary on "Précis of Statistical significance: Rationale, validity, and utility" by S. L. Chow]. *Behavioral and Brain Sciences, 21*, 205–206.

Kihlstrom, J. F. (2002a). Mesmer, the Franklin Commission, and hypnosis: A counterfactual essay. *International Journal of Clinical and Experimental Hypnosis, 50,* 408–419.

Kihlstrom, J. F. (2002b). To honor Kraepelin . . . : From symptoms to pathology in the diagnosis of mental illness. In L. E. Beutler & M. L. Malik (Eds.), *Alternatives to the DSM* (pp. 279–303). Washington, DC: American Psychological Association.

Kihlstrom, J. F., & Kihlstrom, L. C. (1998). Integrating science and practice in an environment of managed care. In D. K. Routh & R. J. DeRubeis (Eds.), *The science of clinical psychology: Accomplishments and future directions* (pp. 281–293). Washington, DC: American Psychological Association.

Kihlstrom, J. F., & McGlynn, S. M. (1991). *Experimental research in clinical psychology, the clinical psychology handbook* (2nd ed., pp. 239–257). New York: Pergamon Press.

Kihlstrom, J. F., & Nasby, W. (1981). Cognitive tasks in clinical assessment: An exercise in applied psychology. In P. C. Kendall & S. D. Hollon (Eds.), *Cognitive–behavioral interventions: Assessment methods* (pp. 287–317). New York: Academic Press.

Klein, D. N., Schwartz, J. E., Santiago, N. J., Vivian, D., Vocisano, C., Castonguay, L. G., et al. (2003). Therapeutic alliance in depression treatment: Controlling for prior change and patient characteristics. *Journal of Consulting and Clinical Psychology, 71,* 997–1006.

Klein, G. (1998). *Sources of power: How people make decisions.* Cambridge, MA: MIT Press.

Kotkin, M., Daviet, C., & Gurin, J. (1996). The *Consumer Reports* mental health survey. *American Psychologist, 51,* 1080–1082.

Lampropoulos, G. K., & Spengler, P. M. (2002). Introduction: Reprioritizing the role of science in a realistic version of the scientist–practitioner model. *Journal of Clinical Psychology, 58,* 1195–1197.

Levant, R. F. (2004). The empirically validated treatments movement: A practitioner/educator perspective. *Clinical Psychology: Science and Practice, 11,* 219–224.

Levant, R. F., Barbanel, L. H., & DeLeon, P. H. (2003). Psychology's response to terrorism. In F. Moghaddam & A. J. Marsella (Eds.), *Understanding terrorism: Psychological roots, consequences and interventions* (pp. 265–282). Washington, DC: American Psychological Association.

Lispey, M. W., & Wilson, D. B. (1993). The efficacy of psychological, educational, and behavioral treatment: Confirmation from meta-analysis. *American Psychologist, 48,* 1181–1209.

Litz, B. T., Gray, M. J., Bryant, R. A., & Adler, A. B. (2002). Early intervention for trauma: Current status and future directions. *Clinical Psychology: Science and Practice, 9,* 112–134.

Lohr, J. M., Lilienfeld, S. O., Tolin, D. F., & Herbert, J. D. (1999). Eye movement desensitization and reprocessing: An analysis of specific versus nonspecific treatment factors. *Journal of Anxiety Disorders, 13*(1–2), 185–207.

Luborsky, L. (1971). Perennial mystery of poor agreement among criteria for psychotherapy outcome. *Journal of Consulting and Clinical Psychology, 37,* 316–319.

Luborsky, L., Diguer, L., Seligman, D. A., Rosenthal, R., Krause, E. D., Johnson, S., et al. (1999). The researcher's own therapy allegiances: A "wild card" in comparisons of treatment efficacy. *Clinical Psychology: Science and Practice, 6*, 95–106.

Luborsky, L., Singer, B. H., & Luborsky, L. (1975). Comparative studies of psychotherapies: Is it true that "everyone has won and all must have prizes"? *Archives of General Psychiatry, 32*, 995–1008.

Magner, L. N. (1992). *A history of medicine.* New York: Dekker Press.

Manson, J. E., Hsia, J., Johnson, K. C., Rossouw, J. E., Assaf, A. R., Lasser, N. L., et al. (2003). Estrogen plus progestin and the risk of coronary heart disease. *New England Journal of Medicine, 349*, 523–534.

Martin, D. J., Garske, J. P., & Davis, M. K. (2000). Relation of the therapeutic alliance with outcome and other variables: A meta-analytic review. *Journal of Consulting and Clinical Psychology, 68*, 438–450.

Maxfield, M., Achman, L., & Cook, A. (2004). *National estimates of mental health insurance benefits* (DHHS Publication No. SMA 04-3872). Rockville, MD: Center for Mental Health Services, Substance Abuse, and Mental Health Services Administration.

Meehl, P. E. (1954). *Clinical vs. statistical prediction.* Minneapolis: University of Minnesota Press.

Mental health: Does therapy help? (1995, November). *Consumer Reports,* 734–739.

Messer, S. B. (2001). Introduction to the Special Issue on assimilative integration. *Journal of Psychotherapy Integration, 11*, 1–4.

Messer, S. B. (2004). Evidence-based practice: Beyond empirically supported treatments. *Professional Psychology, 35*, 580–588.

Messer, S. B., & Woolfolk, P. L. (1998). Philosophical issues in psychotherapy. *Clinical Psychology: Science and Practice, 5*, 251–263.

Meyer, G. J., Finn, S. E., Eyde, L. D., Kay, G. G., Moreland, K. L., Dies, R. R., et al. (2001). Psychological testing and psychological assessment: A review of evidence and issues. *American Psychologist, 56*, 128–165.

Moynihan, D. P. (1993). Defining deviancy down. *American Scholar, 62*(1), 17–30.

Muñoz, R. F., Hollon, S. D., McGrath, E., Rehm, L. P., & VandenBos, G. R. (1994). On the AHCPR depression in primary care guidelines: Further considerations for practitioners. *American Psychologist, 49*, 42–61.

Narrow, W. E., Regier, D. A., Rae, D. S., Manderscheid, R. W., & Locke, B. A. (1993). Use of services by persons with mental and addictive disorders. *Archives of General Psychiatry, 50*, 95–107.

Nasby, W., & Kihlstrom, J. F. (1986). Cognitive assessment in personality and psychopathology. In R. E. Ingram (Ed.), *Information processing approaches to psychopathology and clinical psychology* (pp. 217–239). New York: Academic Press.

Nathan, P. E. (1998). Practice guidelines: Not yet ideal. *American Psychologist, 53*, 290–299.

Nathan, P. E., & Gorman, J. M. (Eds.). (1998). *A guide to treatments that work.* New York: Oxford University Press.

National Institutes of Health. (2004). *State implementation of evidence-based practices: Bridging science and service* (NIMH and SAMHSA Publication No. RFA MH-03-007). Retrieved November 19, 2004, from http://grants1.nih.gov/grants/guide/rfa-files/RFA-MH-03-007.html

Nisbett, R. E., & Ross, L. (1980). *Human inference: Strategies and shortcomings of social judgment.* Englewood Cliffs, NJ: Prentice Hall.

Norcross, J. C. (Ed.). (2002). *Psychotherapy relationships that work.* New York: Oxford University Press.

Norcross, J. C., & Hill, C. E. (2004). Empirically supported therapy relationships. *The Clinical Psychologist, 57*(3), 19–24.

Ogles, B. M., Lambert, M. J., & Sawyer, J. D. (1995). Clinical significance of the National Institute of Mental Health Treatment of Depression Collaborative Research Program data. *Journal of Consulting and Clinical Psychology, 63,* 321–326.

Porter, R. (1997). *The greatest benefit to mankind: A medical history of humanity.* New York: Norton.

Rapaport, D., Gill, M. M., & Schafer, R. (1968). *Diagnostic psychological testing* (Rev. ed. by R. R. Holt). New York: International Universities Press.

Regier, D. A., Narrow, W. E., Rae, D. S., Manderscheid, R. W., Locke, B. Z., & Goodwin, F. K. (1993). The de facto U.S. mental and addictive disorders service system. *Archives of General Psychiatry, 50,* 607–611.

Resick, P. A., & Calhoun, K. S. (2001). Posttraumatic stress disorder. In D. H. Barlow (Ed.), *Clinical handbook of psychological disorders* (3rd ed., pp. 60–113). New York: Guilford Press.

Rosen, G. M., & Davison, G. C. (2003). Psychology should list empirically supported principles of change (ESPs) and not credential trademarked therapies or other treatment packages. *Behavior Modification, 27*(3), 300–312.

Rosenberg, W., & Donald, A. (1995). Evidence based medicine: An approach to clinical problem-solving. *British Medical Journal, 310,* 1122–1126.

Rosenblatt, A., & Attkisson, C. C. (1993). Assessing outcomes for sufferers of severe mental disorder: A conceptual framework and review. *Evaluation and Program Planning, 16,* 347–363.

Rosenthal, D., & Frank, J. D. (1956). Psychotherapy and the placebo effect. *Psychological Bulletin, 55,* 294–302.

Rosenthal, R. (1990). How are we doing in soft psychology? *American Psychologist, 45,* 775–777.

Sackett, D. L., Rosenberg, W. M. C., Muir-Gray, J. A., Haynes, R. B., & Richardson, W. S. (1996). Evidence based medicine: What it is and what it isn't. *British Medical Journal, 312,* 71–72.

Sackett, D. L., Straus, S. E., Richardson, W. S., Rosenberg, W., & Haynes, R. B. (1997). *Evidence-based medicine: How to practise and teach EBM.* Edinburgh, Scotland: Churchill Livingstone.

Sackett, D. L., Straus, S. E., Richardson, W. S., Rosenberg, W., & Haynes, R. B. (2000). *Evidence based medicine: How to practice and teach EBM* (2nd ed.). London: Churchill Livingstone.

Sechrest, L., McKnight, P., & McKnight, K. (1996). Calibration of measures for psychotherapy outcome studies. *American Psychologist, 51,* 1065–1071.

Seligman, M. E. P. (1995). The effectiveness of psychotherapy: The *Consumer Reports* study. *American Psychologist, 50,* 965–974.

Seligman, M. E. P., & Levant, R. F. (1998). Managed care policies rely on inadequate science. *Professional Psychology: Research and Practice, 29,* 211–212.

Smith, M. L., & Glass, G. V. (1977). Meta-analysis of psychotherapy outcome studies. *American Psychologist, 32,* 752–760.

Smith, M. L., Glass, G. V., & Miller, R. L. (1980). *The benefits of psychotherapy.* Baltimore: Johns Hopkins University Press.

Starr, P. (1982). *The social transformation of American medicine: The rise of a sovereign profession and the making of a vast industry.* New York: Basic Books.

Strupp, H. H., & Bergin, A. E. (1969). Some empirical and conceptual bases for coordinated research in psychotherapy: A critical review of issues, trends, and evidence. *International Journal of Psychiatry, 7,* 18–90.

Tanenbaum, S. J. (1999). Evidence and expertise: The challenge of the outcomes movement to medical professionalism. *Academic Medicine, 74,* 757–763.

Tanenbaum, S. J. (2003). Evidence-based practice in mental health: Practical weaknesses meet political strengths. *Journal of Evaluation in Clinical Practice, 9,* 287–301.

Tanenbaum, S. J. (2005). Evidence-based practice as mental health policy: Three controversies and a caveat. *Health Affairs, 24,* 163–173.

Task Force. (1995). Training in and dissemination of empirically validated psychological treatments: Report and recommendations of the Task Force on Promotion and Dissemination of Psychological Procedures of Division 12 (Clinical Psychology) of the American Psychological Association. *Clinical Psychologist, 48,* 3–23.

U.S. Census Bureau News. (2004, August 26). *Income stable, poverty up, numbers of Americans with and without health insurance rise, Census Bureau reports.* Retrieved November 19, 2004, from www.census.gov/Press-Release/www/releases/archives/income_wealth/002484.html

Vedantam, S. (2004, September 9). Journals insist drug manufacturers register all trials. *The Washington Post,* p. A02.

Ventura, J., Liberman, R. P., Green, M. F., Shaner, A., & Mintz, J. (1998). Training and quality assurance with Structured Clinical Interview for *DSM-IV* (SCID-I/P). *Psychiatry Research, 79,* 163–173.

Wampold, B. E. (2001). *The great psychotherapy debate: Model, methods, and findings.* Mahwah, NJ: Erlbaum.

Westen, D., & Morrison, K. (2001). A multidimensional meta-analysis of treatments for depression, panic, and generalized anxiety disorder: An empirical examination of the status of empirically supported therapies. *Journal of Consulting and Clinical Psychology, 60,* 875–899.

Westen, D., Novotny, C., & Thompson-Brenner, H. (2004). The empirical status of empirically supported therapies: Assumptions, methods, and findings. *Psychological Bulletin, 130,* 631–663.

Westen, D., & Weinberger, J. (in press). In praise of clinical judgment: Meehl's forgotten legacy. *American Psychologist.*

Wilson, G. T. (1998). Manual-based treatment and clinical practice. *Clinical Psychology: Science and Practice, 5,* 363–375.

Wilson, G. T., & Davison, G. C. (1971). Processes of fear reduction in systematic desensitization: Animal studies. *Psychological Bulletin, 76,* 1–14.

Wolpe, J. (1958). *Psychotherapy by reciprocal inhibition.* Stanford, CA: Stanford University Press.

Wood, J. M., Nezworski, M. T., Lilienfeld, S. O., & Garb, H. N. (2003). *'What's wrong with the Rorschach? Science confronts the controversial inkblot test.* New York: Jossey-Bass.

World Health Organization. (2001). *The World Health Report 2000; Health systems: Improving performance.* Geneva, Switzerland: Author.

World Health Organization World Mental Health Survey Consortium. (2004). Prevalence, severity, and unmet need for treatment of mental health disorders in the World Health Organization World Mental Health surveys. *Journal of the American Medical Association, 291,* 2581–2590.

Yates, A. J. (1970). *Behavior therapy.* New York: Wiley.

Yehruda, R., Marshall, R., Penkower, A., & Wong, C. M. (2002). Pharmacological treatments for posttraumatic stress disorder. In P. E. Nathan & J. M. Goman (Eds.), *A guide to treatments that work* (2nd ed., pp. 411–445). New York: Oxford University Press.

Zarin, D. A., Young, J. L., & West, J. C. (in press). Challenges to evidence-based medicine: A comparison of patients and treatments in randomized controlled trials with patients and treatments in a practice research network. *Social Psychiatry and Psychiatric Epidemiology.*

2

WHAT QUALIFIES AS RESEARCH ON WHICH TO JUDGE EFFECTIVE PRACTICE?

Case Studies

William B. Stiles

In this position paper, I first discuss how scientific research provides quality control on theory. Then I argue that, for research on psychotherapy, case studies offer an alternative strategy that is as valuable as statistical hypothesis testing. Clinical practice is based on theory—if not a formal, stated theory, then an implicit one drawn from lore, convention, and personal experience. Case studies have some distinct scientific advantages for quality control on the complex, nuanced, context-responsive aspects of

I thank Giancarlo Dimaggio, Hani Henry, Mikael Leiman, James K. Mosher, Katerine Osatuke, and Lisa M. Salvi for comments on drafts of this chapter.

psychotherapy and psychotherapy theories, and they may be more satisfying to clinicians.

THEORY IS THE MAIN PRODUCT OF SCIENCE

Theories are ideas stated in words (or numbers, diagrams, or other signs). Any account or explanation of something could be considered a theory. Commonsense and folk accounts of psychological disturbances and of how people overcome emotional and interpersonal difficulties can be considered theories, though they may be simplistic, internally inconsistent, imprecise, or unrealistic ones. The expectations that people use in daily dealings with each other may be considered as implicit theories. However, to be examined scientifically, a theory must be stated explicitly. In addition, a good theory should be internally consistent, precise, general, and realistic (cf., Levins, 1968).

A statement can be considered as accurate or true if it matches our observations of things or events, that is, if it matches what we see, hear, and feel. Of course, words and things are not the same stuff, but experience can be a common denominator, insofar as both statements and events are experienced. That is, I suggest the experience of an accurate or true statement corresponds in some way to the experience of observing the event it describes. This may be called an experiential correspondence theory of truth (Stiles, 1981, 2003). Such statements may be considered as facts if, additionally, there is agreement—social consensus—that they are accurate. In science, as in law, if people do not agree, then fact has not been established. A good theory, then, is one consistent with the facts, that is, with agreed descriptions of observations.

Research provides quality control on ideas by systematically producing observations and comparing them with the theories. The observations change the ideas and the theories. They may confirm or disconfirm a theory, or, more modestly, strengthen or weaken it. More often, however, the change involves extending, elaborating, refining, modifying, or qualifying the theory.

New observations may be said to permeate the theory. This is a diffusion metaphor; particles of observation spread through theoretical interstices. The ideas change to fit the observations, and aspects of the observations become part of the theory. The theory may be explained differently, for example, using different words that accommodate the new observations along with the previous ones or using the new observations as illustrations. Thus, the theory is modified by the observations to become more general, more precise, and more realistic. Darwin's (1859) theory of the origin of species by natural selection continues to grow as new observations elaborate and refine it. It was extended, for example, by the suggestion that the different nutritional values of the similarly sized bright red berries of dogwood trees (high in lipids and other nutrients) and holly trees (mostly worthless fiber) in eastern deciduous forest may reflect coevolution with different populations of birds (respectively, autumn migrants who take dogwood berries on their way south and local residents who take holly berries in late winter after other resources are exhausted; Stiles, 1980).

Through research, then, observations accumulate in theories. New research results permeate the theory, but earlier thinking and results are retained. The diffusion metaphor offers an alternative to the brick wall metaphor for how science is cumulative. That is, understanding grows not by building a theoretical edifice, stacking fact upon fact, but rather by infusing observations that elaborate and change a theory in subtle (and sometimes not so subtle) ways. A living theory must be able to change, to accommodate this continual infusion of new observations; an impermeable theory is scientifically dead. Thus, permeability is a virtue in theories and in scientists (Stiles, 1993, 2003).

Permeability is a generalization of the traditionally acknowledged virtue of falsifiability. If theories or theoretical tenets were dichotomously true or false, permeability would be equivalent to falsifiability, insofar as the only change that evidence could make would be falsification (cf., Popper, 1934/1959). The concept of permeability, more realistically, I think, suggests that a theory is an approximation that can gradually change to represent scientists' experience more accurately as it accumulates observations.

If theories are informal or implicit, they may remain impermeable to evidence, insofar as the inconsistencies with observations are not exposed. Alternatively, informal theories may be too permeable, changing in response to each new observation and thus undermining any accumulation of understanding. Good theories must balance permeability with coherence and comprehensiveness, respecting previous observations while attending to new ones.

STATISTICAL HYPOTHESIS TESTING VERSUS CASE STUDIES

I meant the foregoing to characterize both hypothesis testing and case studies. Both are strategies of empirical, scientific research, and both provide quality control on theory. Both yield observations that permeate theory, and both inform evidence-based practice (EBP), but they are different strategies.

The statistical hypothesis-testing strategy is to derive one or a few statements from a theory and compare each statement with many observations. If the observations tend to match the statement (in the investigator's experience, as conveyed to readers of the report), then people's confidence in the statement is substantially increased (e.g., not due to chance, $p < .05$). This yields a small increment of confidence in the theory as a whole. For example, in the National Institute of Mental Health (NIMH) Treatment of Depression Collaborative Research Program (Elkin et al., 1989), clients' scores on the Hamilton Rating Scale for Depression (HRSD) showed a statistically significant decrease across 16 sessions of manual-driven interpersonal therapy (IPT). This observation substantially increased confidence in the statement that clients' HRSD scores tend to decrease across 16-session IPT. The finding also added a small increment of confidence to the version of IPT theory from which it was derived (e.g., Klerman, Weissman, Rounsaville, & Chevron, 1984).

The case study strategy is to compare many theoretically based statements with correspondingly many observations. It does this by describing the case observations in theoretical terms. At issue is how well the theory describes details of the case (experiential correspondence of theory and observation). For reasons familiar to people trained in psychological research (selective sampling, low power, investigator biases, etc.), the consequent change in confidence in any one statement may be small, but because many statements are examined, the gain in confidence in the theory may be as large as from a statistical hypothesis-testing study. Campbell (1979) described this as analogous to the multiple degrees of freedom in a statistical hypothesis-testing study.

For example, the assimilation model (Stiles, 2002; Stiles et al., 1990) offers an account of how, in successful psychotherapy, clients assimilate problematic experiences through a sequence of stages. The problem moves from being warded off or dissociated through emerging and becoming understood to being worked through and mastered. The case of Fatima, a refugee (Varvin & Stiles, 1999), helped elaborate the warded-off stage, illustrating how warded-off material could appear initially as film-like memories—in Fatima's case, traumatic memories surrounding the birth and death of a daughter while Fatima was a political prisoner. This case study described how the memories emerged and were assimilated, at least partially. The film-like replaying of warded-off memories was consistent with the theory but not explicitly part of it previously. Incorporating these observations helped point toward similar manifestations of warded-off material in other cases of trauma. The consistency added a small increment of confidence in the theory, whereas the new observations extended it.

Because case studies do not focus on particular variables or hypotheses, the results of case studies are not in the form of decontextualized conclusions. The improvement in generality, precision, or realism is typically spread across the theory rather than concentrated in a sentence. The logic of case studies thus differs from the logic of $n = 1$ designs, in which one or a few targeted dependent variables are examined over time as a function of the introduction or removal of independent variables. Unlike case studies, $n = 1$ designs are meant to yield specific conclusions, stated in terms of the targeted variables.

A few systematically analyzed cases that match a theory in precise or unexpected detail may give people considerable confidence in the theory as a whole, even though each component assertion may remain tentative and uncertain when considered separately. Classic examples of such cases include

Dora for psychoanalysis (Freud, 1905/1953), Little Albert for behaviorism (Watson & Rayner, 1920), and Dibs for nondirective play therapy (Axline, 1964). I think that the degrees-of-freedom logic helps explain why such studies have had such impact. That is, readers were impressed because the studies reported many relevant observations on the cases (details, sequences, context), including some that were consistent with the theory but contrary to intuition or popular wisdom. It is worth noting that, although these cases generally tended to fit a theory that had been articulated previously, they also added or modified details, extending and enriching the theory, rather than merely illustrating it.

The statistical hypothesis-testing strategy can be problematic for studying psychotherapy. For statistical power, hypothesis-testing research must study common features. Common or recurring features of clinical cases are often artificial (e.g., Likert scale responses), global (e.g., efficacy of a treatment), or trivial. Single statements (hypotheses) out of context do not do justice to clinical theory as applied in practice, where it must accommodate variations in people, settings, and circumstances. Clinicians know that an in-session process is so full of nuances and responsive adjustments that researchers' labels or simple descriptions of global variables (e.g., "interpersonal therapy") do not adequately represent clinical reality. Consequently, such research results (increased confidence in isolated statements), even when they are positive, often fail to interest clinicians.

CASE STUDIES TRIANGULATE RATHER THAN REPLICATE

Case studies deal with the perennial tension between generality and uniqueness differently than hypothesis testing as each case includes details not shared with other cases. Statistical hypothesis testing seeks replication, and distinct features are often regarded as irrelevant or as errors in a statistical sense. In contrast, case studies use triangulation, considering distinct and novel features as explicitly informative (see Rosenwald's theory of multiple case research, 1988). Triangulation is a surveying metaphor that refers to the geometrical possibility of fixing a point in space by viewing it from two other locations. Distinctive features inform our understanding of the broader phenomenon of interest. For example, Fatima's film-like memories of her daughter's birth and death (Varvin & Stiles, 1999) offered a new perspective on warded-off material that complemented the assimilation model's previous accounts. Of course, exact replications are never possible, and even traditional replication studies involve alterations or extensions, so what is replicated is the interpretation rather than the observation.

In the Indian parable, as retold by the American poet John Godfrey Saxe (1816–1887), six blind men were each led to a different part of an elephant and asked to describe the beast. The man who felt its side said the elephant was like a wall; the man who felt its tusk, like a spear; the man who felt its trunk, a snake; the man who felt its leg, a tree; the man who felt its ear, a fan; and the man who felt its tail, a rope. Although the men in the story refused to agree or listen to each other, the point of the parable, like multiple case research, is that the beast has many aspects, and understanding it demands multiple, diverse perspectives. A logic that restricts attention to common features is likely to narrow an account of psychotherapy into oblivion or banality. Different cases and different perspectives may be expected to yield different interpretations, and it is the task of theorists to reconcile and integrate them. In this way, allowing the unique aspects of each case to permeate the theory increases the theory's generality.

APPLY THE CASE TO THE THEORY, NOT ONLY THE THEORY TO THE CASE

The logic of permeability suggests that a scientific case study is meant to change the theory, not to understand the case. As in any scientific research, observation is the authority, and a theory that does not converge with observation must be changed. Thus, an investigator must have the confidence to modify the theory—to extend its scope, to change its expression, to add details, and so forth.

A scientific case study thus contrasts with the clinical use of theory, in which the point is to apply theories to understand clinical phenomena. Many case studies miss this distinction, adhering to previously stated theory and ignoring, discounting, or distorting observations that fail to fit. Using the theory to understand the case is an essential first step in research, showing the ways in which the current theoretical account matches the new observations. But investigators must be willing to focus on features of the case that go beyond or differ from the current theoretical account, to turn the observations back on the theory to improve it. A respectful attitude toward theory has a place in clinical applications, insofar as clinicians, and the rest of us, often fail to appreciate phenomena to which the theories are pointing, so that crediting the theory above our own initial impressions or prejudices may open us to things we had overlooked. But case studies that merely apply theories, without putting them at risk of alteration, do not make a scientific contribution.

The logic of permeability also demands a technology of reconciliation. Theories should be internally consistent—logically coherent—as well as consistent with observations. Modifications to theory from different case studies (or any sort of studies) must be reconciled. Changes made to help understand a new case are unhelpful if they discount or distort observations on previous cases. Thus, systematic case studies demand equally systematic conceptual reviews in which inferences on the basis of different cases are compared and reconciled. I suspect that such reconciliation is best accomplished in a dialogical process of statement and response, as well as logical analysis. Perhaps new techniques are needed here, such as systematic ways to reconcile versions of a theory that derive from encompassing different observations.

ADVANTAGES AND DISADVANTAGES

Practitioners have been chronically unhappy with psychotherapy research (e.g., Morrow-Bradley & Elliott, 1986; Talley, Strupp, & Butler, 1994). They often find statistical hypothesis studies narrow, tedious, and too decontexualized to be assimilated into their practice. Many difficulties have contributed to the research–practice gap, of course, but case studies might address some of them.

Case studies can address the complexity and subtlety of psychotherapy. Triangulation allows a case study to encompass nuances and unique context, making research seem more realistic to practitioners while also making productive use of case-to-case and session-to-session variations. By incorporating clients' and therapists' individuality, case studies may also be relatively easily integrated with practitioners' humanitarian values. Case studies may be better suited than hypothesis-testing research to the complex theories practitioners use and the highly contextual material practitioners encounter. Ethical and practical constraints often prevent scientists from exercising the sort of control needed for hypothesis-testing research on psychotherapy, whereas case study research can use practice-based clinical presentations and clinical intervention. In growing recognition of such advantages, several relatively new journals offer outlets for case studies, including *Pragmatic Case Studies in Psychotherapy*, *Journal of Clinical Psychology: In Session*, and *Clinical Case Studies*.

In addition to speaking to practitioners as consumers of research, case studies may offer new opportunities for practitioners to conduct useful research. Practitioners who lack the resources to conduct clinical trials may be able conduct case studies. Anyone who has practiced realizes that, in addition to its potential for healing, psychotherapy can be a marvelous laboratory for observing human experience and behavior. Psychotherapists regularly see aspects of people that others seldom or never see. They thus have an exceptional opportunity to make empirical observations that could bear directly on psychotherapy theory. In principle, case studies offer a way to use this opportunity to improve theory.

Case studies also have disadvantages. Campbell's (1979) degrees-of-freedom argument (i.e., that a study of a single case involves many observations) addresses the argument that case studies lack power, but it does not overcome other familiar objections. Such objections include selective sampling (choice of cases), reliability questions (trustworthiness of observations), the imprecision of measurement, the lack of standard vocabulary, and investigator biases. Case studies also may be more difficult to write about, as they may require more detailed descriptions and rely less on the standardized language of research reports.

The lack of succinct conclusions can make case studies profoundly puzzling to readers used to the results of hypothesis-testing research that can be stated in a sentence. The lack of statistical independence and the associated issues (e.g., collinearity and compounded alpha levels) are not problematic, as independence is not assumed. Indeed, interrelations among observations may make relevant and interesting contributions to descriptions. Different phrases may be needed to characterize how case studies support or fail to support a theory, and questions of validity and alternative explanations must be cast differently when the value of the study depends on many tentative empirical statements, rather than one or a few firm ones. Case studies make the theory-building logic of science more explicit. By offering no context-free conclusions, the case study logic makes it harder to maintain an illusion of context-free knowledge. That is, case studies demand explicit theories, and in my view this is a virtue.

CONCLUSIONS

Both case studies and hypothesis-testing research can provide quality control on theories, which is the main point of scientific research. Both strategies yield observations that permeate the theories, making them more general, precise, and realistic. Case studies use a strategy that is different from hypothesis testing, addressing many theoretical issues in the same study, rather than focusing on only one or a few. Case studies incorporate unique features of cases, emphasizing triangulation rather than replication. Despite familiar drawbacks, case studies have distinctive advantages for research on psychotherapy, particularly their ability to study multifaceted phenomena in context. In summary, case studies are well qualified to provide evidence on the theories that underlie the effective practice of psychotherapy.

Single-Participant (S-P) Design Research

Ruth M. Hurst and Rosemery Nelson-Gray

When a treatment meets all the necessary criteria for empirically supported treatments (ESTs), the practicing clinician can be confident that research has confirmed internal and external validity of the treatment (Chambless et al., 1998). Justifiably, when Chambless and colleagues (1998) established EST criteria, the single-participant (S-P) design experiment was identified as one of the acceptable research methods for assessing treatment validity, and solid criteria for its use in establishing treatment effectiveness were developed.

In this position paper, we review S-P research and argue for its continued use in establishing and guiding EBP in mental health. Because S-P design studies are used to validate treatments, consumers of clinical research should be familiar with the methodology, including when it should be used and the advantages this design offers both the clinician and the researcher. Because S-P research does not typically rely on inferential statistics to assess for treatment effects, which is sometimes a criticism of S-P design research, we also provide information about the analysis of S-P design results.

The core feature of S-P designs when compared to case studies is that they reduce threats to internal validity by controlling for potential confounding variables (Malott & Trojan Suarez, 2004). By definition, S-P design experiments use a small number of participants or even only one participant, repeated measurements of the participant's behavior over time, planned introductions or withdrawals of treatment(s), and evaluations of treatment effects based on the individual's own pretreatment levels of behavior and the replicability of the treatment effect. Inferences about treatment effects are often based on the visual analysis of graphically presented data, although supplemental methods are also available and sometimes encouraged (Fisch, 1998). Valid inferences about treatment effects are possible because of the high degree of experimental control required by S-P design methodology.

S-P design experiments come out of the operant research tradition associated with the experimental analysis of behavior (Baer, Wolf, & Risley, 1968; Kazdin, 1982; Kratochwill, 1978b; Morgan & Morgan, 2003). S-P designs provide an empirical method for understanding the uniqueness of the person (the idiographic approach), and it serves to guide treatment development as a supplement or precursor to research using group design (the nomothetic approach; Kazdin, 1982). It is notable, however, that establishing treatment effectiveness, as defined by the Chambless et al. (1998) criteria, does not necessitate experiments using group design and can be based solely on S-P research. Those utilizing the operant S-P research tradition have a strong interest in understanding functional relationships between the environment and behavior (e.g., Baer & Pinkston, 1997), along with minimal tolerance for inferential statistics (Hopkins, Cole, & Mason, 1998); however, the use of the S-P design is not limited to questions from the operant framework.

TYPES OF S-P DESIGNS

The *simple baseline* (AB) *design* is the most basic of the S-P designs (see Figure 2.1, Panel A; note that Figures 2.1 and 2.2 show stylized graphs of data as they would typically be presented for each of the designs described here). This design requires that data be collected prior to beginning an intervention during what is typically referred to as the baseline phase (A). When the treatment phase (B) is begun, the data collection is continued. To assess for the treatment effect, treatment phase data are compared to baseline data. Following intervention, an immediate and obvious change in the dependent variable is necessary in order to be confident that the treatment is responsible for the change. If a change occurs but is not immediate, then internal validity is questioned with the suspicion that one or more confounding variables could be responsible for the change. This design is useful in the early stages of treatment research, especially for low-incidence problems and new treatment approaches, when refining the treatment and making initial determinations about whether or not the treatment works. This design is similar to the case study in that its internal validity is weak.

The *reversal (ABA or ABAB) design* includes at least three phases to assess the effect of the intervention on the dependent variable (see Figure 2.1, Panel B; Kazdin, 2001; Malott & Trojan Suarez, 2004). The initial phase (A) is a baseline phase and is followed by the treatment phase (B), which is then withdrawn and a return to the baseline phase (A) occurs. If changes in the dependent variable closely correspond to the implementation and withdrawal of treatment, this is taken as evidence that the treatment is responsible for the change. The reversal design can be replicated multiple times (ABABABA) to reduce threats to internal validity. If the dependent variable changes consistently with the implementation and withdrawal of treatment, internal validity is improved. The reversal design is used only if a return to baseline levels of behavior is considered acceptable based on ethical grounds. For example, a reversal design would not typically be used when evaluating a treatment for self-harmful or aggressive behavior. A temporary reversal for behaviors that are not harmful can also be used so that participants experience only a brief loss of gains. The reversal design may not be useful if behavior learned during the treatment phase is likely to endure even when the treatment conditions are withdrawn. For example, if the newly established behavior contacts naturally occurring reinforcers, it is likely to endure even when treatment is withdrawn.

The *alternating-treatments design* (ATD), sometimes referred to as the multi-element design, is useful if two or more treatments are to be compared within the same participant (see Figure 2.1, Panel C; Hayes, Barlow, & Nelson-Gray, 1999; Malott & Trojan Suarez, 2004). The alternating treatments are presented one at a time, more than once, and the presentations occur rapidly, often within the same day, in random or semirandom order. Internal validity is thus established by the random assignment of treatment conditions to treatment sessions (Barlow & Hayes, 1979). Each data set from the different treatment conditions is treated as a separate series, and the mul-

A. Simple Baseline Design

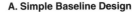
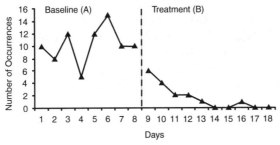

B. Reversal Design

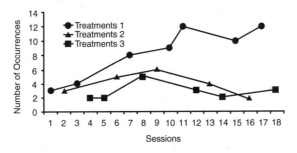

C. Alternating Treatments Design

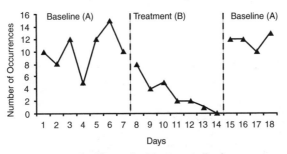

D. Changing Criterion Design

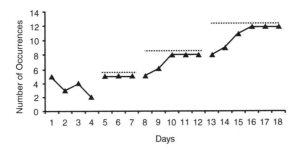

Figure 2.1. S-P research designs depicted using fictional data. Panels A and B show the number of occurrences of a target behavior as a function of baseline and treatment conditions. Panel C shows the number of occurrences of a target behavior as a function of the treatment condition. Panel D shows the number of occurrences of a target behavior as a function of the treatment criterion.

tiple series are then compared to determine differential effects of the randomly presented treatments.

One major problem with the ATD is the inability to rule out effects due to interactions between treatments. However, as part of a total research program, it can serve as a useful step toward the validation of a treatment. Also, it addresses the EST criterion that requires that an intervention be compared to another treatment (Hayes et al., 1999; Malott & Trojan Suarez, 2004). The ATD could also be useful for research on psychological treatments of rare disorders, which are difficult to assess using a group design.

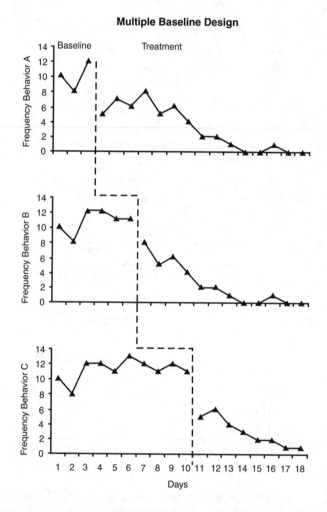

Multiple Baseline Design

Figure 2.2. Multiple baseline design depicted using fictional data. The graphs illustrate the frequency of each of three target behaviors as a function of the baseline and treatment condition.

The *multiple baseline design* replicates treatments across more than one baseline (see Figure 2.2; Kazdin, 2001; Malott & Trojan Suarez, 2004). The multiple baselines can consist of multiple behaviors in one individual, the same behavior in multiple individuals, the same behavior in one individual across multiple settings, or the same behavior in one individual across multiple time periods. The changes in behaviors are considered to result from the treatment if the behaviors change when, and only when, the treatment is implemented. An advantage of this design is that no reversal is required; however, for the design to be useful on its own in validating treatment effects, a sufficient number of replications (at least three baselines) must take place, and the behaviors must change only when the intervention is implemented (Kazdin, 2001). Similar to the reversal design, the multiple baseline design is useful when piloting a treatment in which treatment effects are expected to be enduring or in which return-to-baseline conditions would be inappropriate, as in the treatment of dangerous behavior.

The *changing criterion* design is different from the others described thus far in that it incorporates actual criterion levels that behavior must match in order to show that the behavioral change is a result of treatment (see Figure 2.1, Panel D). After the baseline, a behavioral criterion is set. The participant's receipt of a reinforcing or other planned consequence is contingent on meeting this criterion. When the behavior matches that criterion, usually over several sessions or days, the criterion is changed by making it more stringent. If behavior changes only when the criterion changes, if the behavior matches the criterion, and if sufficient numbers of replications of the relationship between behavior change and criterion levels occur, then the change in behavior can be assumed to be tied directly to treatment (Kazdin, 2001; Malott & Trojan Suarez, 2004). Similar to other S-P designs, the changing criterion design may be useful when piloting a treatment, particularly when that treatment is expected to effect change gradually over time. The changing criterion design is also useful when reversal, even short term, is not warranted due not only to potential for loss of gains but also due to disruptions that would not ordinarily be part of the long-term treatment.

EXAMPLES OF ESTS FIRST ESTABLISHED AS VALID USING S-P RESEARCH

The EST list provided by Chambless et al. (1998) and subsequent lists (e.g., Nathan & Gorman, 2002; Ollendick & King, 2004) include numerous examples of validated treatments. However, the design methodology used in the validation research for the treatments was not specified in the lists. Two ESTs, described briefly in this section, were taken from the Chambless et al. (1998) list as exemplars in which S-P research studies were integral in establishing the treatments as empirically supported. These examples are behavior modification of enuresis (Houts, Berman, & Abramson, 1994) and habit control and reversal techniques (Azrin, Nunn, & Frantz-Renshaw, 1980a; Azrin, Nunn, & Frantz-Renshaw, 1980b).

Houts and colleagues (1994) completed a meta-analysis of treatments for enuresis that included data sets from S-P experiments that showed the superior effectiveness of the behavioral modification of enuresis. Included in the meta-analysis by Houts et al. (1994) was S-P design research completed by Azrin, Sneed, and Foxx (1973) that examined the effect of different treatment components on nocturnal enuresis. Azrin et al. used an ABC design (A = baseline, B = urine alarm treatment, C = dry-bed training) with six participants with developmental disabilities and an AC design with another six participants with similar disabilities to determine the effects of the urine alarm alone and the urine alarm with dry-bed training. Azrin et al. showed that dry-bed training was effective in reducing nocturnal enuresis and that the urine alarm, alone, was not. The success of the procedures used in Azrin et al.'s S-P research has had a major effect on the subsequent development of treatment protocols for nocturnal enuresis (Houts, 2003).

Another group of efficacious treatments that relied on S-P research in their development is habit reversal and control (Azrin et al., 1980a, 1980b). Azrin and colleagues (1980b) cited several S-P experiments that contributed to the development of these techniques (Azrin & Nunn, 1973; Foxx & Azrin, 1973). Foxx and Azrin, using a modified reversal design, demonstrated that overcorrection for self-stimulatory behavior was more effective than either contingent punishment or reinforcement for appropriate behaviors alone. Habit reversal and control techniques, as described by Azrin et al. (1980a, 1980b), involved training normal children with a problematic habit, such as thumb-sucking, to engage in a form of self-provided overcorrection, with parental involvement, called habit reversal training. The evolution from simple overcorrection to more comprehensive habit reversal procedures shows how treatment effects found in S-P design research can be useful when developing effective treatment.

ADVANTAGES OF S-P DESIGN IN CLINICAL PRACTICE

The primary advantage of S-P design by the clinician is that it provides him or her with a data-based approach to the assessment of the treatment effect. This data-based approach to treatment, if used as a matter of routine, results in numerous advantages for the clinical practitioner (Hayes et al., 1999; Morgan & Morgan, 2003). First, this approach assists the clinician in meeting the standards of accountability set by third-party payers. Practitioners are now more than ever being held accountable by insurance and governmental standards to show evidence of treatment effects that go beyond clinical impressions.

Second, the use of S-P design assists the clinician in meeting standards of practice set by the profession (see *Ethical Principles of Psychologists and Code of Conduct*, American Psychological Association [APA], 2002). Ethics (APA, 2002) require the clinician to use reliable and valid data, and to attend to scientific knowledge when forming clinical impressions and making decisions, rather than relying solely on their subjective experience of the client to do so. This is an attempt by the field to assure competent decisions and accurate interpretations of assessment results by clinicians. The S-P design, with its emphasis on reliable measurements of behavior and assessments of treatment validity through multiple replications, provides the clinician with a method for verifying treatment effects on one individual. This method can be used to justify decisions about whether or not a person has improved following the implementation of a particular treatment strategy, and this is in keeping with ethical standards. This is especially important because any given EST will not work for all people, so clinicians can be kept aware of client progress via baseline and treatment data, and be prepared to change or adjust the treatment depending on the outcome.

A third advantage of the S-P design by the clinical practitioner is that it can contribute to scientific knowledge in at least two ways. For one, clinicians could report on the EST effect in cases that differ in some way from the original validation cases in order to help establish the generalizability or limits of that method. For example, an EST for adult depression could be tried with an adolescent or several single cases of adolescents, and those results could either support or limit the generalizability of that method to the adolescent population. For another, clinicians could explore the effect of a new treatment across several single cases, one at a time, and then present these results together as a first step in establishing treatment effectiveness.

ADVANTAGES OF S-P DESIGN IN RESEARCH

S-P research is a valuable research tool for evaluating the efficacy of treatments in mental health and it has some advantages over group-based methods such as randomized clinical trials (RCTs). First, S-P designs can be used more easily in applied settings where RCTs may be prohibitive due to lack of a sufficient sample size or a low incidence of the presenting problem (Hayes et al., 1999; Kazdin, 1998). For example, right now no consensual evidence-based treatments exist for either somatoform or dissociative disorder, both low incidence disorders for which S-P research could be useful in establishing effective treatments. Second, S-P research provides the investigator with a high degree of flexibility when examining components of both already established and potential treatments. Specifically, S-P research can be designed to compare treatment components as they are added, subtracted, or combined across different treatment phases.

Third, the flexibility of S-P research extends its ability to be combined with other conventional research designs, such as a group design, often improving experimental control. For example, in a validation study, participants could be assigned randomly to either a control or a treatment group. The control participants could receive only one treatment throughout the experiment, whereas the participants in the treatment condition could receive that treatment plus others via an alternating-treatments S-P design approach (Kratochwill, 1978a). In this example, experimental control is improved by adding randomization to the assignment of participants to groups (a reduced selection bias) and adding a comparison group (reduced threats to internal validity; Kazdin, 1998). Fourth, S-P research is useful when doing exploratory research when an idea of a treatment might be effective for a particular disorder. An S-P design could be used when first trying out the exploratory treatment with a few clients.

ANALYSIS OF S-P DATA

When interpreting S-P results, decisions about whether or not the dependent variables have changed over time is most often completed according to the tradition of the graphical interpretation of time-series data (see Baird & Nelson-Gray, 1999, for a thorough review). Traditionally, the graphic representation of the data tells the complete story about treatment effects, obviating the need for statistical analysis to confirm the treatment effect (Baer et al., 1968; Morgan & Morgan, 2003). However, empirical research has shown that the visual inspection of graphs is not as reliable as contended by Baer et al., and since that time considerable research and attention have been devoted to improving strategies for the visual inspection of graphs (Fisch, 1998; Fisher, Kelley, & Lomas, 2003). These strategies include blocking data to reduce variability, graphing mean data with standard deviations, adjusting the scale or locations of the abscissa and ordinate, and/or including visual aids in the graph such as the conservative dual-criteria (CDC) visual aid (Fisher et al., 2003).

It should be noted that the statistical analysis of data may be justified for use in the interpretation of graphically presented treatment effects (Fisch, 1998; Gottman & Glass, 1978; Hopkins et al., 1998). When graphically presented data are noisy, when no clear trends are present in the data, or when the clinical significance of change is questioned, a visual interpretation may result in either Type I or Type II errors, although Type II errors are considered to predominate in S-P research (Fisch, 1998). Thus, statistical analyses that evaluate time series in a way that accounts for the serial dependency of data or those that measure the clinical significance of change can be useful (Jacobson & Truax, 1991; Kazdin, 2003). Examples of these analyses would be interrupted time-series analysis, mean baseline reduction, the percentage of nonoverlapping data, the percentage of zero data, and regression-based statistics (Campbell, 2004; Crosbie, 1993). However, following the S-P tradition, the primary message here is that statistical outcomes should appear consistent with the experimental design, graphical depiction, and descriptive analyses of treatment effects (Shull, 1999). If the statistical analysis yields statistically significant differences, but graphed data are not compelling, then one should be skeptical of the statistical significance (Baer et al., 1968).

CONCLUSIONS

S-P research is useful in demonstrating and evaluating evidence-based treatments. This form of research has been instrumental in the development of important treatments for a number of clinical disorders (e.g., enuresis and habit disorders), and it continues to be used as a method for evaluating new treatments (e.g., Barreca et al., 2003; Lantz & Gregoire, 2003; Singh & Banerjee, 2002; van de Vliet et al., 2003). Understanding S-P research requires a familiarity with the basic S-P designs and a background in the assessment of time-series data; however, it does not require a behavioral background because the method is theoretically neutral, even though it comes out of the behavioral framework. The basic tenet of S-P research is that a treatment effect can be evaluated through the assessment of a reliable and replicated baseline and treatment data from a single participant. S-P designs are especially useful when completing research in an applied setting where RCTs may not be practical, when evaluating treatments for problems that occur infrequently, and when assessing exploratory or pilot treatment effects. S-P research has a conceptual basis that allows flexibility and creativity when constructing methods for answering questions about treatment effects. Not only are S-P designs useful for research but they are also useful as a matter of routine in clinical practice, providing the clinician with data-based evidence about a treatment's effect on a case-by-case basis. The clinician who uses S-P methods has the distinct advantage of having data to inform clinical impressions, demonstrate accountability, and support treatment decisions. The data-based approach of the S-P design supports the clinician in attempts to meet insurance, governmental, and ethical standards.

Qualitative Research

Clara E. Hill

I assert that qualitative research qualifies as a method for judging effective practice. In this position paper, I describe the reasons for this assertion and provide an example of using qualitative data to evaluate practice. But first, let me talk briefly about qualitative research.

In psychotherapy research, the most frequently used qualitative methods are variations of grounded theory (Glaser & Strauss, 1967; Rennie, Phillips, & Quartaro, 1988; Strauss & Corbin, 1998), phenomenological (Giorgi, 1985), comprehensive process analysis (CPA; Elliott, 1989), and consensual qualitative research (CQR; Hill, Thompson, & Williams, 1997; Hill et al., in press). Related research methods are exploratory, discovery-oriented methods (e.g., Hill, 1990; Mahrer, 1988), which rely on qualitative data-gathering strategies and developing categories from the data, but then require researchers to train a new set of judges to high reliability and then have them reliably categorize the data. Ponterotto (in press) provides a good description of the different qualitative methods and their philosophical bases.

The defining features of qualitative approaches are the use of open-ended, data-gathering methods; the use of words and visual images rather than statistical data to describe psychological events or experiences; the idea that findings are socially constructed rather than "truth" being discovered; and the search for the participants' meaning using a recursive (i.e., going back and forth between inductive and deductive methods) approach (Denzin & Lincoln, 2000; Morrow & Smith, 2000; Taylor & Bogdan, 1998).

One major variation among qualitative methods involves the number of judges who analyze the data. At one extreme, qualitative researchers aligned with constructivism and critical theory (e.g., Sciarra, 1999) argue that it is not possible to separate the judge from the data analysis, because research is essentially an interpretive endeavor. These researchers believe that research involves a rich description of phenomena and thus are not concerned about agreement among judges. At the other extreme, researchers like myself who are closer philosophically to constructivism and post-positivism (e.g., CQR; Hill et al., 1997; Hill et al., in press) believe that it is important to control for bias among judges so that the perspective attained is that of the participants, rather than the researchers. Hence, we argue for using multiple judges and attaining consensus among the judges.

Because it is difficult to speak for all qualitative researchers in this position paper, I want to make it clear up front that my comments apply mostly

I express my appreciation to Beth Haverkamp, Shirley A. Hess, Sarah Knox, Nicholas Ladany, Susan Morrow, Joseph G. Ponterotto, Barbara J. Thompson, and Elizabeth Nutt Williams for reading drafts of this position paper.

to CQR, which involves a semistructured interview protocol to provide for consistent data across participants and use of a primary team of at least three people examining all data and at least one auditor overseeing all judgments to reduce the influence of groupthink and persuasion. Using semistructured data-gathering methods and multiple perspectives makes CQR a rigorous method (in my opinion) that enables us to have confidence in the findings. A rigorous method and confidence in the findings are particularly important when judging effective practice.

WHAT QUALIFIES AS EVIDENCE?

Rychlak (1968, p. 74) defined evidence as the "grounds for belief or judgment which people use in settling on a position." He then posited that two types of evidence exist: procedural and validating. Procedural evidence refers to believing in something because of "its intelligibility, its consistency with common-sense knowledge, or its implicit self-evidence" (p. 75). Validating evidence, on the other hand, relies on "creating an effect, a change in the order of our knowledge through validation, which we have called research. Validating evidence relies on research methods, and obtaining it is the goal of all those disciplines that employ the scientific method" (p. 77).

I assert that qualitative research provides procedural evidence for judging the effectiveness of therapy. We learn in a very experientially rich way about the inner experiences of participants going through therapy. Having a client tell us about a powerful healing experience with a compassionate therapist is typically far more compelling than learning that the average client's changes were clinically significant. When clients and therapists tell their stories about what worked and what did not work in therapy, we make judgments about whether the stories are credible and intelligible, and thusly determine whether the judgments about the effectiveness of therapy are trustworthy and believable (which is procedural evidence).

Qualitative research provides a method for taking these stories and looking at them in a more systematic manner. We carefully construct the questions we ask, carefully select a sample, search for meanings in their words, evaluate our own biases, and return to the data over and over to make sure that we understand the phenomenon and have portrayed it accurately. Thus, qualitative research allows us to have more confidence in the procedural evidence.

ADVANTAGES AND DISADVANTAGES OF QUALITATIVE RESEARCH

A major advantage of a qualitative approach is that researchers can come close to understanding the felt experience from the individual's perspective. Rather than imposing an agenda or worldview on participants, as is frequently the case in quantitative research using standardized instruments that ask specific questions and designate response options, participants in qualitative research are asked to express their inner experiences and reactions in their own words (although the topic is typically chosen for them, which exerts some influence on the data). For example, using a quantitative approach, we might learn that the client moved from a 3 to 4 on a 5-point scale of a depression after treatment. This increase might be clinically significant, but we would not really know what a 3 or 4 represents because we do not know the meaning of the numbers to the individuals completing the measures. Furthermore, we would not know much about the experiences of the individuals at the extremes of the continuum. By contrast, using a qualitative approach, one client might tell us she could not get out of bed before treatment and now has been able to go back to work as well as regain some interest in reading. She attributes all this to her therapist's support and interpretation about her difficulties being related to feeling abandoned when her mother died. Another client might tell us that her depression was more related to negative thoughts and that the treatment helped modify the way she thinks. These examples show that the qualitative approach helps us understand the richness of change from the individual's perspective.

Understanding effectiveness from the participant's perspective is particularly important for psychotherapy research, given the lack of agreement among clients, therapists, and trained judges (Hill & Lambert, 2004). One major explanation of the lack of correlation among perspectives is that participants in the therapy process experience very different things. We know that clients hide negative reactions in therapy and keep secrets (Hill, Thompson, Cogar, & Denman, 1993; Hill, Thompson, & Corbett, 1992; Kelly, 1998; Watson & Rennie, 1994). Similarly, therapists experience the pressure of wanting to feel like they are being helpful and thus ignore contradictory information, whereas clients often want to look needy at the beginning of therapy and like they have been a success at the end of therapy (the "hello–goodbye" effect). Finally, judges might be critical of the process because of their own transference issues. The use of qualitative data might help us understand more about these different perspectives.

A second major advantage of the qualitative approach is that because it is discovery oriented, researchers can find unexpected results (Glaser & Strauss, 1967). By not formulating hypotheses, staying open to hearing what the participants are saying, and being aware of their biases, qualitative researchers can learn from the participants about the nature of their experiences (e.g., they can learn about the helpful components of therapy). This openness to learning from the data is particularly important in areas where little is currently known (e.g., the effectiveness of a new treatment or the links between process and outcome variables). By contrast, in theoretically driven quantitative research, we can only find or not find what we have set out to find, given that our methods and measures do not allow for discovering anything else and because data snooping is frowned on. If you only go looking for depression, you will only find depression; if you open yourself up to looking for other, as yet unknown things, you might find other things. Although hypothesis testing is useful when we have clear theories, I assert that we are at a more preliminary state of knowledge in psychotherapy where we need to start from the bottom up to learn what is effective and then build theories from the empirical data.

Third, we can examine more complicated phenomena using qualitative rather than quantitative methods. In quantitative studies, our heads start hurting when we have three-way interactions, especially if a few covariates are thrown in. And rarely, in quantitative studies, do we even include all the relevant variables because we simply do not have enough participants to attain adequate power, nor do we have the ability to model all the relationships (although path-analytic techniques have improved the situation). In qualitative research, by contrast, we are not constrained to looking at only a few variables at a time; rather, we can examine all the variables in all their complexity, and we can easily examine how variables operate differently for different clients or therapists.

A fourth advantage of qualitative methods is that researchers stay close to the data. When qualitative researchers conduct the interviews and pore over the data to develop categories, they become intimately familiar with every aspect of the data set and know their results in a very personal way. They can discover new things in the data and generate theories about the findings. With quantitative data, by contrast, researchers administer measures, input data into the computer, and then use statistical analyses to crunch the numbers. Inaccurate results can easily be generated (e.g., the wrong numbers entered or the wrong calculations used) and the researchers might never know (because we learn early on to explain either confirming or disconfirming results).

Fifth, qualitative research findings are useful to clinicians in ways that quantitative research findings rarely are. Because of its similarity to clinical practice and case conceptualization where we think deeply about the complexity of client functioning, qualitative research findings often speak more directly to the practicing clinician (Sciarra, 1999). As with case studies, clinicians can look for ideas that apply to them and their clients and discard those that do not. For example, clinicians have told us that the results of our qualitative studies have been very useful to them because the studies reflected their experiences and gave them ideas for practice. To give a feel for the kinds of topics that can be investigated related to effective practice, we have studied misunderstandings and impasses in therapy (Rhodes, Hill, Thompson, & Elliott, 1994), client anger (Hill et al., 2003), transference (Gelso, Hill, Rochlen, Mohr, & Zack, 1999), countertransference (Hayes et al., 1998), therapist self-disclosure (Knox, Hess, Petersen, & Hill, 1997), client internal representations (Knox, Hill, Goldberg, & Woodhouse, 1999), client gift-giving (Knox, Hess, Williams, & Hill, 2003), and therapist silence (Ladany, Hill, Thompson, & O'Brien, 2004).

Finally, qualitative approaches allow participants a chance to tell their story without the constraints we impose on them in quantitative research. All our measures in a quantitative study might be related to depression, whereas the client might want to talk about her experiences of how the therapy influenced her marriage. Thus, participants often feel more connected to the process when they can tell their stories in their own way, which helps build the research alliance and lets participants feel their perspectives are valued.

One major disadvantage of qualitative approaches is the difficulty of combining results across studies. Different qualitative researchers use different words to describe their findings, and words can be used to mean very different things to different people (e.g., do "effectiveness," "helpfulness," and "satisfaction" mean the same thing?). Hence, it is difficult to know if two different researchers actually found the same or different results when they use the same words. Furthermore, we have no methods, such as meta-analyses, for aggregating qualitative findings.

A second disadvantage of qualitative approaches is that judges interpret the data according to their biases and it can be difficult (if not impossible) to separate the judges' from the participants' perspectives. The use of multiple judges and auditors in some qualitative approaches (e.g., in CQR), however, can mitigate this concern, because judges can be aware of the biases and challenge each other. Other ways of minimizing bias include self-reflective journaling, participant checks, and focus groups.

I should also note, however, that quantitative approaches are not free of biases. For example, measures are chosen because they reflect the researcher's worldview. Furthermore, Luborsky et al.'s (1999) review of 29 studies showed that investigator allegiance was related to treatment outcome, suggesting that investigators found what they set out to prove (e.g., cognitive–behavioral researchers found that cognitive–behavioral treatment was more effective than other treatments, whereas psychodynamic researchers found that psychodynamic treatment was more effective than other approaches). Hence, although one can certainly charge that qualitative methods are subject to bias, quantitative approaches are also subject to bias, perhaps just of a different type.

A third disadvantage of qualitative research is the inability to generalize the results. Given the small samples and the use of rich, descriptive data, it is often hard to generalize results beyond the specific sample of participants and researchers (especially if only one judge is used to interpret the data). Of course, some qualitative researchers, especially those coming from the more hermeneutic extreme, are not bothered by the lack of generalizability because their goal is rich description (similar to what might be found in good journalism), rather than generalizing results. Problems with generalizability can be reduced by careful attention to selecting participants randomly from a well-defined population (just as one would with quantitative research). Researchers can also use larger samples (12 to 15 participants) and then apply frequency labels to characterize how often each result occurred in the sample (see Hill et al., 1997; Hill et al., in press). A final point here is that many quantitative studies also experience problems with generalizability given that they use samples of convenience (e.g., clients from one counseling center), rather than samples representative of the population.

A final disadvantage is that qualitative research typically relies on retrospective recall. For example, participants may be asked to recall their experiences of therapy after they have terminated from therapy. These recollections are subject to recall biases; for example, participants may smooth over feelings because they cannot remember exactly how they felt at the time or because feelings change over time. Furthermore, it is important to realize that the experiences are constructed as people talk about them in the interview, given that the very nature of talking about an experience with another person shapes what one says about the experience.

ILLUSTRATIVE EXAMPLE

We (Hill et al., 2000) conducted a study that used both quantitative and qualitative methods (CQR) to examine the question of the differential effectiveness of working with dreams as compared to working with loss in terms of the process and outcome of therapy for adult clients who had both troubling dreams and a recent troubling loss. The same three-stage model (exploration, insight, and action) was used for 8 to 11 sessions of individual psychotherapy with the focus either on dreams (Hill, 1996) or loss (Hill & O'Brien, 1999). I focus here only on the findings related to effective practice and hope to show that the qualitative findings enriched our understanding of the effectiveness of this treatment.

Quantitative measures indicated that clients in the dream treatment gave higher ratings of the working alliance, session evaluation, mastery-insight, exploration-insight gains, and action gains throughout all the therapy than did clients receiving the loss treatment. No differences were found between treatments, however, for outcome measures (symptomatology, impact of the loss, and interpersonal functioning). Hence, there were session-level differences (i.e., clients liked the process of dream-focused therapy better), but overall outcomes were equivalent.

Qualitative data was collected via interviews one week after the termination of therapy and again one month later. Clients in both treatments were interviewed about their experiences, and results were analyzed using CQR (Hill et al., 1997). In terms of facilitative aspects of the therapy, clients in both treatments stated that their therapists were likeable, generally helpful, good at helping them explore thoughts and feelings, good at making connections and interpretations, and good at asking questions. Clients in the loss treatment more often, however, mentioned that they valued therapists' guidance and suggestions, whereas clients in the dream treatment thought that the focus on dreams was facilitative and that the structure of therapy was helpful. In terms of nonfacilitative aspects, clients receiving the loss treatment more often than in the dream treatment mentioned that the therapist did something that they did not like.

In terms of outcomes, the qualitative data revealed that clients in both treatments were not only very satisfied with their therapy experience but they also reported making positive changes in thoughts, feelings, behaviors, feelings about themselves, and interpersonal relationships. They also reported that they planned on continuing to work on their dreams. In addition, dream clients more often than loss clients reported that their dreams became more positive and that they had made positive changes in school or work.

In addition, clients in both treatments reported in the interviews that they gained insight. Clients in the dream treatment, however, reported that their insight was about their dreams, mostly in relation to what their dreams meant in terms of waking life, parts of self, and interpersonal relationships. In contrast, clients in the loss treatment reported gaining insight about the effects of the past on the present and about the loss itself.

Hence, the results showed that the dream and loss treatments yielded many similar results, but distinct differences between them were also noted. The quantitative results provided a picture of the effectiveness for the average client, whereas the qualitative findings provided richer, more individualized information. The qualitative results also suggested a number of new measures (e.g., content of therapy discussion, content of insights, and ratings of dream content) that could be developed for future studies on dreams or loss.

Both the quantitative and qualitative results were useful in helping us understand the effectiveness of dream work and nicely complemented each other. Although it is not necessary to include both types of data in one study, the inclusion of both allowed a comparison of the data generated from the two methods.

CONCLUSIONS

In this position paper, I have argued that qualitative research can provide convincing procedural evidence related to effective practice. More specifically, I have argued that the advantages of qualitative research are that it provides us with a greater understanding of individuals' reactions, leads to unexpected results, allows us to investigate complex phenomena, helps us get close to data and thus represent it accurately, and enables us to be user-friendly for therapists and clients alike. Its disadvantages are the difficulty of aggregating results across studies, the inseparability of the participants' and judges' biases, problems with generalizing results, and concerns in using retrospective recall.

Although using qualitative research at this stage in advancing an effective practice has distinct advantages, I by no means suggest that we should abandon quantitative research. In fact, both quantitative and qualitative methods have both advantages and disadvantages, as Gelso's (1979) bubble hypothesis suggests. The ideal is to collect evidence about effective practices from a number of perspectives using a number of methods. The most compelling evidence is when we have triangulation from a number of sources of evidence.

In sum, I think there is room in our research armamentarium for qualitative approaches because they give us reliable individualized information about effective practice. As we continue to apply qualitative approaches to psychotherapy, they will certainly evolve and become even more applicable in helping us identify what works for each client.

Change Process Research

Leslie S. Greenberg and Jeanne C. Watson

The emphasis placed on RCTs in identifying EBPs overlooks the integral role of psychotherapy process research. Process research is necessary to explicate, test, and revise the theoretical premises and technical ingredients of specific treatments, as well as to enable researchers to identify the active change ingredients. For psychotherapy research to become a true applied science, it needs not only to provide evidence of the general efficacy of a treatment but also to specify the processes of change that produce the effects. To do so effectively, researchers need to identity therapists' contributions, clients' contributions, and the interaction between them. Only converging strands of evidence will provide a convincing evidentiary base for the effectiveness of a treatment.

Change process research is integral to every phase of treatment development, implementation, and modification. Treatment development should first rely on process research to elucidate the change processes responsible for outcome effects. Next, the successful delivery of a treatment requires not only that therapists engage in a set of behaviors but also that these behaviors engage clients in processes known to effect change. Another way in which process research makes a substantial contribution to EBPs is in treatment dissemination. Process research specifies the key ingredients that need to be transported from highly controlled efficacy studies to relatively uncontrolled practice conditions. Transporting treatments from the lab to the clinic, especially when the treatments are multicomponent and responsively delivered to each case, requires that we know the active ingredients to be transported. It is not that the therapist engages in behaviors that determine therapeutic effects as much as it is how the client responds to those behaviors and what processes the behaviors initiate in the client. To implement treatments, clinicians need to know the active processes that lead to change, not just the specific steps to follow in a manual.

Demonstrating that a particular psychotherapy is effective in an RCT, even when therapist interventions are manualized, still does not specify what processes of change have taken place in the psychotherapy. For a convincing scientific argument that a treatment is effective, we need evidence that both what the therapist does (the distal variable) and the processes he or she induces in clients (the proximal variable) relate to outcome. Clinical trials comparing manualized treatments are analogous to studies testing the effects of pills that contain multiple ingredients acting in concert. The fact that the pill relieves headaches better than the alternative, although useful, still does not tell us what is effective. In the 19th century, people knew that the bark of a chinchona tree relieved fever, but it took 20th-century science to extract the active ingredient quinine, an alkaloid found in the bark, to know what worked. Process research is needed to understand what is working in each specific treatment in the trial.

In a recent presentation on the genetic causes of schizophrenia, a leading NIMH investigator emphasized the importance of viable explanatory models. He argued that having at least two studies showing that a gene is significantly related at the .05 level to the occurrence of schizophrenia is not sufficiently persuasive evidence of the causal role of that gene (Weinberger, 2003). Compelling evidence of a gene's role in schizophrenia is that the gene is causally related to some processes involved in the disease, such as increased visual imagination, a process involved in hallucinations. Thus, explaining the process by which an independent variable has its effects on a dependent variable is the *sine qua non* of scientific understanding, and this is similar to psychotherapy research.

The finding of general equivalence between treatments (Luborsky, Singer, & Luborsky, 1975; Stiles, Shapiro, & Elliott, 1986; Wampold 2001) begs the question of the nature of each treatment's active ingredients. How psychotherapy works is a crucial question in need of empirical investigation if we are to establish a scientific understanding of treatment effects. Without knowing the specific processes and causal paths to the outcome, we do not have a scientific understanding of the treatment. Manuals specify how therapists implement specific treatments, but they are not clear on what constitutes competent delivery, nor do they specify the clients' contributions to the process. For a true science, we need to specify the client and therapist processes as well as their interaction.

For example, numerous treatments have been shown to be effective in the treatment of depression. That many forms of treatment that are effective in the alleviation of depression leaves us a little in the dark as to what works. Are all these approaches to be regarded as interchangeable for the treatment of depression? Yet each treatment proposes different etiologies for depression and provides a different method. If we are to solve the puzzle of what is effective in the treatment of depression, we need to know which in-therapy processes in these treatments lead to positive change. Are they therapeutic factors common to all treatments or do the different therapies induce a common client process? Alternatively, does each treatment induce a different change process but all processes follow a common pathway to alleviate the depression? Or is it the combination in each treatment of a general factor and some specific factor? Or perhaps it is the combination of common and specific factors that account for about the same amount of outcome variance, even though each specific factor may be unique to each treatment and induce a different change process. Neglecting to account for hidden, intervening variables is one of the major problems with current clinical trials (Greenberg & Foerster, 1996; Greenberg & Newman, 1996). Without studying the process of change, it is impossible to determine what portion of the outcome is attributable to the specific change process represented by the therapeutic model and what portion is attributable to other factors.

PROBLEMS WITH RCTS

In psychotherapy research, limiting our assessment of what constitutes effective practice to RCTs and ignoring processes lead to a number of problems. First, research shows that different treatments are effective for treating different disorders in spite of apparent differences in theory and technique. Second, in RCTs a questionable assumption of homogeneity exists in terms of the sample of patients used in each study, the delivery of treatment by different therapists, and the delivery of treatment by the same therapist with different clients. Randomization to balance individual differences in general requires a very large N for variation in the population to be studied, and an N much larger than most studies of psychotherapy effects have attained. Process research helps reveal which process is responsible for change, regardless of treatment or individual difference.

Responsiveness

RCTs typically assume homogeneity with respect to the patients included in the study and the delivery of treatment. However, decades of research have shown that the largest amount of variance in outcome is accounted by client factors and, further, that therapist effects are at least as large as treatment differences (Norcross, 2002). Thus, it is inaccurate to assume that manualization will ensure that the therapy is delivered in the same way by every therapist and that each therapist is the same with every client. Research has informed us that competent treatment requires that therapists be responsive to their patients. Therapists thus must vary what they do. The goal of treatment is engaging the client in a change process, not adhering to a manual. Effective psychotherapy is systematically responsive; therapists' and clients' behavior is influenced by emerging contexts, including perceptions of each other's characteristics and behavior (Stiles, Honos-Webb, & Surko, 1998). Context-sensitive process research is the only way to capture moment by process and responsivity.

Responsiveness may be contrasted with ballistic action, action that is determined at its inception and carries through regardless of external events (Stiles et al., 1998). Ballistic action is nonresponsive and insensitive to emerging information. From this perspective, no psychotherapy is ballistic. Nevertheless, psychotherapy research often incorporates this assumption. For example, the assignment of clients to the same treatment condition in a clinical trial is treated as if the clients were given identical treatments. Treatment conditions are often treated inappropriately as unitary, as shown in reports that clients who received Brand X therapy improved significantly on certain outcome indices. Rather, research is needed that shows that this therapist action, at this patient marker, leads to this complex change process, and this relates to outcome.

Differential Client Process

Reports of overall treatment effects that ignore the important role of the client's process of change fail to recognize the two distinct groups in any treatment: those who fully engage in the change processes and those who don't. This factor has a major influence on outcome. For example, intensive analyses of the client's change process in the empty-chair dialogue (Greenberg, Rice, & Elliott, 1993) led to the development of the essential components of resolution of unfinished business with a significant other (Greenberg et al., 1993; Greenberg & Foerster, 1996). In the process of resolution, the person moves through expressing blame, complaint, and hurt to the arousal and expression of the unresolved emotion, to the mobilization of a previously unmet interpersonal need. In more successful empty-chair dialogues, the view of the other shifts and the other is enacted in a new way. Resolution finally occurs by means of the person adopting a more self-affirming stance and understanding and possibly forgiving the imagined other, or by holding the other accountable.

The findings of a study on the resolution of unfinished business (Greenberg & Malcolm, 2002; Paivio & Greenberg, 1995), however, demonstrated that the treatment did not fully engage all the clients in all the active treatment ingredients necessary for resolution. Only some of the clients engaged fully in the specific mechanisms of change, others engaged partially, and others only minimally. This study demonstrated that those who engaged fully in the change processes benefited more than those who did not, and they benefited more than those who experienced the more general effects of a good alliance.

Thus, when we deliver a treatment, if we do not know the active ingredients, we are not able to assess whether the clients fully engaged in the process or not. This is similar to not knowing whether a person in a drug treatment absorbs the medication. In a clinical trial, we have only the crudest index of the treatment's effects because we are lumping together people who absorb the treatment with those who do not.

Common Factors

Although theoretical concepts that frame different treatments still vary, some agreement is occurring across approaches on the general processes that are relevant to success in psychotherapy. Factors such as empathy (Greenberg, Bohart, Elliott, & Watson, 2001), a good working alliance (Horvath & Greenberg, 1994), the depth of experiencing (Hendricks, 2002; Orlinsky & Howard, 1986), and differences in clients' capacity for engaging in treatment (Beutler et al., 2002) have all been shown as important common elements contributing to outcome. Evidence on psychotherapy relationships that work now abounds (Norcross, 2002). More research has been done on the therapy relationship than on any other process in therapy and than on the effectiveness of any type of therapy. Empathy, alliance, and goal agreement have all been shown to be efficacious and specific elements of a therapeutic relationship, but certain questions still remain. Is it the relationship or the other common factors that are the active ingredients in all treatments? Are specific processes unique to each treatment and are they effective at specific times or with specific clients?

CHANGE PROCESSES

To more accurately address the concerns raised previously, psychotherapy research needs to consider sequences or patterns of events, incorporate context, and recognize that critical incidents or significant events may relate to change (Greenberg, 1986; Rice & Greenberg, 1984). To investigate these, a moment-by-moment change process needs to be studied in innovative ways and with sequential analytic methods. When and in what context a particular kind of process appears also needs to be investigated. A manual is a first approximation in a clinical trial, but it is not useful for understanding complex interactions in which given behaviors have different meanings and impacts in different in-session contexts. Change process research is invaluable for this purpose.

Change process researchers have developed a variety of methods that look at complex interactions, sequences, and contexts. Research using task analysis (Greenberg 1984, 1986), assimilation analysis (Honos-Webb, Stiles, Greenberg, & Goldman, 1998; Stiles, Meshot, Anderson, & Sloan, 1992), comprehensive process analysis (Elliott, 1989), and qualitative analysis (Watson & Rennie, 1994) illustrate ways that questions involving complex psychotherapy processes and outcome can be addressed. Task analysis consists of fine-grained descriptions of tape-recorded events representing successful and unsuccessful resolutions of a common feature problem.

For example, Greenberg (1979) studied how clients resolve conflicts and found that a harsh critical voice softening into one of compassion was essential to resolution of the conflict. Joyce, Duncan, and Piper (1995), using this method, found how clients work with an interpretation and contrasted events in which clients did or did not work with an interpretation. They found that the patient's invitation to interpret was an important component of successful episodes. Nonwork episodes were often characterized by an unclear, indirect, or absent patient invitation to interpret. The subsequent interpretation was then invariably experienced as premature, even if regarded as accurate by external judges. Timing or responsiveness thus was more important in determining impact than the accuracy of the interpretation.

Assimilation analysis tracks clients' progress within problematic themes across treatment. Problematic experiences typically pass through a sequence of stages as they become assimilated, from warded off through problem formulation to problem solution and mastery. Passages dealing with particular themes are collected from transcripts of whole treatments, placed in a temporal sequence, and used to assess and elaborate the model.

In comprehensive process analysis, researchers construct "pathways" in which contributing factors and impacts are related to a particular target event. Patterns that are repeated across events of a particular type are identified. For example, in a study of awareness events, Elliott (1989) found that clients needed to avoid painful awareness at times. The pathway suggested that such avoidance may even be a precursor to later successful work with the problematic material. Using qualitative analysis, Watson and Rennie (1994) examined the client's view of change during systematic evocative unfolding. This study highlighted particular aspects of the intervention that were helpful as well as those that contributed to clients becoming resistant and confused. The findings contributed to the refinement of the treatment model and to changes in its implementation. Ultimately, these models are validated and related to outcome.

DESIGNS FOR PROCESS–OUTCOME RESEARCH

Designs investigating the active ingredients of a treatment require that three statistical relationships be established. The first is between the therapist actions and outcome, the second between the client process and outcome, and the third between the therapist actions and the client process. When all three links are established—when the client process is shown to mediate the path between therapist actions and outcome, and when the therapist actions–client process link has been established—we can say that a path to outcome has been found. Ideally, this design logic would also specify differential links between different interventions, processes, and outcomes. To do this, measures of different interventions, different processes, and different outcomes are needed.

RELATING PROCESS TO OUTCOME: AN EXAMPLE

The importance of deepening in-session emotional experience to promote change has become increasingly recognized (Greenberg, 2002; Samoilov & Goldfried, 2000). The reviews of process and outcome studies testing these claims show a strong relationship between in-session emotional experience, as measured by the Experiencing Scale (EXP; Klein, Mathieu, Gendlin, & Kiesler, 1969), and therapeutic gain (Orlinsky & Howard, 1986). This has been demonstrated in psychodynamic, cognitive, and experiential therapies (Castonguay, Goldfried, Wiser, Raue, & Hayes, 1996; Goldman & Greenberg, in press; Pos, Greenberg, Korman, & Goldman, 2003; Silberschatz, Fretter, & Curtis, 1986). This suggests that this variable may be a common factor and a final common pathway that helps explain change across approaches. The EXP measures the degree of focus on currently felt bodily feeling and meaning, as well as the use of these to solve problems and create new meaning.

We engaged in a series of studies to test whether EXP predicted outcome in the treatment of depression in client-centered and process experiential therapy. In addition, we sought to determine if emotional arousal (EA) was an important process of change, hypothesizing that making sense of aroused emotion would be a better predictor of outcome than either arousal or making sense of experience alone.

Failures to demonstrate patterns of change in experiential processing within prior studies may have resulted from the use of random sampling of therapy segments. This assumes that a client process is equally likely to occur at any point in therapy. Individuals, however, manifest very different profiles within and across sessions depending on what is occurring in the moment (Greenberg & Safran, 1987). The events paradigm suggests that the therapeutic process can be more suitably explored by focusing on clinically important events such as therapeutic tasks, core themes, or emotion episodes.

In our first study, the relation between the theme-related depth of experiencing (EXP) and outcome was confirmed, as 35 clients received 16 to 20 weeks of therapy (Goldman & Greenberg, in press). EXP on core themes accounted for outcome variance over and above that accounted for by early EXP and the alliance. EXP therefore mediated between client capacity for early experiencing and positive outcome. Although the formation of a strong working alliance was shown to be an important contributor to outcome, an increase in the depth of emotional experiencing across therapy was found to contribute 8% to 16% of the outcome variance over and above the alliance.

In the next study, Adams & Greenberg (1996) tracked moment-by-moment client–therapist interactions and found that therapist statements high in experiencing influenced client experiencing, and that the depth of therapist experiential focus predicted outcome. More specifically, if the client was externally focused, and the therapist made an intervention that was targeted toward internal experience, the client was more likely to move to a deeper level of experiencing. The study highlights the importance of the therapist's role in deepening emotional processes. Given that client experiencing predicts the outcome, and that the therapist's depth of experiential focus influences both client experiencing and treatment outcome, a path to outcome was established.

Another study suggested that the effect of early emotional processing on outcome was mediated by late emotional processing (Pos et al., 2003). Here, emotional processing was defined as depth of experiencing on emotion episodes, which are in-session segments in which clients express or talk about having experienced an emotion in relation to a real or imagined situation. The EXP variable was now contextualized by being rated only for those in-session episodes that were explicitly on emotionally laden experience. In this study controlling for early emotional processing and therapeutic alliance, late emotional processing still independently added 21% to the explained variance in symptom reduction. An early capacity for emotional processing did not guarantee a good outcome, nor did entering therapy without this capacity guarantee a poor outcome. Therefore, although likely an advantage, early emotional processing skill appeared not as critical as the ability to acquire or increase the depth of emotional processing throughout psychotherapy.

Another study examined midtherapy EA as well as experiencing in the early, middle, and late phases of therapy (Warwar, 2003). EA was measured using the Client Emotional Arousal Scale III (Warwar & Greenberg, 1999).

Clients who had higher EA midtherapy made greater changes at the end of treatment. In addition, it was found that not only did midtherapy arousal predict outcome but that a client's ability to use aroused internal experience to make meaning and solve problems, particularly in the late phase of treatment, added to the outcome variance over and above middle-phase EA. Thus, this process–outcome study showed that emotional arousal in combination with experiencing was a better predictor of outcome than either variable alone.

The previous studies have added links in the explanatory chain and concretely illustrate the value of change process research in guiding EBP. Different therapeutic approaches have been found to be effective in alleviating depression, and the depth of experiencing has been found to mediate the application of different treatment manuals and outcome. This leads a step closer to a scientific understanding of what is working in psychotherapy

CONCLUSIONS

In this position paper, we have argued that the current focus on randomized clinical trials as the sole arbiter of evidence-based treatment has been too simplistic. It has informed us that most clients find psychotherapy useful, but it has not illuminated the active ingredients, nor has it identified which treatment works best for which client. We need information from multiple sources to understand the complex relationship between specific techniques, therapist actions, and client processes that effect changes in psychotherapy. In particular, change process research should be one of those multiple sources in that it reveals the actual mechanisms of change, which is the active ingredient in psychotherapy.

Effectiveness Research

Tom D. Borkovec and Louis G. Castonguay

Effectiveness research attempts to obtain knowledge about psychotherapy outcomes in real-world clinical situations. Its traditional distinction from efficacy research emerged out of concerns that the findings of carefully controlled, laboratory-based outcome investigations, as they are often conducted,

Preparation of this manuscript was supported in part by National Institute of Mental Health Research Grant RO1 MH58593.

may not generalize to the circumstances that characterize actual clinical practice. This lack of generalizability is said to be due to one or more features of efficacy research that differ considerably from the ways in which clinicians customarily practice. These features include (a) the recruitment of clients to participate in the efficacy study; (b) multiple inclusion and exclusion criteria that limit the heterogeneity of the characteristics of the clients admitted to treatment; (c) the careful assessment (often including objective assessors unaware of clients' condition status) of clients before and after therapy and at long-term follow-up; (d) a primary focus on symptoms, as typically defined by the *Diagnostic and Statistical Manual of Mental Disorders, Fourth Edition* (*DSM–IV*; American Psychiatric Association, 1994), which fails to consider fully client complaints, difficulties, and strengths; (e) the random assignment of clients to experimental and control conditions; (f) the use of a specified, and typically small, number of therapy sessions; (g) the use of detailed protocol therapy manuals and objective monitoring of adherence to those manuals; (h) specific training of study therapists in the protocol manual; and (i) careful supervision of therapists by project investigators (e.g., Castonguay et al., 1999; Hoagwood, Hibbs, Brent, & Jensen, 1995; Seligman, 1995).

The previous distinction between effectiveness and efficacy research relates closely to another customary way of speaking about the presumed differences between the two types of research. Efficacy studies are said to emphasize the internal validity of investigations, whereas effectiveness studies emphasize external (or ecological) validity. Internal validity has to do with the number of plausible rival explanations for the results of a study. In therapy research, this broadly refers to whether the experimental therapy causes the observed change, or alternately whether some or all of that change is plausibly due to other factors. A key issue here is that the more alternative explanations that can be ruled out by the design and methodology of the investigation, the greater its internal validity. Strong internal validity gives us greater confidence in our inferences about the causative role of the investigated therapy. External validity most commonly refers to the extent to which a study's findings are likely to generalize to other clients, types of client problems, assessment measures, therapists, and settings other than those represented in the study. The more representative the study is to actual treatment situations as practiced in the community, the more confident we feel about the likely generalizability of its results to such real-world settings.

The purpose of this position paper is to argue that effectiveness research should be used to determine and guide effective practice. However, the extent to which it will be useful in this way depends on how such research is actually conducted. We thus make recommendations for future effectiveness studies that can potentially maximize their value, both for the sake of knowledge acquisition and for the sake of creating increasingly effective forms of psychotherapy. We will accomplish our purposes by making four position statements.

POSITION 1

Both internal and external validity vary along a continuum (how many rival explanations can be ruled out and the number of ways in which the study is representative of the population to which a generalization is to be made, respectively). The degree to which a psychotherapy study has poor internal validity is the degree to which it is of limited value, no matter how much external validity it possesses. If we are unable to draw confident conclusions from an investigation because its scientific methods fail to rule out numerous rival explanations, then the generalization of flawed conclusions becomes a moot issue.

This position argues for the creation of effectiveness studies that maximize internal validity while at the same time possessing external validity (see also Hoagwood et al., 1995). Certainly, pragmatic challenges exist in implementing carefully controlled research in applied settings, and researchers and participating clinicians understandably need to make decisions on the basis of cost–benefit analyses of implementing possible designs and methodologies. As others have recommended, however, the field would greatly benefit from devoting more time and effort into developing creative ways to overcome obstacles and to conduct research with maximized internal validity (e.g., Clarke, 1995).

POSITION 2

The ultimate goal of psychotherapy research as a scientific enterprise is to specify cause-and-effect relationships. Experimental designs allow for the most unambiguous demonstrations of such relationships, and conclusions from such designs are limited to the identification of such relationships.

This position is grounded in the very nature of scientific research. It reminds us of the facts that (a) "efficacy" and "effectiveness" both refer to causation ["This effects or causes that"], and (b) the best that either type of research can do is to increase our understanding of causal relationships. Neither type of research is capable of directly answering the ultimate questions about psychotherapy in the way that society is asking those questions (Borkovec & Castonguay, 1998).

To answer the questions "Is this therapy effective?" and "How effective is this therapy?" one must necessarily ask, "Relative to what?" (e.g., the passage of time or the provision of a sympathetic listener). An investigator can then answer those questions by comparison conditions that hold constant those other possible causes of clinical change (e.g., no-treatment or common factors [frequently called "nonspecific;" see Castonguay, 1993] control conditions). This is the foundation of the criteria used for "empirically supported treatments" (Chambless & Ollendick, 2001). If statistically significant differences between treatment and control conditions are found, the only scientific conclusion possible, depending on the type of comparison condition used, is "This therapy caused that degree of change beyond the degree of change most plausibly attributable to the mere passage of time or the provision of common factors." Notice that this allowable conclusion is not a direct answer to society's question about whether or not a psychotherapy is effective. Moreover, society's question contains additional important elements about which "empirically supported treatments" criteria are silent. These include the degree of clinically significant change generated by the therapy and a cost–benefit analysis in terms of time or financial resources needed to provide the therapy relative to providing what is contained in the comparison condition.

In terms of scientific attempts to answer the other societal question, "What therapy is best for a particular disorder?" it cannot be done in a compelling manner. Comparative designs (e.g., cognitive therapy versus interpersonal therapy for depression), as they are typically conducted, are inherently and fatally flawed (little or no internal validity). This is because the two treatments vary in so many ways, thus making the specification of causal elements impossible. No valid and reliable methods have been established for guaranteeing equivalence in the quality with which the two therapies are provided. The common use of expert therapists administering only their own therapy results in the confounding of the design with therapist factors and therapist-by-therapy interactions. Further, any applied implications of the results after the 3 to 5 years needed to conduct the study are by then ancient history, even if those results were valid.

Our position argues that effectiveness research would most usefully focus its questions on the identification of cause-and-effect relationships and not have its attention diverted away from that focus by unsuccessful attempts to answer directly society's urgent questions about therapy. The frequent use of common factors control conditions is not helpful in this regard. The superiority of a therapy over common factors treatment only shows that causal ingredients (beyond common therapy factors) exist and not what those specific factors are. Consequently, ideal designs for the sake of increasingly specific cause-and-effect conclusions involve dismantling, additive, parametric, and catalytic designs. At the same time, these designs and their control conditions serve the function of controlling for the passage of time and factors common to all therapies (Behar & Borkovec, 2003).

Controlled experimental research using such designs is ideal for the specification of causes. This is not meant to say that other forms of psychotherapy research are of no value. Investigations that, for example, identify what is actually taking place in therapy sessions and how these events are similar or dissimilar across different therapy approaches are valuable indeed. Similarly, studies on how pretreatment variables, moderators, process variables, session outcomes, and ultimate short-term and long-term clinical outcomes interrelate to one another all provide useful, preliminary information on factors likely involved in causal relationships (Castonguay, Schut, & Constantino, 2000; Hill & Lambert, 2004). Particularly useful are studies that include methodologies and measures that allow for mediational models of therapy outcome to be tested. What we are saying is that correlational research of all types is best performed in the context of experimental therapy research, as indeed mediational research actually requires (Kraemer, Wilson, Fairburn, & Agras, 2002).

POSITION 3

Given the previous positions, the primary goal of psychotherapy research is to acquire basic knowledge. Through its ability to specify relationships (ultimately cause-and-effect relationships), scientific research can inform us about the nature of human beings, the mechanisms of the maintenance of psychological problems, and the nature of therapeutic change. The more causes that we can determine, the more we can include those causes in our developing therapies. Those therapies will thus become increasingly effective for more people and more types of psychological problems. In this way, indirectly but very powerfully, scientific research can eventually contribute to answering society's urgent questions.

POSITION 4

One of the best ways to implement the preceding statements and to advance knowledge about psychotherapy is to establish practice research networks (PRNs). Here, practicing clinicians and clinical scientists are brought together in applied settings to collaborate on large-scale therapy investigations that are scientifically rigorous while retaining strong external validity. These studies will focus on the acquisition of basic knowledge within the context of practitioner-guided, clinically meaningful questions.

The first step in creating such PRNs is the recruitment of clinicians to participate in joint research efforts. The second step is the establishment of an infrastructure to support its research activities. A core assessment battery forms the foundation of this infrastructure. It is given to all clients participating in a PRN, and it covers the domains of symptoms, role functioning, and general well-being (as recommended by the APA conference on core batteries; Strupp, Horowitz, & Lambert, 1997). The core battery must also be brief to minimize the burden on client and clinic staff, as it is administered at pretherapy, posttherapy, and follow-up to assess clinical gains. Additional outcome and session measures can be added, depending on the specific questions being asked in a particular investigation. The third step involves bringing participating clinicians and researchers together to formulate questions that are clinically meaningful and that can be rigorously investigated. Together these collaborators determine the design, methodology, and procedures to be used in their study.

Considerable progress is occurring in the creation of PRNs. For example, the Pennsylvania PRN, supported by the Pennsylvania Psychological Association and the APA, was established in the mid-1990s and successfully completed a Phase I pilot investigation designed to create a statewide infrastructure and to obtain experience in the use of a core battery and in the conduct of collaborative research in the applied setting (Borkovec, Echemendia, Ragusea, & Ruiz, 2001). It has recently completed data collection in a Phase II experimental investigation designed to test the causal role of providing feedback to practitioners from session-by-session reports of what their clients found helpful and hindering during their therapy sessions. This study also provides an opportunity to determine what clients see as helpful, how those reports relate to what therapists believe is helpful, and how both these perspectives relate to outcome. This also serves as an example of correlational research within the context of experimental investigation.

As a further example, in collaboration with Behavioral Health Laboratories, the authors, along with Jeremy Safran, are working on the development of a national PRN. Behavioral Health Laboratories has marketed a core battery (Treatment Outcome Package; Krauss, Seligman, & Jordan, in press) that is now being used in 35 states measuring more than 400,000 clients. The primary reason that these agencies have contracted for the use of the battery is that they wish to assess the effectiveness of the services that they provide and to use the data to improve their care. However, it also provides the opportunity for the creation of an enormous PRN. In a recent survey of these agencies, 88% of respondents indicated that their agency would be very (56%) or somewhat (32%) interested in participating in a PRN. Our plan is to collaborate with these agencies in developing several large-scale, experimentally rigorous effectiveness investigations.

A final example involves efforts that are underway to create PRNs among the training clinics of psychology departments across the country. Our own efforts here will involve organizing training clinics that are all using the Treatment Outcome Package as their core assessment battery. This particular type of PRN has several goals: (a) to stimulate, implement, and share ideas among training clinics for better ways to seamlessly integrate science and practice throughout graduate education; (b) to establish an infrastructure in each clinic within which faculty and students can conduct rigorous and clinically meaningful research; and (c) to develop collaborations among clinics that wish to pursue the same research questions. The training clinic PRN is of particular scientific value, given the degree of control that faculty has over the procedures of their clinic. Moreover, collaborations among clinics would mean that even small clinics can join with larger ones or multiple ones, resulting in large numbers of clients and clinicians participating in the research and thus in high levels of statistical power and large ranges of client and therapist characteristics.

The ideal form of PRN studies would be experimental investigations focused on empirical demonstrations of increasingly specific cause-and-effect relationships. In addition to incorporating recommendations for maximizing internal validity within effectiveness studies (e.g., Clarke, 1995) and external validity within rigorously controlled research (e.g., Shadish, Cook, & Campbell, 2001), we would recommend the use of additive designs (and strongly discourage no-treatment, common factors, and comparative designs for their incapability to draw specific causal conclusions). In this type of design, an experimental element of treatment is added to whatever treatments are customarily provided by clinicians and compared to treatment as usual by itself (e.g., the induction of a deeply relaxed state versus its absence during the provision of experiential emotional deepening therapies for emotional problems, or the addition of emotional deepening techniques to CBT for anxiety disorders; see Borkovec, Newman, & Castonguay, 2003; Newman, Castonguay, Borkovec, & Molnar, 2004). Such a design possesses strong internal validity because all is held constant except for the one additional element. Thus, very specific conclusions about the causal status of that element are possible. Moreover, this type of design is likely to be most attractive to clinicians who are understandably resistant to participate in many types of controlled research. They can administer their usual therapies in their customarily flexible manner, and they can learn a new element of therapy and participate in a study designed to determine the clinical utility of that element.

Within the context of PRN effectiveness studies, several additional features can maximize the amount of information acquired. For example, we can collect measures completed at the end of each session to reflect intermediate outcomes; assess hypothesized mediators, moderators, and predictors of outcome; objectively code session tapes for process research; and compare different diagnostic groups on pretherapy measures for the sake of investigating the distinctive characteristics of each group. With the large numbers of clients and clinicians in PRNs, highly powered investigations of a wide range of therapist and client characteristics become possible in a way not previously available to the field.

CONCLUSIONS

Effectiveness research is extremely important for improving clinical practice because its findings have direct relevance to the real world in which clinicians work. We have argued, however, that its success in accomplishing this goal depends on the use of scientifically rigorous investigations on clinically meaningful questions focused on increasing our understanding of the nature of psychological problems and change mechanisms, as well as on the development of increasingly effective psychotherapies on the basis of that knowledge. The implementation of such recommendations within the context of PRNs provides a unique opportunity for very large, rigorous, and externally valid psychotherapy research that can accomplish those goals and, at the same time, establish an infrastructure whose essence involves a true integration of science and practice.

Randomized Clinical Trials

Steven D. Hollon

I have a long-standing interest in depression. Job was my favorite story in the Bible, and I was intrigued to learn that two of my personal heroes had histories of depression (Churchill and Lincoln). I come from a family that is loaded with psychologists (my father was a practicing psychotherapist and my wife is a developmental psychopathologist) and even more so with depression (I have more relatives with histories of depression than with professional degrees). I have a long-standing interest in its treatment (even before graduate school I got a job working in a community mental health center), and I went to Philadelphia for my internship (against the advice of my clinical program) to see first-hand the wonderful new things that Beck and colleagues were doing with respect to its treatment.

I am a clinician to the core who loves to play at science. Jonas Salk was the first hero of my youth (other than Hopalong Cassidy), and it is my life-long dream to rid the species of depression. I have no allusions that I will succeed, but I do intend to die trying. I have maintained an ongoing clinical practice throughout my career, and the greatest pleasure of my professional life is to help people learn how not to be depressed. When I went to Philadelphia, I had the great fortune of walking into a group that had largely completed the first study to suggest that any psychosocial treatment could hold its own with medications in the treatment of depression (Rush, Beck, Kovacs, & Hollon, 1977). I had the further good fortune to parlay that reflected glory into an academic job at the University of Minnesota to which I had no right to aspire. I met a superb graduate student at Minnesota named Rob DeRubeis (now the department chair at Penn) who shared my interest in depression. We laid out a series of studies that we are still working to complete. Grants and tenure followed, and friends and colleagues joined who made the process of doing clinical research so enjoyable that it was hard to believe we were getting paid.

All this is my way of saying that I care about what I do and whether or not it works. I am no rocket scientist, but I know enough to know that I do not want to make claims I cannot support. Paul Meehl (1987, p. 9) used to say that the basic attribute that ought to distinguish psychologists from the other helping professions is "the general scientific commitment not to be fooled or to fool anybody else." My goal in doing science is to ensure that I do neither.

HOW DO WE KNOW WHETHER A TREATMENT WORKS?

The first and most important question we can ask about any treatment is, does it work (that is, is it better than its absence)? Other interesting and important questions follow: Does it work better than alternative interventions (relative efficacy)? How does it work when it works (mediation)? For whom does it work and under what conditions (moderation)? The first question of interest is one of causal agency, and that is a question I take seriously. As a clinician, I want to know if what I do makes a difference. Life is too short not to be efficacious.

I do not defend controlled trials because I do them; I do controlled trials because I can defend them. One of the seminal experiences of my graduate training came when Lee Sechrest arrived to teach at Florida State and offered a seminar on research design. He had us read a superb primer on experimental and quasi-experimental design by Campbell and Stanley (1963). In that treatise, and particularly in the 30 pages of text surrounding Table 1 (pp. 5–34), the authors laid out the interpretative risks inherent in a variety of different empirical designs and the logic of ruling out rival plausible alternatives with such clarity and grace that I was literally transformed (like Paul on the road to Damascus). I came to understand in the course of a single afternoon how to draw a causal inference with regard to treatment efficacy. Armed with this knowledge, I set forth to Philadelphia (where I presented myself as a research methodologist), traveled from there to Minnesota (where I continued to do clinical trials), and then went on to various adventures as a grant reviewer, a journal editor, and an author of this text. It was the most valuable 30 pages of text I ever read.

Campbell and Stanley (1963) described two types of validity and a number of threats to each. Internal validity refers to the certainty with which an observed event can be attributed to an earlier intervention. External validity refers to the extent to which the effects observed could be generalized to the populations and settings of interest. Internal validity is essential; if you want to know whether something works, you are asking whether you can attribute an observed effect to a cause. At the same time, external validity is also important. It does little good to say that a treatment is efficacious if the people sampled are unrepresentative of the patients you really want to treat. Therapist and setting variables are also important, but somewhat less problematic, for reasons we will return to later.

Internal Validity and the Threats to Causal Inference

How do we know that what we do works? If problems did not wax and wane and if patients did not sometimes improve spontaneously for reasons unrelated to treatment, then drawing causal inferences would be relatively simple. In the vernacular, if you can get a pig to fly, then you do not need a control group (or statistics) to tell you that you have had an effect. Pigs do not fly of their own accord and, if you can overcome the laws of God and nature, then you have done something to write home about. But in the face of heterogeneity in course and outcome, cause and effect are not so easy to discern. Observing change following a clinical intervention does not necessarily prove causal agency, because change could have come about as a consequence of other influences that were independent of the treatment manipulation. Other events could have intervened (history) or the changes might have taken place anyway as a consequence of development (maturation). Practice tends to alter the way people respond to an assessment (testing) or changes may have occurred in the way observations are registered (instrumentation). People selected on the basis of extreme scores tend to exhibit lower scores the next time they are assessed (statistical regression), and because people tend to seek treatment at their worst, things are likely to get better as time goes on (spontaneous remission). Increasing the number of people that we study does little to decrease these threats, but it does increase the certainty with which we misinterpret our data.

RCTs seek to control for such extraneous factors by randomly assigning patients to two or more conditions and comparing the results on some common measure(s) of interest. In essence, randomization is used to equate the groups with respect to patient characteristics and the occurrence of extraneous influences. There is nothing magical about randomization, but it does afford a way to control for individual differences in severity and course, and that is a very important thing to do when drawing a causal inference. This is because differences in outcome could be a product of patients (and the extraneous events that happen to them) or procedures (including the treatment itself and the people who implement it). As a consequence, randomization increases the certainty with which any differences observed could be attributed to the treatment, as opposed to other rival plausible alternatives (patients and extraneous influences). In essence, RCTs provide a way to protect the internal validity of the inferences that can be drawn with respect to causal agency.

RCTs are not the only basis for drawing causal inferences with respect to treatment efficacy. Single-subject designs can do at least as good a job of ruling out rival plausible alternatives when they can be used (Kazdin, 1981), and the whole thrust of the quasi-experimental approach is to build an inter-lacing set of multiple controls to rule out as many interpretative threats as possible (Campbell & Stanley, 1963). RCTs are no panacea. Randomization sometimes fails, and it can be undermined by subsequent attrition (differential mortality). Moreover, some believe that a tradeoff exists between internal and external validity (Seligman, 1995), although this need not always be the case (Hollon, 1996). Nonetheless, when RCTs are adequately implemented, they remain the best single means of drawing a causal inference. I am reminded of Churchill's famous quote about democracy: "No one pretends that democracy is perfect or all-wise . . . indeed, it has been said that democracy is the worst form of Government except all those other forms that have been tried from time to time."

The Consequences of Failing to Randomize

But why must we control treatment assignment? Why not let patients select whatever treatments they prefer and see what happens? That would be a good way to find out what happens to those people who pursue a particular treatment. However, it would not be a good way to determine whether that treatment had a causal effect, that is, whether that treatment was responsible for the changes observed. The recent controversy over hormone replacement therapy (HRT) illustrates why this is so (Barlow, 2004). For close to two decades, women going through menopause were advised to take estrogen to reduce aversive symptoms such as hot flashes and to prevent osteoporosis and coronary heart disease. The common consensus was that this was good medical practice. Indeed, considerable evidence from uncontrolled trials showed that women who took estrogen fared better than those who did not. However, the results of a recent series of RCTs told a very different story. In those trials, in which women were randomly assigned to either active medication or placebo, HRT increased both cardiovascular risk (Manson et al., 2003) and the incidence of breast cancer (Chlebowski et al., 2003).

How could we have been so wrong? How could 20 years of clinical observation have led to conclusions that were so at variance with the RCTs? The current understanding in the field is that differences in patient characteristics obscured the negative effects of treatment. That is, women who exercised better self-care in most respects were more likely to pursue or receive HRT than women who did not, and the former patients would have done better than the latter within either level of treatment (HRT or no HRT). In essence, by relying on clinical observation and uncontrolled trials, we inadvertently confounded individual differences with the effects of treatment. Women who would have done better anyway (or for other reasons) were more likely to receive a treatment that put them at risk than women who would otherwise have had poorer health outcomes. Both women with good health trajectories and women with poor health trajectories would have done worse on HRT than in its absence. But before we did the RCTs, all we saw were women on HRT with good health trajectories compared to women not on HRT with poor health trajectories. Individual differences prevailed and the adverse effects of HRT for all women were obscured by the greater but unrelated propensity for better health in the women who were more likely to receive the treatment.

Other examples can also be examined. When I was an undergraduate, virtually every introductory psychology textbook reprinted a picture of two monkeys sitting side by side in separate chairs with electrodes attached to their bodies. This was Brady's (1958) executive monkey study in which both monkeys were yoked together such that they were shocked on exactly the same schedule, but one monkey (the executive) could turn off the shock, whereas the other could not. The finding from this classic study was that it was the executive monkey who was more likely to develop ulcers under stress, or to quote *Henry IV*, "uneasy lies the head that wears a crown." These findings were used to justify both the larger salaries paid to executives and the greater rewards given by society to those who stood higher in the social hierarchy.

The problem with this interpretation was that it simply was not true. Brady did not randomize his monkeys to the different conditions. What he did instead was to pilot test his subjects to determine which responded fastest and then assigned the more responsive monkeys to be the executive condition (perhaps to reduce the amount of time that each pair would be exposed to shocks). The problem was that this strategy confounded individual differences with his experimental manipulation. It turned out that monkeys with more reactive nervous systems tended both to respond faster to electric stimulation and to have a greater risk for ulceration. It was Jay Weiss (1971) who figured this out. He replicated and extended Brady's study by testing mice to ascertain their level of reactivity and then randomly assigning them to condition. It resulted that, when the effects of individual differences are made independent from the experimental manipulation, you obtain a main effect for each, but the main effect for individual differences in reactivity is greater than the main effect for the manipulated variable of control. That is, mice with more reactive nervous systems are more likely to develop ulcers than less reactive mice in either experimental condition. All mice do better when they have control than when they do not, regardless of how reactive their nervous system happens to be, but reactive mice in the more benign executive condition end up doing worse than less reactive mice in the more stressful subordinate role (Weiss, 1971). Once again, allowing patient characteristics to determine who got put in which condition obscured the true effects of the manipulation. Shakespeare notwithstanding, it turns out that "it is good to be king."

Numerous examples are prevalent in the field of psychotherapy in which good theory and strong opinion have led to the adoption of treatments that have later proven to be ineffective or dangerous. Treatments such as reprogramming therapy, rebirthing therapy, critical incident stress debriefing, and memory recovery therapy have all had their adherents and have all subsequently faded from the scene. In fact, this has happened so often throughout the history of psychology and medicine that we do not have to justify withholding a treatment that derives its support only from the beliefs of its adherents. What we have to justify ethically is failing to determine whether a treatment truly has an effect and whether that effect is benign or malignant.

Of course, certain examples go the other way. Over half a century after Freud first described the basic principles of psychoanalysis, Eysenck (1952) published a major critique in which he claimed that no good evidence proved that psychotherapy had any beneficial effect. In that polemic, he compared outcomes for patients who had received psychotherapy with outcomes for people who had not and found no differences. This created considerable consternation in the field and led to a major debate on the value of psychotherapy. Although no RCTs were available at the time that Eysenck formulated his critique, the firestorm he set off led to the publication of several dozen controlled trials over the next decade, the vast majority of which showed that psychotherapy was better than its absence (Luborsky et al., 1975).

Once again, the problem was that the people in the studies reviewed by Eysenck were free to seek or not to seek treatment as they chose, and it is likely that those who did seek treatment did so for a reason. When individual differences in levels of distress and problem difficulty were uncontrolled, it is likely that those with greater problems went to the additional trouble of seeking treatment and ended up no worse off than those with lesser needs who sought no such help. Subsequent studies that controlled for individual differences via randomization did not share this source of bias and clearly showed that treatment worked better than its absence, regardless of level of distress. Had we relied on uncontrolled observation, we would have erroneously concluded that treatment had no effect, when in fact it does.

Good intentions are not enough, and consensus expert opinion is no protection against the biasing effects of allowing individual differences to determine who gets what treatment. Benjamin Rush was the preeminent physician of his day, a signer of the Declaration of Independence and a close friend of George Washington. When he was called in to treat his friend for pneumonia, he did what any good physician of his day would do: He bled Washington to reduce his fever and likely contributed to his death (Flexner, 1974). His intent was to save a life, but his evidential base consisted solely of expert opinion. As a consequence, his treatment was iatrogenic rather than curative. My colleague Jan Fawcett, a leading research psychiatrist, has a plaque in his office that reads, "One good experiment is worth a thousand opinions." That is as true today as it was at the time of the American Revolution.

HEURISTICS AND BIASES IN MISPERCEPTIONS OF TREATMENT EFFICACY

The problem is that we all take shortcuts when we think. That is, we all use logical heuristics that help us process information more efficiently, but these heuristics also lead us to make certain predictable inferential errors (Kahneman, Slovic, & Tversky, 1982; Nisbett & Ross, 1980). It is inherent in the species. When making judgments, we overvalue that which is vivid and easy to remember (availability), and we are unduly influenced by the similarity between events (representativeness). We overvalue joint cooccurrence between events (treatments and outcomes), and we neglect to count the number of times each occurs without the other (confirmatory bias). We do not think this way because we are not intelligent; we think this way because it is the way we are designed to think and because it likely has survival value. We can train ourselves to override our first impressions, but it is a difficult process that requires constant vigilance. When Kahneman and Tversky first began their classic studies on logical heuristics, they made their initial observations on their colleagues between meetings at a convention of cognitive psychologists. We see causal relationships when none exist because it helped our ancestors survive; it is better to err in assuming that a rustle in the bushes is a tiger than to ignore it and wind up as the tiger's lunch.

The reason we need control groups is to serve as a check on our natural inclination to infer causal agency from observed outcome. If we have a patient who gets better in treatment, then we are prepared by eons of evolution to conclude that it was a consequence of something that we did. The reason we randomize patients to treatments is that it keeps us from confounding patient characteristics with the effects of treatment. Good research design protects us from our biases.

CONSTRUCT VALIDITY AND THE LIMITATIONS OF RCTS

RCTs are not designed to accomplish certain things, such as serve as a particularly good source of inspiration. Karl Popper distinguished between the "context of discovery" (the source of new ideas) and the "context of justification" (the process by which we separate the wheat from the chaff). Clinical trials clearly belong to the latter domain. Clinical innovations typically arise from clinical practice (or everyday life events), not from tightly controlled and systematic programs of research. Lightning rarely strikes in a controlled investigation (although basic research can be a fertile source of new ideas). Similarly, RCTs are not a particularly good way of determining what goes on in clinical practice. To quote another great 20th-century philosopher, Yogi Berra, "You can observe a lot by just watching." If you want to see what people are actually doing in practice, you have to go and look. Empiricism is the essence of science, not experimentation (Cronbach, 1957). Jane Goodall never conducted a controlled experiment, yet she told us much about human nature on the basis of observing our primate relatives. But what experiments do better than any other method is protect us from our inherent biases and heuristics when we want to draw a causal inference about whether a treatment has an effect.

Still, there is more to life than drawing causal inferences; it is good to know whether something does work and better still to understand how it works. Cook and Campbell (1979) revisited these issues over a decade later and added two additional kinds of validity. Statistical conclusion validity refers to whether study findings were analyzed appropriately and is sufficiently technical to be of little immediate interest. Construct validity concerns the extent to which we understand which aspects of the treatment manipulation were actually responsible for the changes observed. Treatment packages are often complex, and it is all too easy to mislabel or to misunderstand which ingredients are causally active. Construct validity is often hard to ascertain and disagreements over just which aspects of an efficacious treatment are causally active abound in the literature (see Wampold, 2001). It is easier to detect an effect than it is to explain it; efforts at construct validity fall in the latter domain.

Experiments can be and often are used to address construct validity, such as when we compare an active treatment against a nonspecific control. Such designs address both internal and construct validity; if the active treatment outperforms the nonspecific control, we know both that it works and that it works for specific reasons. Nonexperimental designs sometimes can also be used to distinguish causation from pure correlation, but their use can be treacherous and fraught with interpretive perils. Designs that examine a process or mechanism within the context of a "true" experiment (with random assignment) provide a much more solid basis for detecting causal mediation (Baron & Kenny, 1986).

IS SPECIFICITY NECESSARY?

Conversely, it is sometimes claimed that treatment must work for specific reasons to be efficacious; that is, it must exceed the effects of a nonspecific control. That simply is not true. If a treatment produces more change than its absence, then it is efficacious. This is true whether it exceeds a nonspecific control or not. We may misunderstand the nature of that effect (attributing it to specific mechanisms rather than those common to other interventions), but an effect is an effect regardless of how it is produced. At the same time, we may have little interest in those effects when they come at too high a price. For example, we insist that medications must exceed the efficacy of placebo controls in part because medications often produce noxious side effects or come at an exorbitant price. Similarly, the number of knee surgeries (once widely practiced) dropped drastically when controlled trials indicated that they provided no greater benefit than "sham" operations (Moseley et al., 2002).

However, no one has ever overdosed on an activity schedule, and few people would deny the beneficial effects of sharing personal confidences with someone who is sworn to keep a secret. Psychotherapy has not and should not be held to the same standards as other medical treatments, if only because the healing effects of a therapeutic relationship have been so well established. Even if psychotherapy were to prove to be nothing more than the purchase of friendship (as some have claimed), then time and attention in the context of a confidential relationship is a perfectly reasonable thing to sell. If additional specific mechanisms are mobilized, then so much the better, but they are not necessary to justify the existence of the helping professions. As noted previously, showing that a treatment works better than a nonspecific control not only shows that the treatment works (internal validity) but that it might work for the reasons specified (construct validity). However, specificity is only required to test a causal theory or to support claims of superiority relative to other types of interventions, not to show that an intervention works (internal validity) as practiced in the field (external validity).

SUMMARY AND CONCLUSIONS

I enjoy working with patients and I enjoy testing the treatments that I use. I particularly enjoy testing myself when I use those treatments (DeRubeis et al., in press; Hollon et al., in press). It increases my confidence in my clinical skills when I subject myself to the rigors of controlled evaluation, and RCTs can test the accuracy of my beliefs about the efficacy of my preferred interventions. Some of the things I believe have turned out to be correct, but I have been wrong so often that I have learned to trust my methods more than I trust my a priori judgments.

For example, I was dead wrong about interpersonal psychotherapy (IPT). When I first heard of the approach, I could not imagine how it could be efficacious in the treatment of depression. However, nature was not bound by my lack of imagination, and IPT has been shown to be efficacious in a series of well-controlled trials (see Hollon, Thase, & Markowitz, 2002, for a review). Similarly, when my friend Neil Jacobson (now deceased) first declared his intent to test the purely behavioral components of cognitive therapy, I went along purely out of affection. I could not imagine that behavioral strategies alone could provide more than modest and temporary relief. Again, nature was unimpressed with my predictions, and two recent trials (one still unpublished) have clearly shown that behavioral activation is at least as efficacious as my preferred approach and quite possibly as enduring (Jacobson et al., 1996).

As someone who is often in error but rarely in doubt, I find the power of RCTs both humbling and somewhat reassuring. I do not have to be free of prejudices to come to know the truth; all I have to do is to apply the kinds of controls that protect me from my biases. Doing science is a delightful way of groping toward enlightenment and doing experiments is the most powerful way of determining causal efficacy. For any therapist who wants to have an effect, attending to the results of well-conducted RCTs is one of the best ways to make sure that what he or she does will truly make a difference. For anyone who is dissatisfied with the quality of the current literature with respect to his or her preferred interventions, taking part in such trials is even better as a solution and ultimately far more satisfying.

Dialogue: Convergence and Contention

William B. Stiles

The parable of the blind men and the elephant may as aptly characterize this chapter's alternative positions on what qualifies as research as it does the alternatives that case studies bring to a theory (see my position paper). Understanding the beast demands multiple, diverse perspectives. I concur with Hill's position that there is room in our armamentarium for multiple approaches. That said, this commentary sounds a note of caution about applying some familiar scientific approaches to psychotherapy.

As cogently explained in the position papers by Hurst and Nelson-Gray, Borkovec and Castonguay, and Hollon, the controlled experiment is the closest science has come to a basis for inferring causation. If everything is held constant (controlled) except for one that is independently varied, then any distinctive consequences can be attributed to that independent variable. If one client receives an intervention and an identical client does not but is treated identically in all other respects, then any differences in their outcomes must have been caused by the intervention.

Difficulties arise because no two people are identical and it is impossible to treat two people identically in all respects except one. Many of the practical problems in applying the experimental method—and the correlational method as well—can be traced to the pervasive phenomenon of responsiveness (Stiles et al., 1998; see also Greenberg's position paper). Responsiveness refers to behavior that is affected by emerging context, including others' behavior. For example, therapists are being responsive when they make a treatment assignment on the basis of a client's presenting problems, design homework assignments taking into account a client's abilities, or rephrase an explanation that a client did not seem to understand the first time. Therapists and clients are responsive to each other on time scales that range from months to milliseconds. Though far from perfect, their responsiveness usually aims to be appropriate; they try to promote desired outcomes in ways consistent with their approach. In effect, then, the anticipated outcome (the dependent variable) feeds back to influence the delivery of treatment (the independent variable) on all time scales. This confounds the causal logic of the experiment.

Hollon's telling examples illustrate how responsiveness can undermine causal inferences. Brady's responsiveness in selecting reactive monkeys and HRT patients' differential responsiveness to their own health needs were overlooked and led to years of mistaken inferences. Defeating responsiveness in psychological research is impossible but nevertheless an enjoyable challenge. One can always think of new alternative explanations that must be ruled out.

The RCT is an adaptation of the experimental method that addresses differences among clients statistically. Rather than comparing single clients, investigators randomly assign clients to different treatment groups, assuming that relevant individual differences will be more or less evenly distributed across the groups. Even though outcomes may vary within groups (because clients are not identical), mean differences between groups beyond those due to chance should be attributable to the different treatments.

The point of randomization is unresponsiveness, but the point of psychotherapy is responsiveness, and many of the difficulties in conducting RCTs of psychotherapies can be understood as manifestations of responsiveness (Haaga & Stiles, 2000). As one manifestation, therapists and clients tend to compensate for protocol-imposed restrictions by responsively making different or more extensive use of the tools they are allowed. For example, a therapist told to decrease question-asking may compensate with more evocative reflections or remaining silent, giving clients more space to talk (Cox, Holbrook, & Rutter, 1981; Cox, Rutter, & Holbrook, 1981). In addition, treatment- and control-group clients may seek help outside a research protocol, responding appropriately to their own requirements. But this can turn an RCT into a confounded comparison of a "planned treatment plus some unspecified kinds of outside help" versus "no planned treatment plus different kinds of unspecified outside help."

Even within treatment groups, no two clients receive the same treatment. Therapist competence demands systematically responding to emerging client differences. Hardy, Stiles, Barkham, and Startup (1998) found that therapists tended to use more affective and relationship-oriented interventions with clients who had an overinvolved interpersonal style, but more cognitive and behavioral interventions with clients who had an underinvolved interpersonal style. Although, or perhaps because, they received different mixes of interventions, clients with these different interpersonal styles had equivalent positive outcomes.

Issues of responsiveness may be even greater in effectiveness research, insofar as the latitude for responsiveness is arguably greater in ordinary practice. Outside of formal research protocols, therapists are relatively free to devise a customized intervention plan and to deviate from or amend the plan in response to emerging information.

As Greenberg intimated, the correlational strategy for identifying active ingredients is also blocked by responsiveness. One might think the helpfulness of a process component (interpretations, "mm-hms," homework, relaxation training) could be assessed by correlating its frequency or intensity with outcome. But correlations assume independent observations, implying that the component is delivered ballistically or at least randomly with respect to client requirements. Such a treatment would be absurd. If therapists are responsive to clients' requirements, clients will get the optimum amount of the component. If the level is always optimum, then the outcome will tend to be the same across clients insofar as it depends on that component. Therapists are not perfectly responsive, of course, but any appropriate responsiveness tends to defeat the process–outcome correlation logic and may even reverse it. And, consistently, most common interventions are uncorrelated with outcome (Stiles, 1988; Stiles et al., 1998; Stiles & Shapiro, 1994). The few process components that empirically correlate with outcome, such as the alliance, group cohesion, empathy, and goal consensus (Norcross, 2002), are not discretionary actions but achievements (Stiles & Wolfe, in press), that is, products of responsive action, of doing the right thing at the right time.

Leiman (2004), building on work by Wampold (2001), distinguished three metamodels of psychotherapy research: the medical metamodel, exemplified by RCTs for drugs; the contextual metamodel, exemplified by process–outcome studies; and the developmental metamodel, exemplified by longitudinal case studies. Whereas responsiveness is problematic for the first two, it can be a focal topic for the third.

Ruth M. Hurst and Rosemery Nelson-Gray

The title of chapter 2 is "What Qualifies as Research on Which to Judge Effective Practice?" To answer that question, we would agree with Hollon's position that RCTs are the gold standard upon which to judge effectiveness.

In RCT, the independent variable is clearly identifiable, namely, replicable treatment manuals. The dependent variables are specified and quantified. Clients are randomly assigned to one or more treatment conditions and possibly a waiting list control condition. To reiterate comments by Hollon, according to the terms used by Campbell and Stanley (1963), RCTs have the advantages of both internal and external validity. With internal validity, the causal relationship between the independent and dependent variables can be identified with a great deal of certainty. With external validity, the observed effects can be generalized to the populations and settings of interest.

RCTs are not without their problems, as noted by Borkovec and Castonguay. Effectiveness is judged in relative terms, namely, that a treatment is more effective than another treatment or is more effective than no treatment. The absolute effectiveness of the treatment is not known. Moreover, the results are usually judged on the basis of statistical significance, not clinical significance. Individuals could improve statistically as the result of an effective treatment, in comparison to another treatment, and still not manifest clinically significant change. In addition, the results are typically based on group means, taking into account group variability. The effectiveness for a particular individual is not a major criterion in RCT to determine the overall effectiveness of a treatment.

At this point, the comments made by Stiles regarding the contributions of case studies and the comments by Hill regarding the contributions of qualitative research become pertinent. Case studies and qualitative research do have the advantages of taking into account the individual and his or her situation. In our view, case studies and qualitative research are useful as starting points in initiating clinical innovation. New treatment ideas or modifications of existing treatments can be suggested by working with individuals, either through case studies or through qualitative research. Hollon also makes this point: "Clinical innovations typically arise from clinical practice, not from tightly controlled and systematic programs of research."

In our view, however, neither case studies nor qualitative research qualifies as research on which to judge effective practice because the key ingredients of research—internal and external validity—are missing. In addition, treatment described in a case study or in qualitative research is generally not replicable. The key components are not identified or specified sufficiently to be replicated by a different therapist. Moreover, it is difficult, if not impossible, to judge how similar the client in the case study or in qualitative research is to a different client. Usually, similarity is judged on the basis of a diagnostic category or on the basis of pretreatment scores on a quantified assessment battery. Without clear criteria on which to judge clients as similar or dissimilar, external validity is seriously damaged. Also, recall that the establishment of external validity depends on the presence of internal validity. Unlike single-participant designs, described in our own contribution to this chapter, case studies and qualitative research do not have internal or external validity.

Another limitation of the gold standard, RCT, is that it typically identifies treatment with effective outcomes without identifying the process by which these outcomes are obtained. The points made by Greenberg and Watson are well taken, that process research is helpful in developing, implementing, and modifying treatment. We also agree with Stiles that case studies could enhance psychological theories that form the basis of effective treatments.

It is our view, however, that process research is a second step after outcome research. We need to know if a treatment is effective before concerning ourselves with the mechanisms or processes by which it is effective. Greenberg and Watson provide a nonpsychological example, that the bark of a chinchona tree relieved fever, but a century later the active ingredient, quinine, was identified. We note that, in the meantime, the fever of many individuals was alleviated (outcome research) without knowing the reason why (process research). In a psychological example, both case studies and group studies first established the effectiveness of systematic desensitization. Then process research was conducted using a dismantling process. Was relaxation necessary? Was the hierarchy necessary? Was the pairing of relaxation and hierarchy items necessary? Based on this process research, it was determined that the process mechanism underlying systematic desensitization was more likely extinction than counterconditioning or reciprocal inhibition, as originally proposed by Wolpe (1959; Marks, 1975). Extinction then formed the basis for the development of many other exposure-based therapies, which have also been found to be effective.

Another point made throughout chapter 2 is that traditional clinical outcome research, including the gold standard of RCT, is based on group data and does not take into account the individual. This is the argument made by Stiles regarding the contributions of case studies and by Hill regarding the contributions of qualitative research. We also argue that more needs to be learned about the application of various effective treatments to individuals. For example, several empirically substantiated treatments for depression have been developed, but no guidelines or decision rules have been established about which of these treatments might be effective with which client (Farmer & Nelson-Gray, 2005). A related concern is the external validity of the RCT to everyday clinical practice; that is, a treatment may work under clinical research conditions, but it may not work in everyday clinical practice. In our view, the way to examine the ordinary applicability of effective treatments is through PRNs, as described by Borkovec and Castonguay.

In conclusion, in answering the question of "What qualifies as research on which to judge effective practice?" we would use the criteria of internal and external validity, and conclude that the gold standard is RCT supplemented by single-participant designs. Case studies and qualitative research are useful as starting points, in suggesting innovative treatments and individualized applications, but they do not meet the criteria of internal and external validity. Process research is useful, but as a second step after outcome research. Process research is worthwhile only when an effective treatment has been established through outcome research.

Clara E. Hill

Each of the methods described in this chapter seems suited for examining a different part of the question about effective practice. In my discussion of these approaches, I divide them into descriptive (qualitative, process, change process, case study) and experimental types (randomized clinical trials, effectiveness research, and single-participant research).

Qualitative methods are ideally suited for describing what goes on in therapy and for highlighting the inner events of participants in ways that other approaches cannot. These methods are also ideally suited for discovering new and unexpected things, which is important given that we do not really know the effective components of therapy.

An approach that was left out of this book but that has a grand tradition in psychotherapy research is descriptive process research, which typically relies on codings of therapist and client behavior within sessions (e.g., head nods and therapist interpretations). This approach is ideal for describing what occurs in naturally occurring psychotherapy from the perspective of trained observers.

Change process research differs from more traditional process research by specifying and then testing for specific theoretical sequences within sessions. It thus goes beyond simple global descriptions of therapy to postulating effective sequences of behaviors within session events and then examining whether these sequences occur. Because researchers can examine successful resolutions of events, some evidence for mechanisms of change can be inferred.

Similarly, case study research takes a descriptive approach and tests theoretical propositions within the context of a single case. Focusing on a single case allows the researchers to use more context in understanding the change process. If change occurs in theoretically indicated ways, again we can infer something about the mechanisms of change.

In sum, these naturalistic, descriptive, observational approaches are very good for describing what goes on in the process of therapy and for modifying treatments to make them more effective on the basis of feedback from participants. They are also excellent for creating hypotheses about the mechanisms of change. Thus, these approaches can be considered as constituting the first step in any scientific endeavor. As we all learned, the first step of the scientific process is to describe the phenomenon. Once we have clear descriptions, we can build theory and test hypotheses.

A huge advantage of these naturalistic designs is that therapy is not manipulated; rather, the therapist is allowed to be responsive to the individual client. As soon as we manipulate the therapy experience, we have changed it in crucial ways. Resulting findings may have some application to practice, but we really never know how much the integrity of therapy has been altered by our manipulations.

Of the experimental approaches, RCTs are the most commonly promoted and used. I agree that it is an excellent approach for establishing causality, particularly for establishing that psychotherapy works. Unfortunately, the RCT approach is more limited, I believe, for figuring out how therapy works. Dismantling and additive studies, as well as looking for outcome mediators, are cited as ways of looking for the effective components of treatment, but these approaches are limited in their ability to inform us about the mechanisms of change (which is probably why practitioners get so turned off to this type of psychotherapy research). At this stage of our knowledge development, where we have established that treatments indeed do work, I think we need to go beyond the simple fact of effectiveness and learn more about how treatments work.

It is also important to note that our treatment packages are not simplistic bullets, but omnibus mega-approaches consisting of many untested components. Furthermore, when therapists apply treatments well, they modify them to fit individual clients, such that treatments look quite different when implemented by different therapists for different clients.

Effectiveness research addresses some of RCTs' problems, particularly in terms of the selection of clients and therapists. Challenges remain, however, about testing the effects of omnibus treatment packages. In addition, Borkovec and Castonguay rightly note that it is not possible to compare two alternate forms of treatment because too many uncontrolled variables exist. Similarly, when comparing treatment to no treatment, we have the problem that people who do not seek formal treatment often seek out other help (e.g., self-help or talking to friends).

S-P designs have some of the advantages of both descriptive and experimental methods. Therapists can be more responsive to the needs of individual clients, but at the same time the independent variable can be introduced and tested. S-P approaches, however, are mainly applicable to discrete behavioral interventions that can be implemented and withdrawn.

In sum, these experimental methods are useful for examining causality. My concern is that we need to step back and observe the effective components of therapy before we build the treatment approaches to be tested.

In my opinion, the question of how therapy works is the most crucial question at this time. We need to build treatments on the basis of empirical evidence of what works, rather than simply testing multicomponent treatments. Once we have some better notions about the effective components of treatment and the mechanisms of change, we can develop better treatments that can then be tested through clinical trials. Naturalistic, qualitative approaches can thus serve as a source of inspiration within the context of discovery and can lead to testing to determine causality using experimental approaches within the context of justification.

That said, I personally prefer the discovery-oriented methods. I feel excited about what I learn using these methods and stay close to the phenomenon of therapy. It may be that each of us gravitates to the method that best fits our personality style.

Finally, I suggest that the way our field can progress is by having lots of different researchers studying psychotherapy in many different ways. We should be encouraging creativity, innovation, and openness of thought about methods, given that many approaches can lead us to a better understanding of psychotherapy.

Leslie S. Greenberg and Jeanne C. Watson

In reading these position papers, including our own, there appear to be two fundamental issues that are not being dealt with. The first is the problem of political–economic power in which the whole matter of the EST debate is embedded. The issues here concern conflict between a dominant objectivist narrative and the failed attempts of disempowered groups to have their voices heard. The dominant group, believing in the correctness of their view, claims superior understanding of the issues but typically lacks true understanding of the effects of their power position on minority groups. The dynamics of oppression lead to the marginalization of dissenting voices. In psychotherapy, power involves privileged access to, and control of, resources (grants), communication (publications), and positions (tenure).

The second issue is whether the logic of cause–effect is applicable to human science and psychotherapy research. Although the logic of experimental procedures proposed in these position papers is impeccable, it is not applicable to evaluating the effectiveness of psychotherapy, as Borkovec and Castonguay point out. The arguments for the best designs for making causal inferences, although sound, lack clinical wisdom. Wisdom implies the ability to use knowledge to make sensible decisions by applying knowledge in appropriate contexts. Hollon, for example, argues for the superiority of RCTs with appropriate confidence that they offer the best way to make causal inferences, but he does not face the question of whether we are in a domain in which this logic applies. The debate implicit in a number of the other presentations (Stiles and Hill) is not on how best to infer cause but on how applicable, at this early stage of development of psychotherapy, is causal inference logic to the question of which treatments work best.

On encountering the work of Campbell and Stanley (1963) when I (LSG) came into psychology from graduate work in engineering, I found their proposals on experimental designs inadequate in studying human concerns. Throughout my graduate engineering training I had absorbed a pluralistic view of science. In moving to psychology I found the application of the experimental methods of natural science, based as they are on linear determinism, highly misplaced in studying nonlinear dynamic systems in interaction. Application of the medical model and RCTs to psychotherapy, as though psychotherapy is the administration of a drug rather than a meaning-making task in which two agents interact, is fraught with difficulties that have been explicated frequently elsewhere (Rice & Greenberg, 1984).

It is important to note that the dominant group in psychotherapy is cognitive–behavioral and that most voices that value RCTs come from this group. Why is this? For two reasons, we think. One is their commitment to a naturalistic science model. This is fair and represents a set of theoretical beliefs. The second reason, however, is more problematic: how power is cloaked in terms of objectivity. In their defense, they too are subject to power dynamics in the field, trying as they are to save psychological treatment from the dominance of psychoactive medication.

The biggest problem with current proposals of RCTs is the lack of a level playing field. Until all proposed treatments are given a fair test, claiming the superiority of some approaches that happen, through preparedness as well as the exercise of power and influence, to have been tested is tantamount to control. It is this lack of a level playing field that is the problem and an important cause of the debate, not the logic of causation. The debate rages because of the threat that some treatments may be eliminated due to a lack of opportunity to be tested in an RCT. The fallacy that "absence of evidence means evidence of absence" is currently dominating psychotherapy funding, practice, and education. Yet CBT, and the few non-CBT members on the ESTs list may be among the poorer forms of treatment we have. How do we know they aren't? They haven't been compared with all the others. This is a central problem with the current EST movement.

Probably the biggest implicit control factor operating to prevent a level playing field is that those who set the criterion of what constitutes knowledge wittingly or unwittingly set criteria that select themselves in and select others out. Thus, the criteria of acceptability of design requirements is set only after it has been met by, or is within the reach of, the dominant group. Once a test has been done showing the effects on a specific diagnostic group, only studies on specific diagnostic groups are acceptable as evidence. Once a manual has been written, then only manual-driven treatments are acceptable. Once a dominant group (medication or CBT proponents) has achieved a certain level of statistical power in a study, then this becomes a new criterion. Motivations for advances in rigor may have unwanted side effects, such as exclusion of other effective treatments.

We are strongly in favor of empirically investigated treatments, but as Hill points out, we are at a preliminary state of knowledge in psychotherapy research and we need to start bottom up to learn what is effective. RCT proponents apply the right logic prematurely, wanting to run before we can walk. Over the last decades, we have witnessed too many proclamations of truth in the name of science. These claims ranged from "psychotherapy is no more effective than spontaneous remission," "behavioral change is superior to insight," to "necessary and sufficient conditions of personality change." These have been followed by "CBT is the treatment of choice for depression," "it isn't, but it is for anxiety and eating disorders," and other things on the list. Each proclamation comes in the name of science by groups with an axe to grind and with power to wield. Changing fads on the basis of RCTs in psychotherapy should make all thoughtful people skeptical. Let us not continue to support these power dynamics and call it science.

Tom D. Borkovec and Louis G. Castonguay

We had two reactions to the important contributions of the other authors on their approaches to psychotherapy research.

First, each contribution, in one way or another, emphasized the importance of pursuing cause-and-effect relationships. Except for Hollon's belief (with which we disagree) that the EST criteria are sufficient for demonstrating "efficacy" for applied purposes, the authors did not explicitly address such criteria within their approaches. Instead, their perspectives on evidence for therapy squarely focused on establishing causal relationships among variables. We completely agree with this view and believe that it emerged as consensus due to the very nature of scientific approaches. Identifying causal relationships is the valid endpoint of research. The determination of increasingly specific causal relationships via the scientific method allows the inclusion of more causes in developing therapies. This process ultimately, though indirectly, provides answers to applied questions about efficacy because it results in increasingly effective therapies (containing more causes) for more people with more types of psychological difficulties.

Given that causal relationships are the ultimate goal, we must remember that correlational research does not demonstrate such relationships. Approaches to revealing relationships on the basis of case studies, consensual qualitative research, and investigations of change process mechanisms provide only hints about possible causes and cannot unambiguously demonstrate their existence. This is accomplished through experiments that manipulate variables found in such studies to correlate with process and outcome, as well as process variables found to correlate with outcome. As Hollon indicates, "Experiments are the most powerful way of determining causal efficacy" (p. 105).

As several authors mentioned, we also need to attend to the validity and reliability in our data and create protections against client, therapist, assessor, and investigator biases. This becomes increasingly important as the variables and their relationships become more complex, as in the proposed nonexperimental approaches. Experimental research has the advantage of decades of development in measurement, design, and methodology specifically geared toward these issues. But even in this approach, biases are possible, as Hill mentioned.

A significant way exists to both minimize such biases and maximize knowledge acquisition. Strong inference (in expansion of Stiles's lovely injunction to put theory at risk of falsification) rests on the centrality of devising rival hypotheses, conducting research to reject one or more of these rivals, and recycling this process on whatever rivals are not yet ruled out (Platt, 1964). In experimental psychotherapy research, this approach is best exemplified by component, additive, parametric, and catalytic designs. Strong inference has been associated with the most rapid accumulation of knowledge in the history of science. It additionally reduces the likelihood of investigator bias because more than one hypothesis (in addition to whatever the investigator believes to be true) is required. Consequently, we would encourage psychotherapy researchers, irrespective of methodological approach, to use strong inference in their planning of a study and in programmatic progressions of their studies.

Our second reaction was stimulated by Hill's insightful comment, "The ideal is to collect evidence about effective practices from a number of perspectives using a number of methods" (p. 81). We recommend including several, perhaps all, of the described approaches in any investigation to maximize the amount of useful knowledge obtained. Several reasons exist for suggesting such an integration of methodologies. First, when differing methods (each with its own advantages and disadvantages) yield the same or similar conclusions, we are all the more confident in those conclusions. Second, because each approach is also likely to reveal some unique relationships, we maximize the discovery of the previously unknown (as Hill eloquently stated) for further pursuit. In this regard, the nonexperimental methods described in this chapter provided very useful emphasis on ways to create contextualized, multifaceted, and intensive analyses of relationships among therapy variables. We wish to point out, however, that experimental designs can also include such qualities through moderator–mediator analysis for contextualization, additive designs for multifacets, and intensive case analyses described by Hurst and Nelson-Gray. Finally, some of the most important questions about causes in psychotherapy require, in ideal form, the combination of experimental and process research. For example, and in expansion of Greenberg and Watson's important section on "Designs for Process–Outcome," to maximize the likelihood that a process mediator can be determined to be a causal contributor to outcome (and not just a predictor or correlate), it is necessary to show a differential outcome between two or more comparison conditions in an experimental design, a differential change in the mediator due to the type of therapy, and a relationship between the mediator and outcome.

Wonderful opportunities exist to actuate the previous recommendation for methodological integrations. Several experimental therapy investigations have archived videotapes of their sessions, allowing other investigators to access incredibly rich information for process research. Tapes from our generalized anxiety disorder projects, for example, are being used for process analyses by investigators from the University of Utah and Miami University of Ohio. The integration of experimental and nonexperimental approaches would also be extremely wise in developing practice research networks in the future.

Finally, pondering our own comments and those of the other authors leads us to recommend one further approach: the resurrection of analogue therapy investigations. The primary disadvantage of experimental therapy outcome research is its cost in both time and financial resources. Such studies require years to complete, and the use of ideal designs (component, additive, parametric, and catalytic) require very large N for the sake of statistical power and the relatively small between-group effect sizes associated with the involved comparison conditions. It is very likely that our pursuit of causal agents in therapy can be markedly accelerated through the use of many single-session therapy investigations that experimentally manipulate putative causes in an efficient manner and establish their causal role initially, prior to a full-scale outcome study. Integrating the other nonexperimental approaches described in this chapter within such analogue studies would further increment our rate of knowledge acquisition and thus our development of increasingly effective forms of psychological intervention.

Steven D. Hollon

There is much in the other contributions in this chapter with which I agree and only little that I would question; I am impressed with the quality of the logic on display. Two principles that emerge as I read the position papers are the logical distinction between the context of discovery and the context of justification (Popper) and the methodological distinction between empirical observation and experimental manipulation (Cronbach).

Stiles makes a thoughtful defense of the use of case studies in which he argues that they generate observations that can provide quality control on theories. He further suggests that case studies fit well to the sensibilities and logistics of clinical practice. The approach he champions offers much of value (empirical observation is the basis of all science), and I agree that it can complement a more formal hypothesis-testing approach. I think that uncontrolled case studies are better suited to suggesting new ideas or modifications (discovery) than they are to testing the accuracy of existing beliefs (justification), but I agree that they contribute to the richness of the clinical enterprise.

The single-participant designs described by Hurst and Nelson-Gray allow for the kind of formal hypothesis testing provided by randomized clinical trials (justification). These designs reduce threats to internal validity by manipulating the timing or target of treatment (thereby controlling for potential confounding variables), and they do so with the same economy of subjects as afforded by unsystematic case studies. Such control must be systematic (treatment can be presented and withdrawn or introduced at different times across different targets), but it does not require group designs or inferential statistics. I rarely use such designs in my research (largely because I tend to examine the kinds of treatments that cannot be readily reversed or targeted with sufficient precision), but I consider them to be the logical equivalent of the randomized clinical trials and recognize that they confer some pragmatic advantages over larger group designs.

I think that great value is provided by the qualitative research described by Clara Hill, and I like the distinction she adopts between procedural versus validating evidence. Qualitative research lets the investigator explore complex phenomena in a rich and unfettered fashion and is particularly well suited to understanding the way people structure their subjective experience. However, qualitative research provides little basis for choosing among competing theories or even falsifying any single one and, as such, is better suited for the context of discovery than it is for justification. People often invent explanations for their subjective experiences or actions that bear no objective relation to the actual factors that control their behavior (see classic examples in Nisbett & Ross, 1980). I see nothing in qualitative research that protects against this proclivity. I think of qualitative research as a valuable way of exploring different interpretive systems for the purpose of generating hypotheses (discovery), but I do not see it as a particularly powerful way of resolving differences between existing beliefs (justification).

Greenberg and Watson make a spirited case for the importance of process research in elucidating our understanding of how change comes about. I agree that understanding the causal pathways of what are always mediated processes contributes greatly to both the confidence and power with which we can proceed. However, I do not agree that such knowledge (though desirable) is necessary to determine whether an intervention has a causal effect. RCTs and single-participant designs that use experimental methods to control for rival plausible hypotheses (internal validity) can determine whether a treatment has a causal impact, even if they do not explain how that effect is transmitted. This is a worthy goal in itself, even if it leaves us susceptible to misinterpreting the nature of the intervention (construct validity), something that process research of the kind described by Greenberg and Watson can address. At the same time, studying process in the absence of outcome does not necessarily tell us the extent to which a treatment works and runs the risk of exploring phenomena of little practical importance. The kind of research described by Greenberg and Watson enriches our understanding of the processes involved and contributes to our understanding of how that change is brought about (construct validity), but it is neither necessary nor sufficient to demonstrate that a treatment has an effect.

I have never fully understood the distinction between efficacy and effectiveness and think it is something of a "straw man" used to explain away the findings from controlled trials that are inconsistent with preferred practices or existing beliefs. Nonetheless, I think that research findings should generalize to clinical practice, and I like the way Borkovec and Castonguay recast the categorical distinction in terms of internal and external validity dimensions and give primacy to the former. I would further argue that, of the majority of the elements typically ascribed to, efficacy studies are neither necessary nor always desirable. Issues of recruitment, inclusion–exclusion, assessment, diagnostic status, treatment duration, the use of manuals, training, and supervision are all free to vary. The only requirements for internal validity are that some strategy such as random assignment or its logical equivalent (see Hurst or Nelson-Gray) be used to control for rival plausible alternatives and that some attention be given to the integrity of the manipulation. I do not share with Borkovec and Castonguay the notion that comparative designs are inherently flawed (if you want to see who has the fastest horse, you put them on a track and let them race), but I like the kinds of studies they endorse and I applaud their efforts to develop practice–research networks in applied clinical settings.

I think that controlled experimentation in the context of justification is the best way to determine whether a treatment works, but I recognize the importance of studying mediating processes and the extent to which it generalizes to actual clinical practice. I also suspect that more good ideas for future research will come from case studies and qualitative research than from more controlled and systematic investigations.

REFERENCES

Adams, K. E., & Greenberg, L. S. (1996, June). *Therapists' influence on depressed clients' therapeutic experiencing and outcome*. Paper presented at 43rd annual convention of the Society for Psychotherapy Research, St. Amelia Island, FL.

American Psychiatric Association. (1994). *Diagnostic and statistical manual of mental disorders* (4th ed.). Washington, DC: Author.

American Psychological Association. (2002). *Ethical principles of psychologists and code of conduct*. Retrieved October 3, 2004, from http://www.apa.org/ethics/code2002.pdf

Anderson, T., & Strupp, H. H. (1996). The ecology of psychotherapy research. *Journal of Consulting and Clinical Psychology, 64*, 776–782.

Angus, L., Hardtke, K., & Levitt, H. (1999). The Narrative Processes Coding System: Research applications and implications for psychotherapy practice. *Journal of Clinical Psychology, 55*, 1255–1270.

Axline, V. (1964). *Dibs: In search of self*. Boston: Houghton Mifflin.

Azrin, N., & Nunn, R. (1973). Habit reversal: A method for eliminating nervous habits and tics. *Behaviour Research and Therapy, 11*, 619–628.

Azrin, N., Nunn, R., & Frantz-Renshaw, S. (1980a). Habit reversal vs. negative practice treatment of nailbiting. *Behaviour Research and Therapy, 18*, 281–285.

Azrin, N., Nunn, R., & Frantz-Renshaw, S. (1980b). Habit reversal treatment of thumbsucking. *Behaviour Research and Therapy, 18*, 395–399.

Azrin, N., Sneed, T., & Foxx, R. (1973). Dry bed: A rapid method of eliminating bedwetting (enuresis) of the retarded. *Behaviour Research and Therapy, 11*, 427–434.

Baer, D., & Pinkston, E. (1997). *Environment and behavior*. Boulder: Westview Press.

Baer, D., Wolf, M., & Risley, T. (1968). Some current dimensions of applied behavior analysis. *Journal of Applied Behavior Analysis, 1*, 91–97.

Baird, S., & Nelson-Gray, R. (1999). Direct observation and self-monitoring. In S. Hayes, D. Barlow, & R. Nelson-Gray (Eds.), *The scientist practitioner: Research and accountability in the age of managed care* (pp. 353–386). Boston: Allyn & Bacon.

Barlow, D. H. (2004). Psychological treatments. *American Psychologist, 59*, 869–878.

Barlow, D. H., & Hayes, S. C. (1979). Alternating treatments design: One strategy for comparing the effects of two treatments in a single subject. *Journal of Applied Behavior Analysis, 12*, 199–210.

Baron, R. M., & Kenny, D. A. (1986). The moderator–mediator variable distinction in social psychological research: Conceptual, strategic, and statistical considerations. *Journal of Personality and Social Psychology, 51*, 1173–1182.

Barreca, S., Velikonja, D., Brown, L., Williams, L., Davis, L., & Sigouin, C. S. (2003). Evaluation of the effectiveness of two clinical training procedures to elicit yes/no responses from patients with a severe acquired brain injury: A randomized single-subject design. *Brain Injury, 17*, 1065–75.

Behar, E., & Borkovec, T. D. (2003). Between-group therapy outcome research. In J. A. Schinka & W. Velicer (Eds.), *Comprehensive handbook of psychology: Research methods* (Vol. 2, pp. 213–241). New York: Wiley.

Beutler, L. E., Harwood, T. M., Alimohamed, S., & Malik, M. (2002). Functional impairment and coping style. In J. C. Norcross (Ed.), *Psychotherapy relationships that work: Therapist contributions and responsiveness to patients* (pp. 145–174). New York: Oxford University Press.

Borkovec, T. D., & Castonguay, L. G. (1998). What is the scientific meaning of "empirically supported therapy?" *Journal of Consulting and Clinical Psychology*, 66, 136–142.

Borkovec, T. D., Echemendia, R. J., Ragusea, S. A., & Ruiz, M. (2001). The Pennsylvania Practice Research Network and future possibilities for clinically meaningful and scientifically rigorous psychotherapy research. *Clinical Psychology: Science and Practice*, 8, 155–168.

Borkovec, T. D., Newman, M. G., & Castonguay, L. G. (2003). Cognitive–behavioral therapy for generalized anxiety disorder with internalizations from interpersonal and experiential therapies. *CNS Spectrums*, 8, 382–389.

Brady, J. V. (1958). Ulcers in executive monkeys. *Scientific American*, 199, 95–103.

Burns, D. D. (1990). *The feeling good handbook*. New York: Morrow.

Campbell, D. T. (1979). "Degrees of freedom" and the case study. In T. D. Cook & C. S. Reichardt (Eds.), *Qualitative and quantitative methods in evaluation research* (pp. 49–67). Beverly Hills, CA: Sage.

Campbell, D. T., & Stanley, J. C. (1963). *Experimental and quasi-experimental designs for research and teaching*. Chicago: Rand McNally.

Campbell, J. M. (2004). Statistical comparison of four effect sizes for single-subject designs. *Behavior Modification*, 28, 234–46.

Castonguay, L. G. (1993). "Common factors" and "nonspecific variables": Clarification of the two concepts and recommendations for research. *Journal of Psychotherapy Integration*, 3, 267–286.

Castonguay, L. G., Arnow, B. A., Blatt, S. J., Jones, E. E., Pilkonis, P. A., & Segal, Z. V. (1999). Psychotherapy for depression: Current and future directions in research, theory, practice, and public policy. *Journal of Clinical Psychology: In Session*, 55, 1347–1370.

Castonguay, L. G., Goldfried, M. R., Wiser, S., Rave, P. J., & Hayes, A. M. (1996). Predicting the effect of cognitive therapy for depression: A study of unique and common factors. *Journal of Consulting and Clinical Psychology*, 64, 497–504.

Castonguay, L. G., Schut, A. J., & Constantino, M. J. (2000). Psychotherapy research. In W. E. Craighead & C. B. Nemeroff (Eds.), *The Corsini encyclopedia of psychology and behavioral science* (3rd ed., pp. 778–780). New York: Wiley.

Chambless, D. L., Baker, M., Baucom, D., Beutler, L., Calhoun, K., & Crits-Christoph, P. (1998). Update on empirically validated therapies, II. *The Clinical Psychologist*, 51, 3–16.

Chambless, D. L., & Ollendick, T. H. (2001). Empirically supported psychological interventions: Controversies and evidence. *Annual Review of Psychology, 52,* 685–716.

Chlebowski, R. T., Hendrix, S. L., Langer, R. D., Stefanick, M. L., Gass, M., Lane, D., et al. (2003). Influence of estrogen plus progestin on breast cancer and mammography in healthy postmenopausal women. *Journal of the American Medical Association, 289,* 3243–3253.

Clarke, G. N. (1995). Improving the transition from basic efficacy research to effectiveness studies: Methodological issues and procedures. *Journal of Consulting and Clinical Psychology, 63,* 718–725.

Cook, T. D., & Campbell, D. T. (1979). *Quasi-experimentation: Design and analysis issues for field settings.* Chicago: Rand McNally.

Cox, A., Holbrook, D., & Rutter, M. (1981). Psychiatric interviewing techniques VI. Experimental study: Eliciting feelings. *British Journal of Psychiatry, 139,* 144–152.

Cox, A., Rutter, M., & Holbrook, D. (1981). Psychiatric interviewing techniques V. Experimental study: Eliciting factual information. *British Journal of Psychiatry, 139,* 29–37.

Cronbach, L. J. (1957). Two disciplines of scientific psychology. *American Psychologist, 12,* 671–684.

Crosbie, J. (1993). Interrupted time-series analysis with brief single-subject data. *Journal of Consulting and Clinical Psychology, 61,* 966–974.

Darwin, C. (1859). *On the origin of species by means of natural selection, or the preservation of favoured races in the struggle for life.* London: J. Murray.

Denzin, N. K., & Lincoln, Y. S. (2000). *Handbook of qualitative research.* Thousand Oaks, CA: Sage.

DeRubeis, R. J., Hollon, S. D., Amsterdam, J. D., Shelton, R. C., Young, P. R., Salomon, R. M., et al. (in press). Cognitive therapy vs. medications in the treatment of moderate to severe depression. *Archives of General Psychiatry.*

Elkin, I., Shea, M. T., Watkins, J. T., Imber, S. D., Sotsky, S. M., Collins, J. F., et al. (1989). National Institute of Mental Health Treatment of Depression Collaborative Research Program: General effectiveness of treatments. *Archives of General Psychiatry, 46,* 971–982.

Elliott, R. (1989). Comprehensive process analysis: Understanding the change process in significant therapy events. In M. J. Packer & R. B. Addison (Eds.), *Entering the circle: Hermeneutic investigations in psychology* (pp. 165–184). Albany: State University of New York Press.

Eysenck, H. J. (1952). The effects of psychotherapy: An evaluation. *Journal of Consulting Psychology, 16,* 319–324.

Farmer, R., & Nelson-Gray, R. O. (2005). *Personality-guided behavior therapy.* Washington, DC: American Psychological Association.

Fisch, G. S. (1998). Visual inspection of data revisited: Do the eyes still have it? *The Behavior Analyst, 21,* 111–124.

Fisher, W., Kelley, M., & Lomas, J. (2003). Visual aids and structured criteria for improving visual inspection and interpretation of single-case designs. *Journal of Applied Behavior Analysis, 3,* 387–406.

Flexner, J. T. (1974). *Washington: The indispensable man.* New York: Little & Brown.

Foxx, R., & Azrin, N. (1973). The elimination of autistic self-stimulatory behavior by overcorrection. *Journal of Applied Behavior Analysis, 6,* 1–14.

Freud, S. (1953). Fragment of an analysis of a case of hysteria. In J. Strachey (Ed. & Trans.), *The standard edition of the complete psychological works of Sigmund Freud* (Vol. 7, pp. 3–122). London: Hogarth. (Original work published 1905)

Frijda, N. H. (1986). *The emotions.* New York: Cambridge University Press.

Gelso, C. J. (1979). Research in counseling psychology: Methodological and professional issues. *The Counseling Psychologist, 8,* 7–35.

Gelso, C. J., Hill, C. E., Rochlen, A., Mohr, J., & Zack, J. (1999). Describing the face of transference: Psychodynamic therapists' recollections of transference in successful long-term therapy. *Journal of Counseling Psychology, 46,* 257–267.

Giorgi, A. (1985). Sketch of a psychological phenomenological method. In A. Giorgi (Ed.), *Phenomenology and psychological research* (pp. 8–22). Pittsburgh, PA: Duquesne University Press.

Glaser, B., & Strauss, A. L. (1967). *The discovery of grounded theory: Strategies for qualitative research.* Hawthorne, NY: Aldine de Gruyter.

Goldman, R., & Greenberg, L. S. (in press). Depth of emotional experience and outcome. *Psychotherapy Research.*

Goldman, R., Greenberg, L. S., & Angus, L. (2004). *The effects of adding specific emotion-focused interventions to the therapeutic relationship in the treatment of depression.* Manuscript under review.

Gottman, J., & Glass, G. (1978). Analysis of interrupted time-series experiments. In T. Kratochwill (Ed.), *Single subject research: Strategies for evaluating change* (pp. 197–236). New York: Academic Press.

Greenberg, L. (1979). Resolving splits: Use of the two-chair technique. *Psychotherapy, 16,* 310–318.

Greenberg, L. (1984). Task analysis of intrapersonal conflict. In L. Rice & L. Greenberg (Eds.), *Patterns of change: Intensive analysis of psychotherapy* (pp. 67–123). New York: Guilford Press.

Greenberg, L. (1986). Change process research. *Journal of Consulting and Clinical Psychology, 54,* 4–9.

Greenberg, L. (2002). *Emotion-focused therapy: Coaching clients to work through feelings.* Washington, DC: American Psychological Association.

Greenberg, L., Bohart, A., Elliott, R., & Watson, J. (2001). Empathy. *Psychotherapy, 38,* 380–385.

Greenberg, L., & Foerster, F. (1996). Resolving unfinished business: The process of change. *Journal of Consulting and Clinical Psychology, 64,* 439–446.

Greenberg, L., & Malcolm, W. (2002). Resolving unfinished business: Relating process to outcome. *Journal of Consulting and Clinical Psychology, 70,* 406–416.

Greenberg, L., & Newman, F. (1996). An approach to psychotherapy change process research: Introduction to the special section. *Journal of Consulting and Clinical Psychology, 64,* 435–438.

Greenberg, L., Rice, L., & Elliott, R. (1993). *Facilitating emotional change: The moment-by-moment process.* New York: Guilford Press.

Greenberg, L., & Safran, J. (1987). *Emotion in psychotherapy: Affect, cognition and the process of change.* New York: Guilford Press.

Greenberg, L., & Watson, J. (1998). Experiential therapy of depression: Differential effects of client-centered relationship conditions and process experiential interventions. *Psychotherapy Research, 8*(2), 210–224.

Haaga, D. A. F., & Stiles, W. B. (2000). Randomized clinical trials in psychotherapy research: Methodology, design, and evaluation. In C. R. Snyder & R. E. Ingram (Eds.), *Handbook of psychological change: Psychotherapy processes and practices for the 21st century* (pp. 14–39). New York: Wiley.

Hardy, G., Stiles, W., Barkham, M., & Startup, M. (1998). Therapist responsiveness to client interpersonal style in time-limited treatments for depression. *Journal of Consulting and Clinical Psychology, 66,* 304–312.

Hayes, J. A., McCracken, J. E., McClanahan, M. K., Hill, C. E., Harp, J. S., & Carozzoni, P. (1998). Therapist perspectives on countertransference: Qualitative data in search of a theory. *Journal of Counseling Psychology, 45,* 468–482.

Hayes, S., Barlow, D., & Nelson-Gray, R. (1999). *The scientist practitioner: Research and accountability in the age of managed care.* Boston: Allyn & Bacon.

Hendricks, M. N. (2002). Focusing-oriented/experiential psychotherapy. In D. Cain & J. Seeman (Eds.), *Humanistic psychotherapies: Handbook of research and practice* (pp. 221–252). Washington, DC: American Psychological Association.

Henry, W. P., Strupp, H. H., Butler, S. F., Schacht, T. E., & Binder, J. L. (1993). Effects of training in time-limited dynamic psychotherapy: Changes in therapist behavior. *Journal of Consulting and Clinical Psychology, 61,* 434–440.

Hill, C. E. (1990). A review of exploratory in-session process research. *Journal of Consulting and Clinical Psychology, 58,* 288–294.

Hill, C. E. (1996). *Working with dreams in psychotherapy.* New York: Guilford Press.

Hill, C. E., Kellems, I. S., Kolchakian, M. R., Wonnell, T. L., Davis, T. L., & Nakayama, E. Y. (2003). The therapist experience of being the target of hostile versus suspected-unasserted client anger: Factors associated with resolution. *Psychotherapy Research, 13,* 475–491.

Hill, C. E., Knox, S., Thompson, B. J., Williams, E. N., Hess, S. A., & Ladany, N. (in press). Consensual qualitative research: An update. *Journal of Counseling Psychology.*

Hill, C. E., & Lambert, M. J. (2004). Methodological issues in studying psychotherapy processes and outcomes. In M. J. Lambert (Ed.), *Bergin and Garfield's handbook of psychotherapy and behavior change* (5th ed., pp. 72–113). New York: Wiley.

Hill, C. E., & O'Brien, K. (1999). *Helping skills: Facilitating exploration, insight, and action.* Washington, DC: American Psychological Association.

Hill, C. E., Thompson, B. J., Cogar, M. M., & Denman, D. W. III. (1993). Beneath the surface of long-term therapy: Client and therapist report of their own and each other's covert processes. *Journal of Counseling Psychology, 40,* 278–288.

Hill, C. E., Thompson, B. J., & Corbett, M. M. (1992). The impact of therapist ability to perceive displayed and hidden client reactions on immediate outcome in first sessions of brief therapy. *Psychotherapy Research, 2,* 143–155.

Hill, C. E., Thompson, B. J., & Williams, E. N. (1997). A guide to conducting consensual qualitative research. *Counseling Psychologist, 25,* 517–572.

Hill, C. E., Zack, J. S., Wonnell, T. L., Hoffman, M. A., Rochlen, A. B., Goldberg, J. L., et al. (2000). Structured brief therapy with a focus on dreams or loss for clients with troubling dreams and recent loss. *Journal of Counseling Psychology, 47,* 90–101.

Hoagwood, K., Hibbs, E., Brent, D., & Jensen, P. (1995). Introduction to the special section: Efficacy and effectiveness in studies of child and adolescent psychotherapy. *Journal of Consulting and Clinical Psychology, 63,* 683–688.

Hollon, S. D. (1996). The efficacy and effectiveness of psychotherapy relative to medications. *American Psychologist, 51,* 1025–1030.

Hollon, S. D., DeRubeis, R. J., Shelton, R. C., Amsterdam, J. D., Salomon, R. M., O'Reardon, J. P., et al. (in press). Prevention of relapse following cognitive therapy versus medications in moderate to severe depression. *Archives of General Psychiatry.*

Hollon, S. D., Thase, M. E., & Markowitz, J. C. (2002). Treatment and prevention of depression. *Psychological Science in the Public Interest, 3,* 39–77.

Honos-Webb, L., Stiles, W. B., Greenberg, L. S., & Goldman, R. (1998). Assimilation analysis of process–experiential psychotherapy: A comparison of two cases. *Psychotherapy Research, 8,* 264–286.

Honos-Webb, L., Surko, M., Stiles, W. B., & Greenberg, L. S. (1999). Assimilation of voices in psychotherapy: The case of Jan. *Journal of Counseling Psychology, 46,* 448–460.

Hopkins, B., Cole, B., & Mason, T. (1998). A critique of the usefulness of inferential statistics in applied behavior analysis. *The Behavior Analyst, 21,* 125–138.

Horvath, A., & Greenberg, L. (Eds.). (1994). *The working alliance: Theory, research and practice.* New York: Wiley.

Houts, A. (2003). Behavioral treatment for enuresis. In A. Kazdin & J. Weisz (Eds.), *Evidence-based psychotherapies for children and adolescents* (pp. 389–406). New York: Guilford Press.

Houts, A., Berman, J., & Abramson, H. (1994). The effectiveness of psychological and pharmacological treatments for nocturnal enuresis. *Journal of Consulting and Clinical Psychology, 62,* 737–745.

Jacobson, N. S., Dobson, K. S., Truax, P. A., Addis, M. E., Koerner, K., Gollan, J. K., et al. (1996). A component analysis of cognitive behavioral treatment for depression. *Journal of Consulting and Clinical Psychology, 64,* 295–304.

Jacobson, N. S., & Truax, P. (1991). Clinical significance: A statistical approach to defining meaningful change in psychotherapy research. *Journal of Consulting and Clinical Psychology, 59*, 12–19.

Joyce, A. S., Duncan, S. C., & Piper, W. E. (1995). Responses to dynamic interpretation in short-term individual psychotherapy. *Psychotherapy Research, 5*, 49–62.

Kahneman, D., Slovic, P., & Tversky, A. (1982). *Judgment under uncertainty: Heuristics and biases*. New York: Cambridge University Press.

Kazdin, A. (1981). Drawing valid inferences from case studies. *Journal of Consulting and Clinical Psychology, 49*, 183–192.

Kazdin, A. (1982). *Single-case design research*. New York: Oxford University Press.

Kazdin, A. (1998). *Research design in clinical psychology*. Boston: Allyn & Bacon.

Kazdin, A. (2001). *Behavior modification in applied settings* (6th ed.). Belmont, CA: Wadsworth.

Kazdin, A. (2003). Clinical significance: Measuring whether interventions make a difference. In A. Kazdin (Ed.), *Methodological issues and strategies in clinical research* (3rd ed., pp. 691–710). Washington, DC: American Psychological Association.

Kelly, A. (1998). Clients' secret keeping in outpatient therapy. *Journal of Counseling Psychology, 45*, 50–57.

Klein, M. H., Mathieu, P. L., Gendlin, E. T., & Kiesler, D. J. (1969). *The Experiencing Scale: A research and training manual* (Vol. 1.). Madison: Wisconsin Psychiatric Institute.

Klein, M. H., Mathieu-Coughlan, P., & Kiesler, D. J. (1986). The Experiencing Scales. In L. Greenberg & W. Pinsof (Eds.), *The psychotherapeutic process* (pp. 21–71). New York: Guilford Press.

Klerman, G. L., Weissman, M. M., Rounsaville, B. J., & Chevron, E. S. (1984). *Interpersonal psychotherapy of depression*. New York: Basic Books.

Knox, S., Hess, S., Petersen, D., & Hill, C. E. (1997). A qualitative analysis of client perceptions of the effects of helpful therapist self-disclosure in long-term therapy. *Journal of Counseling Psychology, 44*, 274–283.

Knox, S., Hess, S., Williams, E. N., & Hill, C. E. (2003). Here's a little something for you: How therapists respond to client gifts. *Journal of Counseling Psychology, 50*, 199–210.

Knox, S., Hill, C. E., Goldberg, J., & Woodhouse, S. (1999). Clients' internal representations of their therapists. *Journal of Counseling Psychology, 46*, 244–256.

Kraemer, H. C., Wilson, G. T., Fairburn, C. G., & Agras, W. S. (2002). Mediators and moderators of treatment effects in randomized clinical trials. *Archives of General Psychiatry, 59*, 877–883.

Kratochwill, T. (1978a). Foundations of time-series research. In T. Kratochwill (Ed.), *Single subject research: Strategies for evaluating change* (pp. 1–100). New York: Academic Press.

Kratochwill, T. (1978b). *Single subject research: Strategies for evaluating change*. New York: Academic Press.

Krauss, D. R., Seligman, D. A., & Jordan, J. R. (in press). Validation of a behavioral health treatment outcome and assessment tool designed for naturalistic settings: The treatment outcome package. *Journal of Clinical Psychology*.

Ladany, N., Hill, C. E., Thompson, B. J., & O'Brien, K. M. (2004). Therapist perspectives about using silence in therapy: A qualitative study. *Counselling and Psychotherapy Research, 4*, 80–89.

Lampropoulos, G. K., Goldfried, M. R., Castonguay, L. G., Lambert, M. J., Stiles, W. B., & Nestoros, J. N. (2002) What kind of research can we realistically expect from the practitioner? *Journal of Clinical Psychology, 58*, 1241–1264.

Lantz, J., & Gregoire, T. (2003). Existential trauma therapy with men after a heart attack. *Journal of Contemporary Psychotherapy, 33*, 19–33.

Leiman, M. (2004). Vaikuttavuustutkimuksen pulmallisuus psykoterapiatutkimuksessa [Problems of efficacy studies in psychotherapy research]. *Duodecim, 120*, 2645–2653.

Levins, R. (1968). *Evolution in changing environments: Some theoretical explorations.* Princeton, NJ: Princeton University Press.

Luborsky, L., Diguer, L., Seligman, D. A., Rosenthal, R., Krause, E. D., Johnson, S., et al. (1999). The researcher's own therapy allegiances: A "wild card" in comparisons of treatment efficacy. *Clinical Psychology: Science and Practice, 6*, 95–106.

Luborsky, L., Singer, B., & Luborsky, L. (1975). Comparative studies of psychotherapies: Is it true that "Everyone has won and all must have prizes"? *Archives of General Psychiatry, 32*, 995–1008.

Mahrer, A. R. (1988). Discovery-oriented psychotherapy research. *American Psychologist, 43*, 694–702.

Malott, R., & Trojan Suarez, E. (2004). *Principles of behavior.* Upper Saddle River, NJ: Pearson.

Manson, J. E., Hsia, J., Johnson, K. C., Rossouw, J. E., Assaf, A. R., Lasser, N. L., et al. (2003). Estrogen plus progestin and the risk of coronary heart disease. *New England Journal of Medicine, 349*, 523–534.

Margison, F. R. (1994). Comprehensive process analysis of insight events in cognitive–behavioral and psychodynamic–interpersonal psychotherapies. *Journal of Counseling Psychology, 41*, 449–463.

Marks, I. (1975). Behavioral treatments of phobic and obsessive–compulsive disorders: A critical appraisal. In M. Hersen, R. M. Eisler, & P. M. Miller (Eds.), *Progress in behavior modification* (Vol. 1, pp. 66–158). New York: Academic Press.

Meehl, P. E. (1987). Theory and practice: Reflections of an academic clinician. In E. F. Bourg, R. J. Bent, J. E. Callan, N. F. Jones, J. McHolland, & G. Stricker (Eds.), *Standards and evaluation in the education and training of professional psychologists: Knowledge, attitudes, and skills* (pp. 7–23). Norman, OK: Transcript Press.

Morgan, D., & Morgan, R. (2003). Single-participant research design: Bringing science to managed care. In A. Kazdin (Ed.), *Methodological issues and strategies in clinical research* (3rd ed., pp. 635–654). Washington, DC: American Psychological Association.

Morrow, S. L., & Smith, M. L. (2000). Qualitative research for counseling psychology. In S. D. Brown & R. W. Lent (Eds.), *Handbook of counseling psychology* (3rd ed., pp. 199–230). New York: Wiley.

Morrow-Bradley, C., & Elliott, R. (1986). The utilization of psychotherapy research by practicing psychotherapists. *American Psychologist, 41,* 188–197.

Moseley, J. B., O'Malley, K., Petersen, N. J., Menke, T. J., Brody, B. A., Kuykendall, D. H., et al. (2002). A controlled trial of arthroscopic surgery for osteoarthritis of the knee. *New England Journal of Medicine, 347,* 81–88.

Nathan, P., & Gorman, J. (2002). *A guide to treatments that work.* New York: Oxford University Press.

Newman, M. G., Castonguay, L. G., Borkovec, T. D., & Molnar, C. (2004). Integrative therapy. In R. G. Heimberg, C. L. Turk, D. S. Mennin (Eds.), *Generalized anxiety disorder* (pp. 320–350). New York: Guilford Press.

Nisbett, R., & Ross, L. (1980). *Human inference: Strategies and shortcomings of social judgment.* Englewood Cliffs, NJ: Prentice Hall.

Norcross, J. C. (2002). Empirically supported therapy relationships. In J. C. Norcross (Ed.), *Psychotherapy relationships that work: Therapist contributions and responsiveness to patients* (pp. 3–16). New York: Oxford University Press.

Norcross, J. C. (Ed.). (2002). *Psychotherapy relationships that work: Therapist contributions and responsiveness to patient needs.* New York: Oxford University Press.

Ollendick, T., & King, N. (2004). Empirically supported treatments for children and adolescents: Advances toward evidence-based practice. In R. Barrett & T. Ollendick (Eds.), *Handbook of interventions that work with children and adolescents: Prevention and treatment* (pp. 3–25). New York: Wiley.

Orlinsky, D. E., & Howard, K. I. (1986). Process and outcome in psychotherapy. In S. Garfield & A. Bergin (Eds.), *Handbook of psychotherapy and behavior change.* New York: Wiley.

Paivio, S., & Greenberg, L. (1995). Resolving unfinished business: Experiential therapy using empty chair dialogue. *Journal of Consulting and Clinical Psychology, 63,* 419–425.

Platt, J. R. (1964). Strong inference. *Science, 146,* 347–353.

Ponterotto, J. G. (in press). Qualitative research in counseling psychology: A primer on research paradigms, philosophy of science, and some quantitative/qualitative distinctions. *Journal of Counseling Psychology.*

Popper, K. (1959). *The logic of scientific discovery.* New York: Basic Books. (Original work published 1934)

Pos, A. E., Greenberg, L. S., Korman, L. M., & Goldman, R. N. (2003). Emotional processing during experiential treatment of depression. *Journal of Consulting and Clinical Psychology, 71,* 1007–1016.

Rennie, D. L., Phillips, J. R., & Quartaro, G. K. (1988). Grounded theory: A promising approach to conceptualization in psychology? *Canadian Psychology, 29,* 138–150.

Rhodes, R., Hill, C. E., Thompson, B. J., & Elliott, R. (1994). Client retrospective recall of resolved and unresolved misunderstanding events. *Journal of Counseling Psychology, 41*, 473–483.

Rice, L., & Greenberg, L. (Eds.). (1984). *Patterns of change: An intensive analysis of psychotherapeutic process.* New York: Guilford Press.

Rosenwald, G. C. (1988). A theory of multiple case research. *Journal of Personality, 56*, 239–264.

Rush, A. J., Beck, A. T., Kovacs, M., & Hollon, S. D. (1977). Comparative efficacy of cognitive therapy and imipramine in the treatment of depressed patients. *Cognitive Therapy and Research, 1*, 17–37.

Rychlak, J. F. (1968). *A philosophy of science for personality theory.* Boston: Houghton Mifflin.

Samoilov, A., & Goldfried, M. (2000). Role of emotion in cognitive behavior therapy. *Clinical Psychology: Science and Practice, 7*, 373–385.

Sciarra, D. (1999). The role of the qualitative researcher. In M. Kopala & L. A. Suzuki (Eds.), *Using qualitative methods in psychology* (pp. 37–48). Thousand Oaks, CA: Sage.

Seligman, M. E. P. (1995). The effectiveness of psychotherapy: The *Consumer Reports* study. *American Psychologist, 50*, 965–974.

Shadish, W. R., Cook, T. D., & Campbell, D. T. (2001). *Experimental and quasi-experimental designs for generalized causal inference.* Boston: Houghton Mifflin.

Shull, R. (1999). Statistical inference in behavior analysis: Discussant's remarks. *The Behavior Analyst, 22*, 117–121.

Silberschatz, G., Fretter, P. B., & Curtis, J. T. (1986). How do interpretations influence the process of psychotherapy? *Journal of Consulting and Clinical Psychology, 54*, 646–652.

Singh, A., & Banerjee, K. (2002). Treating panic attack with hypnosis in combination with rational emotive therapy—a case report. *Journal of Projective Psychology and Mental Health, 9*, 105–108.

Stiles, E. W. (1980). Patterns of fruit presentation and seed dispersal in bird-disseminated woody plants in the eastern deciduous forest. *The American Naturalist, 116*, 670–688.

Stiles, W. B. (1981). Science, experience, and truth: A conversation with myself. *Teaching of Psychology, 8*, 227–230.

Stiles, W. B. (1988). Psychotherapy process-outcome correlations may be misleading. *Psychotherapy, 25*, 27–35.

Stiles, W. B. (1993). Quality control in qualitative research. *Clinical Psychology Review, 13*, 593–618.

Stiles, W. B. (2002). Assimilation of problematic experiences. In J. C. Norcross (Ed.), *Psychotherapy relationships that work: Therapist contributions and responsiveness to patients* (pp. 357–365). New York: Oxford University Press.

Stiles, W. B. (2003). Qualitative research: Evaluating the process and the product. In S. P. Llewelyn & P. Kennedy (Eds.), *Handbook of clinical health psychology* (pp. 477–499). London: Wiley.

Stiles, W. B., Elliott, R., Llewelyn, S. P., Firth-Cozens, J. A., Margison, F. R., Shapiro, D. A., et al. (1990). Assimilation of problematic experiences by clients in psychotherapy. *Psychotherapy, 27*, 411–420.

Stiles, W. B., Honos-Webb, L., & Surko, M. (1998). Responsiveness in psychotherapy. *Clinical Psychology: Science and Practice, 5*, 439–458.

Stiles, W. B., Meshot, C. M., Anderson, T. M., & Sloan, W. W., Jr. (1992). Assimilation of problematic experiences: The case of John Jones. *Psychotherapy Research, 2*, 81–101.

Stiles, W. B., & Shapiro, D. A. (1994). Disabuse of the drug metaphor: Psychotherapy process-outcome correlations. *Journal of Consulting and Clinical Psychology, 62*, 942–948.

Stiles, W. B., Shapiro, D. A., & Elliott, R. (1986). "Are all psychotherapies equivalent?" *American Psychologist, 41*, 165–180.

Stiles, W. B., & Wolfe, B. E. (in press). Relationship contributions to the treatment of anxiety disorders: Empirically supported principles. In L. G. Castonguay & L. E. Beutler (Eds.), *Principles of change in psychotherapy*. New York: Oxford University Press.

Strauss, A., & Corbin, J. (1998). *Basics of qualitative research: Grounded theory procedures and techniques* (2nd ed.). Newbury Park, CA: Sage.

Strupp, H. H., Horowitz, L. M., & Lambert, M. J. (Eds.). (1997). *Measuring patient changes in mood, anxiety, and personality disorders: Toward a core battery*. Washington, DC: American Psychological Association.

Talley, P. F., Strupp, H. H., & Butler, S. F. (Eds.). (1994). *Psychotherapy research and practice: Bridging the gap*. New York: Basic Books.

Taylor, S. T., & Bogdan, R. (1998). *Introduction to qualitative research methods: A guidebook and resource* (3rd ed.). New York: Wiley.

van de Vliet, P., Onghena, P., Knapen, J., Fox, K. R., Probst, M., van Coppenolle, H., et al. (2003). Assessing the additional impact of fitness training in depressed psychiatric patients receiving multifaceted treatment: A replicated single-subject design. *Disability and Rehabilitation, 25*, 1344–1353.

Varvin, S., & Stiles, W. B. (1999). Emergence of severe traumatic experiences: An assimilation analysis of psychoanalytic therapy with a political refugee. *Psychotherapy Research, 9*, 381–404.

Wampold, B. E. (2001). *The great psychotherapy debate: Models, methods, and findings*. Mahwah, NJ: Erlbaum.

Wampold, B. E., Mondin, G. W., Moody, M., Stich, F., Benson, K., & Ahn, H. (1997). A meta-analysis of outcome studies comparing bona fide psychotherapies: Empirically, "all must have prizes." *Psychological Bulletin, 122*, 203–215.

Warwar, S. (2003). *Relating emotional processes to outcome in experiential psychotherapy of depression*. Unpublished doctoral dissertation, York University, Toronto, Canada.

Warwar, N., & Greenberg, L. (1999, June). *Emotional processing and therapeutic change*. Paper presented at the International Society for Psychotherapy Research annual meeting, Braga, Portugal.

Watson, J. B., & Rayner, R. (1920). Conditioned emotional reactions. *Journal of Experimental Psychology, 3*, 1–14.

Watson, J. C., Gordon, L. B., Stermac, L., Kalogerakos, F., & Steckley, P. (2003). Comparing the effectiveness of process–experiential with cognitive–behavioral psychotherapy in the treatment of depression. *Journal of Consulting and Clinical Psychology, 71*, 773–781.

Watson, J. C., & Rennie, D. L. (1994). Qualitative analysis of clients' subjective experience of significant moments during the exploration of problematic reactions. *Journal of Counseling Psychology, 41*, 500–509.

Weinberger, D. (2003, July). *Evolution of the sites of molecular action for the treatment of psychosis*. Paper presented at the International Conference on Constructivism, Bari, Italy.

Weiss, J. M. (1971). Effects of coping behavior with and without a feedback signal on stress pathology in rats. *Journal of Comparative and Physiological Psychology, 77*, 22–30.

Wolpe, J. (1959). *Psychotherapy by reciprocal inhibition*. Stanford, CA: Stanford University Press.

3

DOES MANUALIZATION IMPROVE THERAPY OUTCOMES?

Psychotherapy Manuals Can Improve Outcomes

Michael E. Addis and Esteban V. Cardemil

Debates over the value of psychotherapy manuals for research and clinical practice have now continued for over a decade. In some respects, it is remarkable that something as straightforward as a book describing the components of psychotherapy could generate such heated controversy. It does not take an expert psychotherapist, however, to intuit that these debates involve much more than treatment manuals alone. Manuals themselves, and the treatments they describe, are only the manifest point of debate. At stake are much deeper conflicts over professional identity, territory, decision-making power, and access to resources in the increasingly embattled field of clinical practice. These deeper and perennial conflicts in the research–practice relationship are probably the reasons that balanced perspectives on the assets of manual-based treatments for clinical practice have been conspicuously lacking in the literature. We consider some of these larger issues at the end of this position paper. For now, we provide an argument in favor of the use of treatment manuals in clinical practice.

Our argument is based on the following five premises:

- Treatment manuals, evidence-based treatments, and manual-based treatments are not one and the same, although they have been repeatedly treated as such in the literature.
- Treatment manuals are widely mischaracterized as overly structured, step-by-step, how-to guides that rob practitioners of their therapeutic creativity and skill.
- Despite widespread assumptions to the contrary, numerous studies have shown that evidence-based treatments are effective in clinical practice.
- Treatment manuals themselves are nothing more than attempts to delineate the conceptual and structural boundaries of an evidence-based treatment. As such, a manual's usefulness lies in the degree to which it helps therapists monitor their own adherence to strategies and techniques that facilitate the assumed active ingredients.
- Our current empirical database on the utility of treatment manuals per se (as opposed to the treatments they describe) is woefully inadequate for drawing any firm conclusions about the specific effectiveness of manuals one way or the other.

WHAT ARE TREATMENT MANUALS?

Treatment manuals evolved in the context of psychotherapy outcome research (Luborsky & DeRubeis, 1984). In a research context, their primary function is to describe an intervention in sufficient detail such that a test of treatment integrity can be performed to document whether the independent variable (i.e., the treatment under consideration) was successfully manipulated in an experimental paradigm. Over time, as evidence accumulated supporting the efficacy of various psychotherapies, treatment manuals began to be disseminated to clinical practice (Wilson, 1996, 1998). The emphasis on treatment manuals as a means of dissemination was, and is, driven more by convenience than by the conviction on the part of treatment developers that manuals alone are sufficient to provide quality care to clients (Addis, 1997; Henggeler & Schoenwald, 2002). Practitioners are typically hungry for new research-supported interventions, and treatment manuals are a relatively low-cost and easily available means of educating oneself in a particular treatment.

Treatment manuals in their current forms vary considerably from relatively structured guidelines for session-by-session interventions (e.g., Craske, Meadows, & Barlow, 1994) to more general outlines of therapeutic strategies that can be implemented flexibly by clinicians according to the needs of individual clients (e.g., Martell, Addis, & Jacobson, 2001; Strupp & Binder, 1984). Although the structure of psychotherapy treatment manuals varies considerably, all manuals attempt to describe an intervention in enough detail that a practitioner can implement the core ingredients in the treatment.

Early arguments against manual-based treatments often ignored this variability in degree of detail and structure. Manuals were typically painted as step-by-step (or "paint by numbers;" see Silverman, 1996) guides that overly emphasized therapeutic techniques at the expense of attention to the therapeutic relationship (Fensterheim & Raw, 1996; Garfield, 1996). As a result, early critics of treatment manuals often created a straw-person argument in which psychotherapy manuals were characterized as not all that different than manuals for hooking up a VCR or installing a garbage disposal (see Kendall, 1998). Obviously, such an extreme degree of rigidity that prohibits any form of deviation on the basis of clinical judgment would be useless (or worse than useless) in clinical practice, where patients are varied along many different dimensions (e.g., comorbidity, race–ethnicity, and individual life circumstances).

In contrast to the impressions painted by early critics of treatment manuals, numerous authors who have developed and evaluated manual-based treatments have identified therapist flexibility and creativity as essential components of successful treatment. For example, Addis and colleagues (1999) described a number of dialectics in manual-based treatment, including adherence to the manual versus flexibility, attention to the therapeutic relationship versus attention to therapeutic techniques, and others. They suggest that the goal in using a treatment manual is to find a creative synthesis among various oppositions rather than to adhere rigidly to one end of the therapeutic spectrum. Other authors have identified similar creative ways to remain flexible and tailor treatment to the needs of individual clients while adhering to therapeutic methods that have been evaluated in controlled research (Goebel-Fabbri, Fikkan, & Franko, 2003; Hembree, Rauch, & Foa, 2003; Huppert & Baker-Morrisette, 2003; Kendall, Chu, Gifford, Hayes, & Nauta, 1998).

In fact, the importance of flexibility was highlighted over 25 years ago by Beck and colleagues (1979), who warned that novice therapists may rigidly adhere to techniques at the expense of the therapeutic alliance. In their view, this would be poorly delivered therapy. Some empirical research has supported the concern that the overly rigid application of manual-based interventions would be associated with the poor delivery of psychotherapy and worse clinical outcome (Castonguay, Goldfried, Wiser, Raue, & Hayes, 1996; Henry, Strupp, Butler, Schacht, & Binder, 1993; Vakoch & Strupp, 2000). And yet what often goes unacknowledged by critics of treatment manuals is the variability in therapist competence in the implementation of treatment (e.g., Dobson & Shaw, 1988; Waltz, Addis, Koerner, & Jacobson, 1993; Weissman, Markowitz, & Klerman, 2000). Thus, early criticisms of treatment manuals took concerns that were relevant to less experienced therapists and extrapolated them to critique the entire enterprise of using a treatment manual in therapy. These criticisms have been further undermined by recent evidence suggesting that therapists who conduct manual-based treatments typically do so in a flexible client-responsive fashion (e.g., Gibbons, Crits-Christoph, Levinson, & Barber, 2003).

EVIDENCE-BASED TREATMENTS, TREATMENT MANUALS, AND MANUAL-BASED TREATMENTS

It is easier to assess the potential assets of treatment manuals per se if they are clearly distinguished from evidence-based treatments and so-called manual-based treatments. The three have often been conflated in the literature. For example, in considering problems associated with linking treatment to Axis I *Diagnostic and Statistical Manual of Mental Disorders, Fourth Edition* (*DSM–IV*; American Psychiatric Association, 1994) diagnoses, Westen, Novotony, and Thompson-Brenner (2004, p. 634) argued that, "the sheer number of disorders in the *DSM–IV* renders the notion of clinicians learning disorder-specific manuals for more than a handful of disorders unrealistic." The central issue here is not learning specific manuals. The goal of evidence-based practice (EBP) is learning and implementing treatments that have garnered empirical support.

Evidence-based treatments are those treatments that have been tested in controlled clinical research and found to be efficacious. Treatment manuals are written documents intended to aid in the evaluation, dissemination, and implementation of some evidence-based treatments (Addis, 1997). The term "manual-based treatments" originally emerged in the literature as a description of treatments that had an accompanying treatment manual; such manuals, as we described previously, vary considerably in their structure and content. At no time did proponents of treatment manuals claim that the treatment was to be literally "based" on the manual, as if the manual were the treatment. Rather, the manual was considered an important and helpful part of the treatment. Unfortunately, the term "manual-based treatment" now seems to refer to a hypothetical treatment that follows some highly structured manual page by page, utterance by utterance, to such a degree that the therapist is essentially replaced by the manual. We have never seen such a treatment and doubt that one exists.

CAN TREATMENT MANUALS ENHANCE CLINICAL OUTCOMES?

Once manuals have been distinguished from the treatments they describe, it is possible to ask a series of more specific questions. One such question is whether evidence-based treatments can enhance clinical outcomes. This question is addressed elsewhere in this book. A second question is whether treatment manuals can enhance psychotherapy outcomes. A few authors have attempted to answer this question by examining the empirical literature on various indirect connections between treatment manuals and treatment outcome (e.g., Miller & Binder, 2002; Westen, Novotony, & Thompson-Brenner, 2004). For example, some studies have demonstrated relationships between therapist training, of which one component is typically a treatment manual, and therapist adherence to a treatment (see Miller & Binder, 2002). Other studies have examined correlations between adherence to a manual and treatment outcome, with some studies documenting a positive correlation and others finding no correlation (see Westen et al., 2004).

From our perspective, none of this research bears directly on the value of treatment manuals per se. The function of a treatment manual is not to replace the sensitive, creative, and flexible clinician but to assist in the dissemination and implementation of an evidence-based treatment. Viewed this way, treatment manuals have several potential benefits to offer to practitioners of evidence-based interventions. First, treatment manuals articulate the conceptual and structural boundaries of a given treatment. Conceptual boundaries delineate a theory of both the therapeutic change process and the etiological or maintaining factors underlying a particular problem or disorder. For example, within a psychodynamic or interpersonal approach to the treatment of depression (e.g., Klerman, Weissman, Rounsaville, & Chevron, 1984), the assumption that a client's automatic thoughts are the core determinants of his or her mood would be conceptually outside the boundaries of treatment. Structural boundaries are more concrete and include such things as the typical length of treatment, the amount of training required of therapists, critical interventions or treatment strategies, and so on. For example, dream interpretation would be outside the structural boundaries of cognitive–behavioral treatment for panic disorder (Craske, Meadows, & Barlow, 1994), whereas interoceptive exposure interventions would be critical to the treatment.

Of course, one could ask, why have boundaries at all? Many practitioners prefer an eclectic or integrative approach where they take into consideration the perceived needs of individual clients and then blend together the conceptual models and structural aspects of treatment. The question of eclecticism versus relatively "pure-form" intervention runs right to the center of the broader debate over EBP. With few exceptions (e.g., Beutler, Clarkin, & Bongar, 2000; Beutler, Malik, Talebi, Fleming, & Moleiro, 2004), the majority of evidence-based treatments proceed from a single, coherent, conceptual framework or therapeutic orientation and are targeted toward a particular problem or disorder (typically defined according to the *DSM–IV*). This is because an adequate, internally valid test of a treatment requires the specification of a finite number of ingredients that can be reasonably replicated, with flexibility according to the needs of individual clients, across different cases. In other words, it needs to be clear when the treatment is being conducted and when it is not (Waltz, Addis, Koerner, & Jacobson, 1993; Yeaton & Sechrest, 1981).

The advantage of therapists being able to monitor their degree of adherence to a well-defined treatment is not limited to research contexts. In clinical practice, adhering to any intervention strategy long enough to receive systematic feedback on client improvement is essential for helping individual clients and for facilitating learning from experience (Dawes, 1994). How can a therapist know whether a particular approach is effective with a given client unless the therapist is confident that he or she is actually delivering the treatment? Thus, another asset of treatment manuals is their ability to serve as beacons that help therapists remain on course and provide an adequate "dose" of treatment with clients.

An objection could be raised here that the emphasis on adherence and "dose" overly focuses on therapeutic techniques and obscures the importance of therapeutic relationships as change processes. This is an artificial distinction. In practice, therapeutic techniques are always embedded in the context of a therapeutic relationship and vice versa. It is simply impossible to introduce a particular technique or strategy without invoking a particular relational context with a client. Similarly, it is impossible to create a therapeutic relationship with a client without doing something, even if that something is as simple as listening empathically, which is a therapeutic technique in and of itself. Treatment manuals can help delineate and monitor the presence of active change ingredients in a treatment regardless of whether they are more "technique" or "relationship" focused (Addis, 1997). For example, there is no reason a researcher or clinician from a humanistic tradition could not develop a treatment manual that explicitly targets the therapeutic alliance, making theoretically driven recommendations. In addition, treatment manuals could just as easily focus on principles of therapeutic change as much as they may focus on techniques (Castonguay & Beutler, in press). What is critical is that the assumed active-change ingredients are well described and that therapists have a reliable way of knowing whether these ingredients are present in the therapy.

Finally, for better or worse, treatment manuals often help link a particular *DSM–IV* diagnosis to an etiological theory and a set of treatments. Considering the advantages and disadvantages of working within the *DSM–IV* as a nosological system is beyond the scope of this position paper. However, assuming that some sort of nosological system matching problem to treatment is helpful, and recognizing that the *DSM–IV* is currently the dominant such system, manuals explicitly linking disorders to specific treatment techniques offer practical advantages to clinicians. It should be clear, however, that nothing about the manuals per se requires linkage to the *DSM–IV*.

THE ONGOING DEBATE: MORE HEAT THAN LIGHT

In general, the debates over psychotherapy treatment manuals have been unnecessarily polarized and have included, on both sides, an excess of hyperbolic rhetoric and a dearth of balanced critical analysis. Consider the current position paper. So far we have argued the following points:

- Treatment manuals are nothing more or less than books that attempt to describe the conceptual and structural boundaries of a treatment.
- Very little research attests to the effectiveness of manuals per se versus the treatments they describe.
- Nonetheless, there are good reasons to hypothesize that treatment manuals can, under the right conditions, enhance the EBP of psychotherapy.

We have also not argued in favor of any of the following conclusions:

- The best psychotherapy outcomes will be achieved through rigid step-by-step adherence to a treatment manual.
- Treatment manuals by themselves should be the major, and possibly the only, medium through which EBP is achieved.
- Treatment manuals remove the need for practitioner skill, creativity, and clinical judgment.
- The function of treatment manuals is to standardize psychotherapy such that each client with a particular diagnosis receives the same treatment.

The first set of arguments seems, to us, much more reasonable and balanced. We also believe it reflects the general view held by many advocates of psychotherapy manuals, although we cannot be sure. The second set of arguments includes those often invoked by opponents of treatment manuals to characterize a simple-minded, scientistic, and antihumanistic approach to psychotherapy. They are also arguments that we have never seen put forth in the literature by proponents of treatment manuals. Why do the debates continue in this way?

Here are three possible causes. First, the very word "manual" itself may have been a costly historical mistake. Manuals are typically designed to walk people through a linear process in a step-by-step fashion. Their function is to enhance efficiency by breaking a complex process down into manageable steps. Neither of these are necessarily bad things, but they tend to conjure up mechanistic and other sterile or restrictive associations that simply do not "feel" like the way we typically think about psychotherapy. Perhaps "guide," "outline," or "framework" would have been better choices. For now, the field could, and in our opinion should, make a concerted effort to move discussion away from manuals per se and toward the treatments they describe.

A second source of fuel for the unnecessarily heated debates comes from a lack of familiarity with manuals and significant misunderstandings about what treatment manuals are and are not. In a national survey of psychotherapists' attitudes toward treatment manuals, Addis and Krasnow (2000) found that 63% of respondents rated themselves as having a reasonably (46%) or very (17%) clear idea of what a treatment manual is. In addition, 65% of respondents reported having somewhat to very strong attitudes about the role of psychotherapy manuals in clinical practice.

On the basis of these data alone, one might conclude that practitioners were well informed about the nature of treatment manuals and had thought through their advantages and disadvantages. However, only 16% of the respondents indicated that they had ever helped create a treatment manual. Moreover, when asked to describe treatment manuals, several misconceptions emerged. On average, respondents rated the description "a treatment protocol imposed by a third-party payer" at 3.3 on a 4-point scale from not at all characteristic to very characteristic of treatment manuals. The description, "a 'cookbook' of therapeutic techniques," received a mean rating of 3.7. Not surprisingly, those who tended to agree with the previous descriptions were more likely to endorse items emphasizing negative effects of treatment manuals on the therapeutic process. If a significant number of practitioners think treatment manuals are protocols imposed by insurance companies or HMOs, it is not surprising that the debates continue to generate so much heat!

Finally, the debates over treatment manuals can be seen as manifest expressions of two substantially deeper conflicts (Fongay, 1999). One is longstanding in the field and one is more recent, although both essentially boil down to questions of professional identity and access to resources: Who defines the practice of psychotherapy, and who decides whether and how it should be paid for? Considering the first question, it is perfectly clear to all involved, though rarely acknowledged directly, that the majority of treatment manuals describe cognitive–behavioral interventions. To the degree that adherence to a theoretical orientation is associated with a wide range of tangible aspects of professional identity, it is likely that treatment manuals are perceived by cognitive and behaviorally oriented practitioners as a resource, and by more dynamically, interpersonally, or humanistically oriented practitioners as a threat to their roles as psychotherapists.

Some evidence supports this perspective. For example, in their national survey of psychotherapists' attitudes toward treatment manuals, Addis and Krasnow (2000) found that psychodynamically oriented clinicians reported significantly more negative attitudes toward treatment manuals than did cognitive–behavioral clinicians. Similarly, in a multisite cocaine treatment trial, Najavits and colleagues (2004) found that psychodynamic (supportive–expressive) therapists consistently reported less satisfaction with their manual-based experience than the other therapists in the study (i.e., cognitive–behavioral, individual drug counseling, and group drug counseling). Others who have examined therapist satisfaction among cognitive–behavioral therapists have also found positive support for their manual experiences (e.g., Morgenstern, Morgan, McCrady, Keller, & Carroll, 2001; Najavits, Weiss, Shaw, & Dierberger, 2000).

In effect, treatment manuals may be seen as contributing to the perceived marginalization of noncognitive–behavioral therapies and therapists. This is unfortunate because several excellent psychodynamic and interpersonal treatment manuals are widely available (e.g., Klerman et al., 1984; Luborsky, 1984). It would do the field a tremendous disservice if such treatments did not continue to be developed and described in ways that facilitate their evaluation, and then ultimately lead to EBP.

Treatment manuals have also found themselves caught in a crossfire between traditional psychotherapy practices and the reformation of third-party compensation for mental health services in the form of managed care. Contemporary practitioners are rightly sensitive to arbitrary or financially motivated constraints on client care put forth by managed care companies and other third-party payers. Unfortunately, and possibly as a result of such sensitivity, treatment manuals have often been confused with arbitrary session limits or other treatment constraints that have little to do with their ability to assist clients. This is unfortunate because, in fact, the existence of evidence-based psychotherapies (of which treatment manuals are one part) can provide practitioners with a strong argument for more treatment than might typically be provided to a client. In point of fact, many cognitive–behavioral treatments for mood and anxiety disorders require approximately 12 to 20 sessions, far beyond the limits imposed by some managed care companies and third-party payers.

CONCLUSIONS

We have argued that existing debates about treatment manuals largely miss the mark by (a) stereotyping treatment manuals as overly rigid; (b) misrepresenting the intended function of treatment manuals as replacing therapist skill, creativity, and judgment; and (c) conflating treatment manuals with the treatments they describe. In support of manuals, we have argued that (a) they are a good way to describe the structural and conceptual boundaries of a treatment, (b) they may aid in the dissemination and implementation of evidence-based psychotherapies, (c) they are not limited to therapeutic techniques at the expense of the process or the therapy relationship, and (d) they can provide a guide for therapists to monitor their own adherence to a set of treatment principles and interventions. It is well time to progress from debates over treatment manuals to a consideration of the pros and cons and ins and outs of EBP. The current volume is a welcome move in that direction.

Treatment Manuals Do Not Improve Outcomes

Barry L. Duncan and Scott D. Miller

> You can't do cognitive therapy from a manual any more than you can do surgery from a manual.
> —Aaron T. Beck, *New York Times*

Although manuals date back to the 1960's (Lang & Lasovik, 1963), the trend toward describing, researching, teaching, practicing, and regulating psychotherapy in terms of the medical model began much earlier. Albee (2000) suggested that psychology made a Faustian deal with the medical model when it uncritically accepted the call to provide psychiatric services to returning veterans of World War II, and perhaps permanently inscribed it at the historic Boulder conference in 1949, under protest by many, when the scientist–practitioner model incorporated medical language and the concept of "mental disease."

Later, with the passing of freedom of choice legislation guaranteeing reimbursement parity with psychiatrists, psychologists learned to collect from third-party payers by providing a psychiatric diagnosis. Soon thereafter, the National Institute of Mental Health (NIMH) decided to apply the same methodology used in drug research to evaluate psychotherapy—the randomized clinical trial (RCT). This meant that a study must include manualized therapies and *DSM–IV*-defined disorders to be eligible for an NIMH-sponsored grant (Goldfried & Wolfe, 1998).

Manualization, however, reached its zenith with the advent of EBP. Following the trend in medicine toward diagnostic-related groups, in 1993 the American Psychiatric Association first developed practice guidelines for major depression and eating disorders, and followed with many other diagnoses. Psychiatry's imprimatur gave an aura of scientific legitimacy to what was primarily an agreement among psychiatrists about their preferred practices, with an emphasis on biological treatment (Duncan, 2001).

Arguing that clients have a right to empirically validated treatments, a task force of the APA's Division 12 (Society of Clinical Psychology) derided psychiatry's practice guidelines as medically biased and unrepresentative of the literature and set forth its decision rules about what constituted scientifically valid treatments (Task Force, 1993). Instead of a clinical consensus, the task force adopted decision rules that favored manualized therapies and research demonstrations that a particular treatment has proven beneficial for clients in RCTs. An explosion of manualized therapies ensued: Drawing on 8 of the 12 overlapping lists of empirically supported therapies, Chambless and Ollendick (2001) noted that 108 different manualized treatments have met the specific criteria of empirical support, a daunting number for any clinician to consider.

Although the move to manualize psychotherapy emerges from its increasing medicalization, this position paper seeks not to demonize manuals as the "evil accomplice" of the medical model. Manuals have a positive role to play. They enhance the internal validity of comparative outcome studies, facilitate treatment integrity as well as therapists' technical competence, ensure the possibility of replication, and provide a systematic way of training and supervising therapists in specific models (Lambert & Ogles, 2004). Rather, this position paper focuses on two critical disadvantages: Manuals provide an inadequate map of the psychotherapy territory, and their use does not improve the outcome of psychotherapy. Manuals emphasize specific technical operations in the face of evidence that psychotherapies demonstrate few, if any, specific effects and very little differential efficacy. Moreover, in direct contrast to the move to transfer manualized therapies to clinical settings, manuals have demonstrated little relationship to outcome and perhaps detract from positive results. In fact, manualizing psychological interventions as if they were independent of those administering and receiving them does not reflect what is known about psychotherapy outcome.

MANUALS AND SPECIFIC EFFECTS

> The great tragedy of science—the slaying of a beautiful hypothesis by an ugly fact.
> —Thomas Henry Huxley, presidential address to the British Association for the Advancement of Science

One probable assumption that underlies the manualization of psychotherapy is that specific technical operations are largely responsible for client improvement, that active (unique) ingredients of a given approach produce different effects with different disorders. In effect, this assumption likens psychotherapy to a pill, with discernable, unique ingredients that can be shown to have more potency than other active ingredients of other drugs.

Three empirical arguments cast doubt on this assumption. First is the dodo bird verdict, which colorfully summarizes the robust finding that specific therapy approaches do not show specific effects or relative efficacy. In

1936, Saul Rosenzweig first invoked the dodo's words from *Alice's Adventures in Wonderland*, "Everybody has won and all must have prizes," to illustrate his observation of the equivalent success of diverse psychotherapies. Almost 40 years later, Luborsky, Singer, and Luborsky (1975) empirically validated Rozenzweig's conclusion in their now classic review of comparative clinical trials. The dodo bird verdict has since become perhaps the most replicated finding in the psychological literature, encompassing a broad array of research designs, problems, and clinical settings.

A meta-analysis, designed specifically to test the dodo bird verdict (Wampold et al., 1997), included some 277 studies conducted from 1970 to 1995. This analysis verified that no approach has reliably demonstrated superiority over any other. At most, the effect size (ES) of treatment differences was a weak .2. "Why," Wampold et al. asked, "[do] researchers persist in attempts to find treatment differences, when they know that these effects are small?" (p. 211). Finally, an enormous real-world study conducted by Human Affairs International of over 2,000 therapists and 20,000 clients revealed no differences in outcome among 13 approaches, including medication as well as family therapy approaches (Brown, Dreis, & Nace, 1999).

Although Lambert and Ogles (2004) concluded that decades of research have not produced support for one superior treatment or set of techniques, Lambert, Garfield, and Bergin (2004) suggested that some specific and superior effects can be attributed to cognitive and behavioral methods for problems of greater severity. To address the severity issue, Wampold, Mondin, Moody, and Ahn (1997) reanalyzed the 1997 data and separated out the studies addressing severe disorders. The dodo bird verdict remained the best description of the data. The preponderance of the data therefore indicates a lack of specific effects and refutes any claim of superiority when two or more bona fide treatments fully intended to be therapeutic are compared. If no specific technical operations can be reliably shown to produce a specific effect, then manualizing psychotherapy seems to make little sense.

The second argument shining a light on the empirical pitfalls of manuals emerges from estimates regarding the impact of specific technique on outcome. After an extensive but nonstatistical analysis of decades of outcome research, Lambert (1992) suggested that model–technique factors account for about 15% of outcome variance. Wampold (2001) proposed an even smaller role for specific technical operations of various psychotherapy approaches. His meta-analysis assigned only a 13% contribution to the impact of therapy, with both general and specific factors combined. Of that 13%, a mere 8% was portioned to the contribution of model effects. Of the total variance of change, only 1% can be assigned to specific technique. This surprising low number is derived from the 1997 meta-analytic study, in which the most liberally defined effect size for treatment differences was .2, indicating that only 1% of the variance in outcomes can be attributed to specific treatment factors. A consideration of Lambert's and Wampold's estimates of variance reveals that manuals arise from factors that do not account for 85% and 99%, respectively, of the variance of outcome. Manuals, because of the limited amount of variance accounted for by specific therapist technical operations, simply do not map enough of the landscape to make them worthwhile guides to the psychotherapy territory.

Finally, component studies, which dismantle approaches to tease out unique ingredients, have similarly found little evidence to support any specific effects of therapy. A prototypic component study can be found in an investigation by Jacobson et al. (1996) of cognitive–behavioral therapy (CBT) and depression. Clients were randomly assigned to (a) behavioral activation treatment, (b) behavioral activation treatment plus coping skills related to automatic thoughts, or (c) the complete cognitive treatment (the previous two conditions plus the identification and modification of core dysfunctional schemas). Results generally indicated no differences at termination and follow-up. Perhaps putting this issue to rest, a recent meta-analytic investigation of component studies (Ahn & Wampold, 2001) located 27 comparisons in the literature between 1970 and 1998 that tested an approach against itself but without a specific component. The results revealed no differences. These studies have shown that it doesn't matter what component you leave out; the approach still works as well as the treatment containing all of its parts. When taken in total, comparative clinical trials, meta-analytic investigations, and component studies point in the same direction. Therapy approaches have no unique ingredients and little empirical justification exists for manualizing psychotherapies for clinical use.

MANUALS, TRANSPORTABILITY, AND OUTCOME

Seek facts and classify them and you will be the workmen of science. Conceive or accept theories and you will be their politicians.

—Nicholas Maurice Arthus, *De l'Anaphylaxie à l'immunité*

When manualized psychotherapy is portrayed in the literature, it is easy to form the impression that it has a technological precision. The illusion is that the manual is like a silver bullet, potent and transferable from research setting to clinical practice. Any therapist need only to load the silver bullet into any psychotherapy revolver and shoot the psychic werewolf terrorizing the client. Some studies support this perspective. For example, Wade, Treat, and Stuart (1998) examined the "transportability" of manualized CBT for panic disorder with 110 clients in a community mental health center (CMHC). Outcomes were compared with two clinical trials of CBT for panic disorder using a benchmarking strategy. The clients who received manualized therapy in the CMHC improved on every measure comparable to the clinical trials. Confounding any direct conclusions of this study, no control group or measures of treatment integrity were used.

Other better controlled studies argue the opposite point. Henry and colleagues (Henry, Schacht, Strupp, Butler, & Binder, 1993; Henry, Strupp, et al., 1993) found that therapist interpersonal skills were negatively correlated with the ability to learn a manual in the Vanderbilt II project, which examined the effects of training in time-limited dynamic psychotherapy (TLDP) for 16 therapists. These therapists provided services to two clients prior to the training, one client during training, and two clients in the year following training. The treatment was brief (25 sessions) conducted in the therapists' usual fashion prior to training and according to the TLDP model following training. During the year of training, therapists participated in weekly group supervision and attended workshops teaching the manualized approach. Evaluation of the training revealed that the therapists learned the manualized protocol (Henry, Schacht, et al., 1993; Henry, Strupp, et al., 1993). The extensive training, however, did not result in improved treatment outcomes. Clients prior to their therapists' manualized training were as likely to improve as those seen after training (Bein et al., 2000).

This study and others indicate that manuals can effectively train therapists in a given psychotherapy approach. Not withstanding, the same research shows no resulting improvement in outcome and the strong possibility of untoward negative consequences (Beutler et al., 2004; Lambert & Ogles, 2004). With regard to the former, researchers Shadish, Matt, Navarro, and Phillips (2000) found nonmanualized psychotherapy as effective as manualized in a meta-analysis of 90 studies. Comparing an individualized cognitive therapy to a manualized cognitive therapy, Emmelkamp, Bouman, and Blaauw (1994) found a modest, mean negative effect of manualization at treatment's end and at follow-up. On the other hand, Schulte, Kunzel, Pepping, and Schulte-Bahrenberg (1992) found small positive effects of manualization. Finally, a mega-analysis of 302 meta-analyses of various forms of psychotherapy and psychoeducation (Lipsey & Wilson, 1993) also revealed very similar outcomes between highly structured research treatments and those applied in naturalistic settings. The consistency of these results suggests few differences in outcome following the use of manuals in clinical settings.

Regarding detrimental effects, Addis, Wade, and Hatgis (1999) showed that practitioners believe that manuals negatively impact the quality of the therapeutic relationship, unnecessarily and inadvertently curtail the scope of treatment, and decrease the likelihood of clinical innovation. Clinicians' beliefs appear well founded: High levels of adherence to specific technical procedures interfere with the development of a good relationship (Henry, Strupp, et al., 1993) and with positive outcomes (Castonguay et al., 1996). In a study of 30 depressed clients, Castonguay and colleagues (1996) compared the impact of a technique specific to cognitive therapy—the focus on correcting distorted cognitions—with two other nonspecific factors: the alliance and the client's emotional involvement with the therapist. Results revealed that although the two common factors were highly related to progress, the technique unique to CBT—eliminating negative emotions by changing distorted cognitions—was negatively related to successful outcome. In effect, therapists who do therapy by the book develop better relationships with their manuals than with clients and seem to lose the ability to respond creatively. Little evidence, therefore, exists that manualized treatments have any impact on outcome, although some indication of negative effects is present.

MANUALS AND THE KNOWN SOURCES OF VARIANCE

Whoever acquires knowledge and does not practice it resembles him who ploughs his land and leaves it unsown.

—Sa'di, *Gulistan*

The idea of making psychological interventions dummy-proof has a certain seductive appeal, where the users—the client and the therapist—are basically irrelevant. This product view of therapy is perhaps the most empirically vacuous aspect of manualization because the treatment itself accounts for so little of outcome variance, whereas the client and the therapist, and their relationship, account for so much.

Starting with the variance attributed to the alliance, a partnership between the client and therapist to achieve the client's goals (Bordin, 1979), researchers repeatedly find that a positive alliance is one of the best predictors of outcome (Horvath & Symonds, 1991; Martin, Garske, & Davis, 2000). Research on the power of the alliance reflects over 1,000 findings and counting (Orlinsky, Rønnestad, & Willutzki, 2004). For example, Krupnick et al. (1996) analyzed data from the landmark Treatment of Depression Collaborative Research Program (TDCRP) and found that the alliance was predictive of success for all conditions; the treatment model was not. In another large study of diverse therapies for alcoholism, the alliance was also significantly predictive of success (sobriety), even at one year follow-up (Connors, DiClemente, Carroll, Longabaugh, & Donovan, 1997).

On the basis of the Horvath and Symonds (1991) meta-analysis, Wampold (2001) portioned 7% of the overall variance of outcome to the alliance. Putting this into perspective, the amount of change attributable to the alliance is about seven times that of specific model or technique. As another point of comparison, in the TDCRP, mean alliance scores accounted for up to 21% of the variance, whereas treatment differences accounted for at most 2% of outcome variance (Krupnick et al., 1996; Wampold, 2001) over a tenfold difference. The recognition of this disparity led to the creation of a counterbalancing movement by the APA Division of Psychotherapy to identify elements of effective therapy relationships (Norcross, 2001).

Turning to variance attributed to the therapist, the explosion of manuals has not eliminated the influence of the individual therapist on outcomes. Treatment still varies significantly by therapist. Once again, the TDCRP offers a case in point. Blatt, Sanislow, Zuroff, and Pilkonis (1996) reanalyzed the data to determine the characteristics of effective therapists. This is a telling investigation because the TDCRP was well controlled, and it used manuals as well as a nested design in which the therapists were committed to and skilled in the treatments they delivered. A significant variation among the therapists emerged in this study, related not to the type of treatment provided or the therapist's level of experience but rather to his or her orientation toward a psychological versus biological perspective and longer-term treatment.

Substantial evidence shows differences in effectiveness between clinicians and treatment settings (Lambert et al., 2003; Miller, Duncan, Brown, Sorrell, & Chalk, in preparation). Conservative estimates indicate that between 6% (Crits-Christoph et al., 1991) and 9% (Project MATCH Research Group, 1998) of the variance in outcomes is attributable to therapist effects, whereas treatment context accounts for up to 3% to 4% (Wampold, 2001). These percentages are particularly noteworthy when compared with the variability among treatments (1%).

Finally, the largest source of variance, virtually ignored by the move to manualize, is accounted for by the so-called extratherapeutic factors, those variables associated with the client, including unexplained (and error) variance. These variables are incidental to the treatment model and idiosyncratic to the specific client, factors that are part of the client and his or her environment that aid in recovery regardless of participation in therapy (Lambert, 1992). What clients bring to the process—their attributes, struggles, motivations, and social supports—accounts for 40% of the variance (Lambert, 1992); clients are the engine of change (Bohart & Tallman, 1999). Wampold's (2001) meta-analytic perspective assigns an 87% contribution to extratherapeutic factors and unexplained variance.

Among the client variables frequently mentioned are the severity of the disturbance, motivation, the capacity to relate, ego strength, psychological mindedness, and the ability to identify a focal problem (Assay & Lambert, 1999). In the absence of compelling evidence for any of the specific client variables to predict outcome or account for the unexplained variance, this most potent source of variance remains largely uncharted. This suggests that the largest source of variance cannot be generalized because these factors differ with each client. These unpredictable differences can only emerge one client at a time, one alliance at a time, one therapist at a time, and one treatment at a time. Although specific treatments do not have unique ingredients, the data seem to suggest that clients do.

Manualization neither explains nor capitalizes on the sources of variance known to effect treatment outcome. Indeed, as Wampold (2001) notes, "manuals focus attention toward a wasteland and away from the fertile ground" (p. 212). Given the data, we believe that continuing to invest precious time and resources in the development and dissemination of treatment manuals is misguided. A simpler path to effective, efficient, and accountable intervention exists. Rather than attempting to fit clients into manualized treatments via EBP, we recommend that therapists and systems of care tailor their work to individual clients through practice-based evidence.

FROM EBP TO PRACTICE-BASED EVIDENCE

The proof of the pudding is in the eating.

—Cervantes, *Don Quixote*

Early treatment benefit has emerged as a robust predictor of eventual outcome (e.g., Brown et al., 1999; Hansen & Lambert, 2003; Howard, Kopte, Krause, & Orlinsky, 1986). In recent years, researchers have been using data about client progress generated during treatment to enhance the quality and outcome of care (Howard, Moras, Brill, Martinovich, & Lutz, 1996; Lambert et al., 2001; Whipple et al., 2003). Unlike treatment manuals, such approaches actively use the known sources of variance in psychotherapy outcome. For example, in one representative study of 6,224 clients, Miller et al. (in press) provided therapists with ongoing, real-time feedback regarding two potent factors affecting outcome: the client's experience of the alliance and progress in treatment. The availability of this practice-based evidence not only resulted in higher retention rates but also doubled the overall effect size of services offered (baseline ES = .37 versus final phase ES = .79; $p < .001$). Germane to the controversy of treatment manuals, the findings were obtained without any attempt to control the treatment process; clinicians were not trained in any new techniques or diagnostic procedures. Rather, they were completely free to engage their individual clients in the manner they saw fit.

Paradoxically, practice-based evidence, at least when judged on the basis of measurable improvements in outcome alone, may be the most effective EBP identified to date. Indeed, Lambert et al. (2003, p. 296) pointed out, "those advocating the use of empirically supported psychotherapies do so on the basis of much smaller treatment effects." Other advantages exist as well. For example, Miller, Duncan, Sorrell, and Brown (2005) showed how practice-based evidence could be used to identify reliable differences in outcome among clinicians. Such differences, it will be recalled, account for several times more of the variance in outcomes than method (Wampold, 2001). Ongoing research is currently examining the ways such information can be used to enhance training, supervision, and quality assurance. Preliminary data from one site document a slow but progressive decrease in the variability of outcomes among clinicians when they are provided with ongoing, real-time feedback regarding their effectiveness as compared to the average effectiveness of the agency as a whole (Miller, Duncan, Sorrell, & Chalk, in preparation).

CONCLUSIONS: THE MANUAL IS NOT THE TERRITORY

> At bottom every man knows well enough that he is a unique being, only once on this earth; and by no extraordinary chance will such a marvelously picturesque piece of diversity in unity as he is, ever be put together a second time.
> —Friedrich Nietzsche, *Schopenhauer as Educator*

Manuals provide an empirically incorrect map of the psychotherapy terrain that sends both research and practice in the wrong direction. The evidence does not support the assumption that specific therapist technical operations result in client change. Although training in manualized psychotherapies does enhance therapist learning of and technical competence in a given approach, no relationship exists between such manuals and outcome. Because of the emphasis on specific or unique ingredients, manuals ignore the known sources of variance. The manual simply is not the psychotherapy territory.

Manuals equate the client with a *DSM–IV* diagnosis and the therapist with a treatment technology, both interchangeable and insignificant to the procedure at hand. Consequently, manuals lose sight of the idiographic analysis of single cases (Davison, 1998). Given the amount of variance attributed to unidentified client variables and unexplained variance, there is no way to know a priori which factors will emerge as salient for a given client–therapist pairing. Specific treatments are not unique, but clients are. From this perspective, manuals fall flat. Experienced therapists know that the work requires the tailoring of any approach to a particular client's unique circumstances. The nuances and creativity of an actual encounter flow from the moment-to-moment interaction of the participants—from the client, relational, and therapist idiographic mix, not from step A to step B on page 39. Monitoring the client's progress and view of the alliance using practice-based evidence and altering treatment accordingly is one way to manage the complexity and wonderful uncertainty that accompanies the process of psychotherapy (Duncan, Miller, & Sparks, 2004).

Psychotherapy is not an uninhabited terrain of technical procedures. It is not the sterile, stepwise process of surgery, nor the predictable path of diagnosis, prescription, and cure. It cannot be described without the client and therapist, coadventurers in a journey across largely uncharted territory. The psychotherapy landscape is intensely interpersonal and ultimately idiographic.

Dialogue: Convergence and Contention

Michael E. Addis and Esteban V. Cardemil

We found some common ground for agreement with Duncan and Miller, particularly when they briefly noted the positive role that treatment manuals could play. Additionally, we found that they continued the unfortunate trend of assuming that treatment manuals are direct threats to the creativity and decision-making processes of individual clinicians. Here we respond to Duncan and Miller's two primary criticisms of treatment manuals.

Duncan and Miller's first argument is that manuals emphasize specific technical operations when little evidence supports the differential efficacy of psychotherapies. Without extensively revisiting the "dodo bird" debate (Luborsky et al., 1975), we note that this highly controversial claim (e.g., Beutler, 2002; Chambless, 2002) is covered in chapter 7 of this book. One pertinent criticism of the dodo bird verdict is that considerable evidence exists for the superiority of specific treatment approaches in the treatment of certain disorders (e.g., the treatment of anxiety disorders with behavioral treatments). Thus, it is unclear why meta-analytic approaches that aggregate across both disorders and therapies would be an appropriate methodological approach.

Rather than reopen the debate about the utility of specific techniques, we are puzzled as to why Duncan and Miller, like many other treatment manual critics, seem unable to disentangle treatment manuals from therapeutic techniques. The value of manuals lies in their ability to specify and operationalize the assumedly critical ingredients of a therapeutic approach, be they "technical" or otherwise. We do agree with Duncan and Miller that the therapy alliance is an important ingredient in treatment outcome and may be particularly critical in the treatment of certain disorders (e.g., depression). Thus, we would be interested in seeing a treatment manual for depression that focused on the therapy alliance; it would likely include a set of prescribed behaviors that therapists would use to enhance the therapist–client relationship and a set of proscribed behaviors that therapists should avoid to develop a strong therapy alliance.

Duncan and Miller's second critique is that little evidence indicates that treatment manuals improve outcomes in clinical practice. They selectively reference a few studies that found no outcome differences between "manualized" and "nonmanualized" treatments. Duncan and Miller did not reference a growing body of effectiveness research demonstrating that manual-based treatments can produce outcomes comparable to those demonstrated in controlled clinical trials (Addis et al., 2004; Franklin, Abramowitz, Kozak, Levitt, & Foa, 2000; Hahlweg, Feigenbaum, Frank, Shroeder, & von Witzleben, 2001; Lincoln et al., 2003; Persons, Bostrom, & Bertagnolli, 1999; Tuschen-Caffier, Pook, & Frank, 2001; Wade, Treat, & Stuart, 1998; Warren, 1995; Warren & Thomas, 2001). Also, more recent studies directly comparing manual-based treatments to "treatment as usual" have found support for the superiority of manual-based treatments. For example, Turkington, Kingdon, and Turner (2002) found that a brief, manualized CBT intervention for schizophrenia produced superior changes in depression, insight, and schizophrenic symptoms compared to treatment as usual. Addis and colleagues (2004) found that training masters-level practitioners in a managed care setting in a manualized psychotherapy for panic disorder produced greater statistically and clinically significant levels of change in clients compared to those receiving usual care. Thus, contrary to Duncan and Miller's suggestion, the limited evidence that exists actually suggests that manual-based treatments produce outcomes superior to usual nonmanualized treatment in real-world clinical settings, at least for the client populations studied.

Duncan and Miller next reference three studies that purportedly found negative effects of manuals on outcome (Addis, Wade, & Hatgis, 1999; Castonguay et al., 1996; Henry, Strupp, et al., 1993). A close reading of each of these studies yields little support for this notion. For example, Duncan and Miller claimed that Addis et al. (1999) found that practitioners believe that manuals negatively impact the quality of the therapeutic relationship, unnecessarily and inadvertently curtail the scope of treatment, and decrease the likelihood of clinical innovation. Yet the Addis et al. article they cite was not an empirical study. Rather, the authors discussed a number of possible barriers to EBP. In fact, in an empirical study on practitioner attitudes toward manual-based treatments, Addis and Krasnow (2000) found considerable variation in practitioner attitudes.

The findings from two other studies purportedly demonstrating that high levels of adherence to treatment manuals may lead to negative outcomes are much more nuanced than Duncan and Miller suggest. For instance, few of the "striking findings" noted by Duncan and Miller in the Henry, Strupp, et al. (1993) study were actually statistically significant, and there also existed many positive findings that Duncan and Miller did not present. For example, following training, therapists were more likely to encourage patients to experience and express affect in sessions, maintain an optimal participant–observer stance, and use open-ended questions (Henry, Strupp, et al., 1993). Similarly, Castonguay and associates (1996) highlighted poor implementation of manual-based treatments, not the treatments themselves, to account for the correlational findings (no evidence suggested that high adherence caused poor outcomes). An example in which a therapist attempts to force-feed the cognitive model to a client, ignoring the client's wish to discuss her pain, seems to us like a good example of poorly delivered psychotherapy, rather than a criticism of treatment manuals.

Why are we stuck in the same old arguments? We speculate that critics of treatment manuals may be responding to an unstated fear that manual-based treatments will lead to the loss of both therapist and client individuality. Duncan and Miller articulate this fear when they say, "Manuals equate the client with a *DSM–IV* diagnosis and the therapist with a treatment technology, both interchangeable and insignificant to the procedure at hand" (p. 148). This description puzzles us. We know of no manual-based therapy proponents who believe that manuals should or do eliminate therapist and client individuality.

Throughout this chapter, we have tried to present a balanced perspective on the value of treatment manuals. Because treatment manuals vary tremendously in their emphasis on theory, technique, and flexibility, their use is likely more helpful in some situations than in others. We remain hopeful that this chapter will shift the field's attention away from polarizing debates over treatment manuals and instead help us refocus our energies on the more relevant questions of how and under what conditions EBP can enhance clinical outcomes

Barry L. Duncan and Scott D. Miller

Addis and Cardemil have written a rational and balanced position paper supporting the use of treatment manuals in which we find much with which to agree. They rightfully argue that the polemics and hyperbole surrounding the use of manuals has served to cloud the issues at hand. They reasonably propose that manuals are a good way to describe the structural and conceptual boundaries of treatment, that they aid in the dissemination and implementation of so-called evidence-based psychotherapies, and that manuals can provide a guide for therapists to monitor their own adherence to a set of treatment principles and interventions. Their fine paper also captures the essence of some of the tensions that underlie the differences between pro- and antimanualization (and EBP) positions. And we heartily agree that relationship and technique are impossible to separate, that any technical operation of the therapist necessarily occurs in the context of the relationship. From this view, technique is an instance of the alliance in action.

We agree with two other points, but come to entirely different conclusions. First, Addis and Cardemil assert "a manual's usefulness lies in the degree to which it helps therapists monitor their own adherence to strategies and techniques that facilitate the *assumed* active ingredients" (p. 132, emphasis added). The authors' use of "assumed" active ingredients is accurate and reflects the main point of our position paper. As we argued, these ingredients are assumed and are not empirically demonstrated, and they should be so indicated in manuals (see the following) to prevent misunderstandings. Other ingredients are research demonstrated and are not assumed, such as client, relationship, and therapist variables. Consequently, it doesn't make sense to manualize what is assumed when we already know what actually does improve outcome.

Second, Addis and Cardemil argue, "At no time did proponents assume the treatment was to be literally 'based' on the manual, as if the manual were the treatment" (p. 134) and "existing debates about treatment manuals largely miss the mark by . . . (c) conflating treatment manuals with the treatments they describe" (p. 139). In other words, Addis and Cardemil make our point that manuals are not the treatment. Manuals simply do not reflect the idiographic or relational nuances of the therapeutic process. As we concluded in our position paper, the manual is not the psychotherapy territory.

Where we disagree completely with Addis and Cardemil is in the issue of intent. They argue that therapists misunderstand the intent of manuals and that existing debates misrepresent the intended function of treatment manuals as replacing therapist skill, creativity, and judgment while limiting treatment to technique at the expense of the relationship. In addition, Addis and Cardemil insist that it is *not* a function of manuals to standardize psychotherapy such that each client with a particular diagnosis receives the same treatment.

The reality on the ground regarding the intent of treatment manuals is quite different than that described by Addis and Cardemil. Consider three examples, two of which are from noted visionaries of psychological health care policy. Nicholas Cummings, a premiere soothsayer of psychology who predicted the sweeping changes ushered by managed care, suggested that therapists of the future will spend most of their time in medical settings "leading time-limited, protocol-based psychoeducational groups" (as cited in Simon, 2001, p. 39). Similarly, Charles Kiesler (2000), who, like Cummings, predicted the age of managed care, forecasted that the psychotherapist of the future will intervene with specific disorders in integrated care settings with standardized treatment protocols. Finally, and not a prediction of the future, an editorial (Scott, 2000) in the *New England Journal of Medicine* advised physicians to refer patients to therapists proficient at manualized cognitive–behavioral therapy for chronic depression.

These are but three of countless statements that confirm the fears of those critical of manualized treatments: Clients are reduced to a diagnosis and psychotherapists to technicians, while psychotherapy is administered like a pill at the request of the referring physician. A significant gap exists between what Addis and Cardemil propose as the intent and function of manuals and the reality suggested by these examples. The "misunderstandings" seem not to arise from "misrepresentations" but rather are accurate appraisals of where things are and where they are going. No wonder so many see manuals as tangible representations of the death of psychotherapy as we know it.

While tempted to compare the intent of manuals and the intent and actual impact of handguns, we will instead take Addis and Cardemil at their word regarding the intent of manuals and suggest a possible prophylaxis against future misunderstandings. We propose a black box warning printed on each and every manual, akin to the recent black box warning imposed by the FDA concerning antidepressant use with children:

> **Warning:** Following the suggestions in this manual has not been shown by research to improve treatment outcomes. Rigid adherence to this treatment manual may damage the alliance and be hazardous to a positive outcome.

- The "assumed active ingredients" herein have not been supported by research, nor has their superiority to other "assumed active ingredients" been demonstrated.
- Client, alliance, and therapist variables account for far more of the effects of treatment than the "assumed active ingredients" proposed in this manual.
- Do not lose sight of the fact that this manual is but a representation of the evidence-based practice under question; it is not the treatment per se. The manual is not the psychotherapy territory.

REFERENCES

Addis, M. E. (1997). Evaluating the treatment manual as a means of disseminating empirically validated psychotherapies. *Clinical Psychology: Science and Practice, 4*, 1–11.

Addis, M. E. (2002). Methods for disseminating research products and increasing evidence-based practice: Promises, obstacles, and future directions. *Clinical Psychology: Science and Practice, 9*, 381–392.

Addis, M. E., Hatgis, C., Krasnow, A. D., Jacob, K., Bourne, L., & Mansfield, A. (2004). Effectiveness of cognitive–behavioral treatment for panic disorder versus treatment as usual in a managed care setting. *Journal of Consulting and Clinical Psychology, 72*, 625–635.

Addis, M. E., Hatgis, C., Soysa, C., Zaslavsky, I., & Bourne, L. S. (1999). The dialectics of manual-based psychotherapy. *The Behavior Therapist, 22*, 130–132.

Addis, M. E., & Krasnow, A. D. (2000). A national survey of practicing psychologists' attitudes toward psychotherapy treatment manuals. *Journal of Consulting and Clinical Psychology, 68*, 331–339.

Addis, M. E., Wade, W. A., & Hatgis, C. (1999). Barriers to the dissemination of evidence-based practices: Addressing practitioners' concerns about manual-based therapies. *Clinical Psychology: Science and Practice, 6*, 430–441.

Ahn, H., & Wampold, B. (2001). Where oh where are the specific ingredients? A meta-analysis of component studies in counseling and psychotherapy. *Journal of Counseling Psychology, 38*, 251–257.

Albee, G. (2000). The Boulder model's fatal flaw. *American Psychologist, 55*, 247–248.

American Psychiatric Association. (1994). *Diagnostic and statistical manual of mental disorders* (4th ed.). Washington, DC: Author.

Assay, T. P., & Lambert, M. J. (1999). The empirical case for the common factors in therapy: Quantitative findings. In M. A. Hubble, B. L. Duncan, & S. D. Miller (Eds.), *The heart and soul of change: What works in therapy* (pp. 33–56). Washington, DC: American Psychological Association.

Beck, A.T., Rush, J., Shaw, B., & Emery, G. (1979). *Cognitive therapy of depression.* New York: Guilford Press.

Bein, E., Anderson, T., Strupp, H. H., Henry, W. P., Schacht, T. E., Binder, J. L., & Butler, S. F. (2000). The effects of training in Time-Limited Dynamic Psychotherapy: Change in therapeutic outcome. *Psychotherapy Research, 10*, 119–132.

Beutler, L. E. (2002). The dodo bird is extinct. *Clinical Psychology: Science and Practice, 9*, 30–34.

Beutler, L. E., Clarkin, J., & Bongar, B. (2000). *Guidelines for the systematic treatment of the depressed patient.* New York: Oxford University Press.

Beutler, L. E., Malik, M., Alimohamed, S., Harwood, T. M., Talebi, H., Noble, S., & Wong, E. (2004). Therapist effects. In M. J. Lambert (Ed.), *Bergin and Garfield's handbook of psychotherapy and behavior change* (5th ed., pp. 227–306). New York: Wiley.

Beutler, L. E., Malik, M., Talebi, H., Fleming, J., & Moleiro, C. (2004). Use of psychological tests/instruments for treatment planning. In M. E. Maruish (Ed.), *The use of psychological tests for treatment planning and outcome assessment* (Vol. 1, 3rd ed., pp. 111–145). Hillsdale, NJ: Erlbaum.

Blatt, S. J., Sanislow, C.A., Zuroff, D. C., & Pilkonis, P. (1996). Characteristics of effective therapists. Further analyses of the NIMH Treatment of Depression Collaborative Research Program. *Journal of Consulting and Clinical Psychology, 64*, 1276–1284.

Bohart, A., & Tallman, K. (1999). *What clients do to make therapy work.* Washington, DC: American Psychological Association.

Bordin, E. S. (1979). The generalizability of the psychoanalytic concept of the working alliance. *Psychotherapy, 16*, 252–260.

Brown, J., Dreis, S., & Nace, D. K. (1999). What really makes a difference in psychotherapy outcome? Why does managed care want to know? In M. A. Hubble, B. L. Duncan, & S. D. Miller (Eds.), *The heart and soul of change: What works in therapy* (pp. 389–406). Washington, DC: American Psychological Association.

Castonguay, L. G., & Beutler, L. E. (Eds.). (in press). *Principles of therapeutic change that work.* New York: Oxford University Press.

Castonguay, L. G., Goldfried, M. R., Wiser, S., Raue, P. J., & Hayes, A. M. (1996). Predicting the effect of cognitive therapy for depression: A study of unique and common factors. *Journal of Consulting and Clinical Psychology, 64*, 497–504.

Chambless, D. L. (2002). Beware the dodo bird: The dangers of overgeneralization. *Clinical Psychology: Science and Practice, 9*, 13–16.

Chambless, D. L., & Ollendick, T. H. (2001). Empirically supported psychological interventions: Controversies and evidence. *Annual Review of Psychology, 52*, 685–716.

Connors, G. J., DiClemente, C. C., Carroll, K. M., Longabaugh, R., & Donovan, D. M. (1997). The therapeutic alliance and its relationship to alcoholism treatment participation and outcome. *Journal of Consulting and Clinical Psychology, 65*, 588–598.

Craske, M. G., Meadows, E., & Barlow, D. H. (1994). *Therapist's guide for the mastery of your anxiety and panic II and agoraphobia supplement.* New York: Graywind Press.

Crits-Christoph, P., Barancackie, K., Kurcias, J. S., Beck, A. T., Carroll, K., Perry, K., et al. (1991). Meta-analysis of therapist effects in psychotherapy outcome studies. *Psychotherapy Research, 1*, 81–91.

Davison, G. C. (1998). Being bolder with the Boulder model: The challenge of education and training in empirically supported treatments. *Journal of Consulting and Clinical Psychology, 66*, 163–167.

Dawes, R. M. (1994). *House of cards: Psychology and psychotherapy built on myth.* New York: Free Press.

Dobson, K. S., & Shaw, B. F. (1988). The use of treatment manuals in cognitive therapy: Experience and issues. *Journal of Consulting and Clinical Psychology, 56*, 1–8.

Duncan, B. (2001, July/August). The future of psychotherapy: Beware the siren call of integrated care. *Psychotherapy Networker*, 24–33, 52–53.

Duncan, B. L., Miller. S. D., & Sparks, J. (2004). *The heroic client: A revolutionary way to improve effectiveness through client directed outcome informed therapy* (revised ed.). San Francisco: Jossey-Bass.

Emmelkamp, P. M., Bouman, T. K., & Blaauw, E. (1994). Individualized versus standardized therapy: A comparative evaluation with obsessive–compulsive patients. *Clinical Psychology and Psychotherapy, 1*, 95–100.

Fensterheim, H., & Raw, S. D. (1996). Psychotherapy research is not psychotherapy practice. *Clinical Psychology: Science and Practice, 3*, 168–171.

Fongay, P. (1999). Achieving evidence-based psychotherapy practice: A psychodynamic perspective on the general acceptance of treatment manuals. *Clinical Psychology: Science and Practice, 6*, 442–444.

Franklin, M. E., Abramowitz, J. S., Kozak, M. J., Levitt, J. T., & Foa, E. B. (2000). Effectiveness of exposure and ritual prevention for obsessive–compulsive disorder: Randomized compared with nonrandomized samples. *Journal of Consulting and Clinical Psychology, 68*, 594–602.

Garfield, S. L. (1996). Some problems associated with "validated" forms of psychotherapy. *Clinical Psychology: Science and Practice, 3*, 218–229.

Gibbons, M. B. C., Crits-Christoph, P., Levinson, J., & Barber, J. (2003). Flexibility in manual-based psychotherapies: Predictors of therapist interventions in interpersonal and cognitive–behavioral therapy. *Psychotherapy Research, 13*, 169–185.

Goebel-Fabbri, A. E., Fikkan, J., & Franko, D. L. (2003). Beyond the manual: The flexible use of cognitive behavioral therapy. *Cognitive and Behavioral Practice, 10*, 41–50.

Goldfried, M. R., & Wolfe, B. E. (1998). Toward a more clinically valid approach to therapy research. *American Psychologist, 66*, 143–150.

Hahlweg, K., Feigenbaum, W., Frank, M., Shroeder, B., & von Witzleben, I. (2001). Short- and long-term effectiveness of an empirically supported treatment for agoraphobia. *Journal of Consulting and Clinical Psychology, 69*, 375–382.

Hansen, N. B., & Lambert, M. J. (2003). An evaluation of the dose–response relationship in naturalistic treatment settings using survival analysis. *Mental Health Services Research, 5*, 1–12.

Hembree, E. A., Rauch, S. A. M., & Foa, E. B. (2003). Beyond the manual: The insider's guide to prolonged exposure therapy for PTSD. *Cognitive and Behavioral Practice, 10*, 22–30.

Henggeler, S. W., & Schoenwald, S. (2002). Treatment manuals: Necessary, but far from sufficient: Commentary. *Clinical Psychology: Science and Practice, 9*, 419–420.

Henry, W. P., Schacht, T. E., Strupp, H. H., Butler, S. F., & Binder, J. L. (1993). Effects of training in time-limited psychotherapy: Mediators of therapists' response to training. *Journal of Consulting and Clinical Psychology, 61*, 441–447.

Henry, W. P., Strupp, H. H., Butler, S. F., Schacht, T. E., & Binder, J. L. (1993). Effects of training in time-limited dynamic psychotherapy: Changes in therapist behavior. *Journal of Consulting and Clinical Psychology, 61*, 434–440.

Horvath, A. O., & Symonds, B. D. (1991). Relation between working alliance and outcome in psychotherapy: A meta-analysis. *Journal of Counseling Psychology, 38*, 139–149.

Howard, K. I., Kopte, S. M., Krause, M. S., & Orlinsky, D. E. (1986). The dose–effect relationship in psychotherapy. *American Psychologist, 41*, 159–164.

Howard, K. I, Moras, K., Brill, P. L., Martinovich, Z., & Lutz, W. (1996). Evaluation of psychotherapy: Efficacy, effectiveness, and patient progress. *American Psychologist, 51*, 1059–1064.

Huppert, J. D., & Baker-Morrisette, S. L. (2003). Beyond the manual: The insider's guide to panic control treatment. *Cognitive and Behavioral Practice, 10*, 2–13.

Jacobson, N., Dobson, K., Truax, P., Addis, M., Koerner, K., Gollan, J., et al. (1996). A component analysis of cognitive–behavioral treatment for depression. *Journal of Consulting and Clinical Psychology, 64*, 295–304.

Kendall, P. C. (1998). Directing misperceptions: Researching the issues facing manual-based treatments. *Clinical Psychology: Science and Practice, 5*, 396–399.

Kendall, P. C., Chu, B., Gifford, A., Hayes, C., & Nauta, A. (1998). Breathing life into a manual: Flexibility and creativity with manual-based treatments. *Cognitive and Behavioral Practice, 5,* 177–198.

Kiesler, C. (2000). The next wave of change for psychology and mental health services in the health care revolution. *American Psychologist, 55,* 481–487.

Klerman, G. L., Weissman, M. M., Rounsaville, B. J., & Chevron, E. S. (1984). *Interpersonal psychotherapy of depression.* New York: Basic Books.

Krupnick, J. L., Sotsky, S. M., Simmens, S., Moyher, J., Elkin, I., Watkins, J., et al. (1996). The role of the therapeutic alliance in psychotherapy and pharmacotherapy outcome: Findings in the National Institute of Mental Health Treatment of Depression Collaborative Research Program. *Journal of Consulting and Clinical Psychology, 64,* 532–539.

Lambert, M. J. (1992). Psychotherapy outcome research: Implications for integrative and eclectic therapists. In J. C. Norcross & M. R. Goldfried (Eds.), *Handbook of psychotherapy integration* (pp. 94–129). New York: Basic Books.

Lambert, M. J., Garfield, S. L., & Bergin, A. E. (2004). Overview, trends, and future issues. In M. J. Lambert (Ed.), *Bergin and Garfield's handbook of psychotherapy and behavior change* (5th ed., pp. 805–819). New York: Wiley.

Lambert, M. J., & Ogles, B. (2004). The efficacy and effectiveness of psychotherapy. In M. J. Lambert (Ed.), *Bergin and Garfield's handbook of psychotherapy and behavior change* (5th ed., pp. 139–193). New York: Wiley.

Lambert, M. J., Whipple, J. L., Hawkins, E. J., Vermeersch, D. A., Nielsen, S. L., & Smart, D. W. (2003). Is it time for clinicians routinely to track patient outcome? A meta-analysis. *Clinical Psychology, 10,* 288–301.

Lambert, M. J., Whipple, J., Smart, D., Vermeersch, D., Nielsen, S., & Hawkins, E. (2001). The effects of providing therapists with feedback on patient progress during psychotherapy: Are outcomes enhanced? *Psychotherapy Research, 11,* 49–68.

Lang, P. J., & Lasovik, A. D. (1963). Experimental desensitization of a phobia. *Journal of Abnormal and Social Psychology, 66,* 519–525.

Lincoln, T. M., Rief, W., Hahlweg, K., Frank, M., von Witzleben, I., Shroeder, B., et al. (2003). Effectiveness of an empirically supported treatment for social phobia in the field. *Behaviour Research and Therapy, 41,* 1251–1269.

Lipsey, M. W., & Wilson, D. B. (1993). The efficacy of psychological, educational, and behavioral treatment: Confirmation from meta-analyses. *American Psychologist, 48,* 1181–1209.

Luborsky, L. (1984). *Principles of psychoanalytic psychotherapy: A manual for supportive–expressive treatment.* New York: Basic Books.

Luborsky, L., & DeRubeis, R. J. (1984). The use of psychotherapy treatment manuals: A small revolution in psychotherapy research style. *Clinical Psychology Review, 4,* 5–14.

Luborsky, L., Singer, B., & Luborsky, L. (1975). Comparative studies of psychotherapies: Is it true that "Everyone has won and all must have prizes"? *Archives of General Psychiatry, 32,* 995–1008.

Martin, D. J., Garske, J. P., & Davis, K. M. (2000). Relation of the therapeutic alliance with outcome and other variables: A meta-analytic review. *Journal of Consulting and Clinical Psychology, 68,* 438–450.

Martell, C. R., Addis, M. E., & Jacobson, N. S. (2001). *Depression in context: Strategies for guided action.* New York: Norton.

Miller, S. J., & Binder, J. L. (2002). The effects of manual-based training on treatment fidelity and outcome: A review of the literature on adult individual psychotherapy. *Psychotherapy, 39,* 184–198.

Miller, S. D., Duncan, B. L., Brown, J., Sorrell, R., & Chalk, M. B. (in press). Using outcome to inform and improve treatment outcomes. *Journal of Brief Therapy.*

Miller, S. D., Duncan, B. L., Sorrell, R., & Brown, J. (2005). The partners for change outcome management system. *Journal of Clinical Psychology: In Session, 61,* 199–208.

Miller, S. D., Duncan, B. L., Sorrell, R., & Chalk, M. B. (in preparation). *The effects of feedback on therapist variability over time.*

Morgenstern, J., Morgan, T. J., McCrady, B. S., Keller, D. S., & Carroll, K. M. (2001). Manual-guided cognitive–behavioral therapy training: A promising method for disseminating empirically supported substance abuse treatments to the practicing community. *Psychology of Addictive Behaviors, 15,* 83–88.

Najavits, L. M., Ghinassi, F., Van Horn, A., Weiss, R. D., Siqueland, L., Frank, A., et al. (2004). Therapist satisfaction with four manual-based treatments on a national multisite trial: An exploratory study. *Psychotherapy, 41,* 26–37.

Najavits, L. M., Weiss, R. D., Shaw, S. R., & Dierberger, A. E. (2000). Psychotherapists' views of treatment manuals. *Professional Psychology: Research and Practice, 31,* 404–408.

Norcross, J. C. (Ed.). (2001). Empirically supported therapy relationships: Summary Report of the Division 29 Task Force. *Psychotherapy, 38,* 345–497.

Orlinsky, D. E., Rønnestad, M. H., & Willutzki, U. (2004). Fifty years of process–outcome research: Continuity and change. In M. J. Lambert (Ed.), *Bergin and Garfield's handbook of psychotherapy and behavior change* (5th ed., pp. 307–390). New York: Wiley.

Persons, J. B., Bostrom, A., & Bertagnolli, A. (1999). Results of randomized controlled trials of cognitive therapy for depression generalize to private practice. *Cognitive Therapy and Research, 23,* 535–548.

Project MATCH Research Group. (1998). Therapist effects in three treatments for alcohol problems. *Psychotherapy Research, 8,* 455–474.

Rosenzweig, S. (1936). Some implicit common factors in diverse methods of psychotherapy. *American Journal of Orthopsychiatry, 6,* 412–415.

Schulte, D., Kunzel, R., Pepping, G., & Schulte-Bahrenberg, T. (1992). Tailor-made versus standardized therapy of phobic patients. *Advanced Behavior Research and Therapy, 14,* 67–92.

Scott, J. (2000). Treatment of chronic depression. *New England Journal of Medicine, 342,* 1518–1520.

Shadish, W. R., Matt, G. E., Navarro, A. M., & Phillips, G. (2000). The effects of psychological therapies under clinically representative conditions: A meta-analysis. *Psychological Bulletin, 126*, 512–529.

Silverman, W. H. (1996). Cookbooks, manuals, and paint-by-numbers: Psychotherapy in the 90's. *Psychotherapy, 33*, 207–215.

Simon, R. (2001, July/August). Psychotherapy's soothsayer. *Psychotherapy Networker*, 34–39, 62.

Strupp, H. H., & Binder, J. L. (1984). *Psychotherapy in a new key: A guide to time-limited dynamic psychotherapy.* New York: Basic Books.

Task Force Report on Promotion and Dissemination of Psychological Practices. (1993). Training in and dissemination of empirically-validated psychological treatment: Report and recommendations. *The Clinical Psychologist, 48*, 2–23.

Turkington, D., Kingdon, D., & Turner, T. (2002). Effectiveness of a brief cognitive–behavioural therapy intervention in the treatment of schizophrenia. *British Journal of Psychiatry, 180*, 523–527.

Tuschen-Caffier, B., Pook, M., & Frank, M. (2001). Evaluation of manual-based cognitive–behavioral therapy for bulimia nervosa in a service setting. *Behavioral Research and Therapy, 39*, 299–308.

Vakoch, D. A., & Strupp, H. H. (2000). The evolution of psychotherapy training: Reflections on manual-based learning and future alternatives. *Journal of Clinical Psychology, 56*, 309–318.

Wade, W. A., Treat, T. A., & Stuart, G. L. (1998). Transporting an empirically supported treatment for panic disorder to a service clinic setting: A benchmarking strategy. *Journal of Consulting and Clinical Psychology, 66*, 231–239.

Waltz, J., Addis, M., Koerner, K., & Jacobson, N. S. (1993). Testing the integrity of a psychotherapy protocol: Assessing therapist adherence and competence. *Journal of Consulting and Clinical Psychology, 61*, 620–630.

Wampold, B. E. (2001). *The great psychotherapy debate: Models, methods, and findings.* Mahwah, NJ: Erlbaum.

Wampold, B. E., Mondin, G. W., Moody, M., & Ahn, H. (1997). The flat earth as a metaphor for the evidence of uniform efficacy of bona fide psychotherapies: Reply to Crits-Christoph (1997) and Howard et al. (1997). *Psychological Bulletin, 122*, 226–230.

Wampold, B. E., Mondin, G. W., Moody, M., Stich, F., Benson, K., & Ahn, H. (1997). A meta-analysis of outcome studies comparing bona fide psychotherapies: Empirically, "All Must Have Prizes." *Psychological Bulletin, 122*, 203–215.

Warren, R. (1995). Panic control treatment of panic disorder with agoraphobia and comorbid major depression: A private practice case. *Journal of Cognitive Psychotherapy, 9*, 123–134.

Warren, R., & Thomas, J. C. (2001). Cognitive–behavior therapy of obsessive–compulsive disorder in private practice: An effectiveness study. *Journal of Anxiety Disorders, 15*, 277–285.

Weissman, M. M., Markowitz, J. C., & Klerman, G. L. (2000). *Comprehensive guide to interpersonal psychotherapy.* New York: Basic Books.

Westen, D., Novotny, C. M., & Thompson-Brenner, H. (2004). The empirical status of empirically supported psychotherapies: Assumptions, findings, and reporting in controlled clinical trials. *Psychological Bulletin, 130,* 631–663.

Whipple, J. L., Lambert, M. J., Vermeersch, D. A., Smart, D. W., Nielsen, S. L., & Hawkins, E. J. (2003). Improving the effects of psychotherapy: The use of early identification of treatment and problem-solving strategies in routine practice. *Journal of Counseling Psychology, 50,* 59–68.

Wilson, G. T. (1996). Manual-based treatments: The clinical application of research findings. *Behavior Research and Therapy, 34,* 1–59.

Wilson, G. T. (1998). Manual-based treatment and clinical practice. *Clinical Psychology: Science and Practice, 5,* 363–375.

Yeaton, W. H., & Sechrest, L. (1981). Critical dimensions in the choice and maintenance of successful treatments: Strength, integrity, and effectiveness. *Journal of Consulting and Clinical Psychology, 49,* 156–167.

4

ARE RESEARCH PATIENTS AND CLINICAL TRIALS REPRESENTATIVE OF CLINICAL PRACTICE?

Patients and Treatments in Clinical Trials Are Not Adequately Representative of Clinical Practice

Drew I. Westen

One of the issues at the heart of the debate over evidence-based practice (EBP) is the question of generalizability of laboratory treatments to patients and treatments in the community. It is a truism that internal validity (the adequacy of the research design) and external validity (generalizability of the results) always involve tradeoffs. A demand for absolute representativeness in psychotherapy research would cripple the scientific enterprise and leave clinicians with a far more imperfect sample from which to generalize than most randomized clinical trials (RCTs), namely their own patients (assessed and treated by a single, nonblind assessor). On the other hand, dramatic shifts in clinical training and reimbursement over the last

161

decade reflect an implicit if not explicit assumption that the samples and techniques used in laboratory trials of psychotherapy do indeed generalize to the community.

In this position paper I argue, first, that patients treated in the laboratory have not been adequately representative of patients treated in the community, and second, that treatments tested in the laboratory have not been adequately representative of treatments as practiced in the community.

ARE PATIENTS IN CLINICAL TRIALS REPRESENTATIVE OF PATIENTS IN THE COMMUNITY?

In considering the representativeness of patients in RCTs, I address two issues: how researchers have addressed representativeness and generalizability in presenting and interpreting their results, and how they have addressed these issues in sampling decisions.

Interpretation and Presentation of Results

The representativeness of a sample is always relative to the population to which the investigators intend the results to generalize. Depression researchers do not need to assume or demonstrate that their treatments generalize to all patients with depression. However, if they intend the treatments to generalize to only a subset, they need to specify that subset clearly and use the same inclusion and exclusion criteria across multiple experiments to develop a replicable body of evidence. Although treatment researchers explicitly understand this aspect of generalizability, their explicit knowledge is not, by and large, reflected in the way they summarize their data in the titles, abstracts, or even the text of most primary studies or reviews of the scientific evidence (Westen, Novotny, & Thompson-Brenner, 2004a, 2004b).

For example, if researchers use major depression as defined by the *Diagnostic and Statistical Manual of Mental Disorders, Fourth Edition* (DSM–IV; American Psychiatric Association, 1994), as their inclusion criterion in a study of depression, they cannot generalize to "depression." Treatments that work well for major depression may or may not be optimal for treating less severe but nonetheless clinically significant depressive symptomatology and vice versa. Similarly, if researchers consistently impose exclusion criteria that exclude patients with suicidality or borderline personality disorder (BPD) from studies of major depression (explicitly or de facto, e.g., by excluding patients with suicidality and substance abuse), they need to qualify their conclusions appropriately, given the prevalence of suicidality and BPD among patients with major depression.

Unfortunately, such qualifications are rare in the literature. Consider a study recently completed, which is arguably the most impressive, ecologically valid RCT of depression ever conducted: the National Institute of Mental Health (NIMH) Treatment of Adolescent Depression Study (TADS; March et al., 2004). (I will use this example throughout the chapter because of its strengths relative to other studies.) In brief, the investigators compared fluoxetine (Prozac), cognitive–behavioral therapy, and their combination to a placebo control condition. They found that Prozac with and without cognitive–behavior therapy (CBT) was highly effective (approximately 70% and 60% of participants responded in the two conditions, respectively), whereas CBT alone and a placebo produced similar response rates (approximately 35% and 40%, respectively). Although the authors were generally careful in limiting their conclusions to adolescents with major depressive disorder (MDD), at the end of the article describing their results in the *Journal of the American Medical Association* they concluded (as did most media reports of the study) that CBT "should be readily available as part of comprehensive treatment for *depressed adolescents*" (emphasis added) as opposed to the minority of depressed adolescents who meet criteria for MDD.

Even limiting the generalizability of this study to MDD may, however, be problematic. The investigators conclude that the "TADS succeeded in recruiting a sample that includes the full range of treatment-seeking patients with MDD. Accordingly, we conclude that the results of the study should be broadly applicable to youth with MDD seen in clinical practice." Yet the TADS excluded 85% of the adolescents who were screened for participation, in part for perfectly legitimate reasons (e.g., they did not meet MDD criteria or they chose not to participate once they learned the full details of the study) and in part because of exclusion criteria that may render this an atypical sample of adolescents with major depression.

The TADS excluded adolescents if they were abusing drugs or if they had missed 25% or more of school days in the prior 2 months. This would effectively eliminate many adolescents with externalizing pathology (who were further excluded by virtue of another exclusion criterion, severe conduct disorder), adolescents who were debilitated by their depression, or adolescents with chaotic families or neglectful parents who did not ensure they went to school every day. The investigators also excluded patients with a current or past diagnosis of bipolar disorder. This is appropriate in studies of adult MDD, where bipolar diagnoses are generally clearer, but it can be problematic in a study of depressed adolescents, for whom the bipolar diagnosis is often applied inappropriately to teenagers with personality disorders or a history of childhood sexual abuse because of their "mood swings." The researchers also excluded adolescents who had been hospitalized for any psychiatric reason within the past 3 months or had not resided with a primary caretaker for the last 6 months, effectively excluding many troubled adolescents and those from troubled homes.

Another exclusion criterion is perhaps the most problematic, particularly in light of the justification for the study in the introduction to the paper, that "Depression . . . is an important contributor to adolescent suicidal behavior and to completed suicide, which is the third leading cause of death among depressed adolescents." As in virtually every clinical trial of psychotherapy and medication for adult and adolescent depression conducted over the last two decades, the investigators excluded patients if they were deemed to be at high risk for suicide attempts, whether because they had recently made one, had an active plan, or had "suicidal ideation with a disorganized family unable to guarantee adequate safety monitoring." Aside from suicidality being a common symptom in adolescent major depression, a combination of exclusion criteria—substance abuse, problematic school attendance, bipolar diagnosis, psychiatric hospitalizations, residence with someone other than a primary caretaker, and suicidality—virtually assured the absence of adolescents with BPD in the sample. This personality disorder is, however, highly prevalent among both adolescents and adults with MDD and often moderates treatment outcome (see Wixom, Ludolph, & Westen, 1993).

The investigators made one other decision that likely rendered this an atypical sample (and might actually explain in part why CBT fared so poorly): They required that the patient meet MDD criteria continuously over the course of multiple screenings, producing a sample of adolescents who on average were in the midst of a 40- to 50-week major depressive episode. Although their goal was to ensure that the patient had "stable and continuous" major depression, this criterion would likely rule out the kinds of "reactive" depressions characteristic of many adolescents with depression (major or otherwise), including those with significant personality pathology.

Again, my goal is not to criticize this particular study, which had much less restrictive exclusion criteria than the average study of adolescent depression. Indeed, the modal study of adolescent depression enrolls nontreatment-seeking adolescents in clinically unrepresentative group settings (e.g., classroom sessions) and does not report crucial information relevant to generalizability, such as patients' socioeconomic status (SES) and ethnicity, setting characteristics (e.g., school, community mental health center [CMHC], outpatient clinic), or clinician characteristics (e.g., whether clinicians were graduate students or experienced clinicians, and whether they treated participants in both experimental and control conditions; Weisz, Jensen Doss, & Hawley, 2005). My point is that even the best studies published in the best journals make statements about generalizability that may confuse their intended consumers (clinicians deciding whether to use the treatment under investigation, third-party payers, public policy makers, and consumers), and that researchers need to be more careful in the conclusions they draw about the populations to whom they expect their treatments to generalize.

Sampling Decisions and Generalizability

Aside from the way researchers report and interpret their findings, a second and related issue pertains to design decisions that render most of the psychotherapies tested in RCTs over the last 20 years of unknown generalizability. I am not arguing that the data from these studies are not generalizable. Generalizability is a continuous variable, not a dichotomous one (i.e., studies vary on the extent to which they apply to various populations and subpopulations). Many of us have expressed concern about the widespread assumption that treatments identified as empirically supported therapies (ESTs) are more efficacious than widely practiced treatments that have never been tested in RCTs (Roth & Fonagy, 1996), and the same is true for the generalizability of RCTs: The absence of evidence does not imply the evidence of absence. My argument is that we do not know, because researchers have consistently used selection criteria for entry into RCTs that differ substantially from the selection criteria in clinical settings, that is, the reasons patients seek treatment in the community and the reasons clinicians choose either to treat or refer them.

Some differences between the patients who present for treatment in the community and those who present in research settings are unavoidable, such as their willingness to enter into a study (and often one with a placebo condition in which they can expect not to receive help). In such cases, however, the burden of proof lies as much with the critic to explain how this might have led to the obtained results (e.g., a difference between exposure versus exposure plus cognitive restructuring for a specific anxiety disorder) as with the investigator to make a case for generalizability.

Two other issues, however, are potentially much more problematic for generalizability: differences in the problems with which patients present in research and practice, and differences between the exclusion criteria used by researchers and clinicians in everyday practice. A major change in clinical trials since the 1970s and early 1980s is the specificity of patient diagnosis. Virtually all RCTs today study patients who meet *DSM–IV* thresholds for specific disorders. Indeed, in the United States, researchers seeking funding have no choice but to fit their patients into the procrustean bed of the *DSM–IV*. This has many advantages vis-à-vis the comparability of samples across research settings, but it has serious drawbacks as well. From an empirical standpoint, we have surprisingly little data on the reasons the average patient seeks treatment in the community (particularly in private practice), but we know that neither patients in the community nor patients studied in basic science research on psychopathology typically present with a single, primary Axis I disorder. Unfortunately, this is the modal inclusion criterion for participating in an RCT (see Westen et al., 2004a). Indeed, clinicians report that most of their patients present with personality pathology requiring treatment that does not cross the threshold for an Axis II diagnosis (Westen &

Arkowitz-Westen, 1998), and research consistently finds "subthreshold" Axis I pathology (e.g., anxiety, depression, eating pathology, or drug use that does not cross *DSM–IV* thresholds) to be of both high prevalence and high impact on life satisfaction and public health (e.g., Fava & Mangelli, 2001).

In my own experience, most patients present in private practice complaining of problems such as the following: "My life is a mess. I can't decide if I want to stay in my marriage, I sometimes feeling panicky, and I don't find my work satisfying anymore." A moment's reflection suggests that such a presentation is not just the lament of the "worried well." Few of us could maintain our mental health while in turmoil about our most central relationship and our work. Yet such a patient would be excluded from virtually every potentially relevant RCT conducted over the last two decades, unless his or her panicky feelings happened to rise to the level of panic disorder (in which case the patient would be randomized to a treatment that might not address the other equally burning problems with which he or she presented, for which ESTs are not available).

For some disorders, such as panic, we may well be able to make some inroads in treating the disorder decontextualized from the person who happens to have it (or the life circumstances in which the patient finds herself). This is particularly likely to be the case for symptoms or syndromes that can take on functional autonomy (Westen et al., 2004a), such as when panic patients develop conditioned fear responses to their own internal sensations and experience shortness of breath (Barlow, 2002). Even for these disorders, however, treating the broader systemic and personality context may reduce or eliminate the *DSM–IV* symptoms, or, as in this example, the patient may have many other problems for which she is seeking help. Indeed, nearly half of the patients treated in RCTs for the most prevalent disorders report seeking treatment again within two years when researchers collect data on posttreatment treatment seeking (Westen & Morrison, 2001).

Perhaps more troubling, a plethora of taxonomic studies has now documented that personality variables, notably negative affectivity or internalizing pathology, account for much of the variance in mood and anxiety syndromes, and they explain why comorbidity among these disorders is so high (e.g., Brown, Chorpita, & Barlow, 1998; Krueger & Piasecki, 2002). If we are to develop treatments for specific forms of pathology, we might do well to develop treatments for broadband personality variables such as negative affectivity, with additional techniques designed to address the specific symptoms or syndromes with which the patient may present at any given time. In this respect, a promising development, just under way, is the development of treatments that cut across *DSM–IV* diagnostic groupings (Barlow, Allen, & Choate, 2004; Fairburn, Cooper, & Shafran, 2003). What remains to be seen is how researchers will maintain the brevity of these treatments while expanding the targets of intervention.

Even if we accept the focus on single (primarily Axis I) diagnoses, the data on the representativeness of RCT patients are not encouraging. Across a range of disorders, from depression to posttraumatic stress disorder (PTSD), researchers routinely exclude most patients who present for treatment using exclusion criteria that vary from study to study and hence render generalizations across studies difficult (see Bradley, Greene, Russ, Dutra, & Westen, in press; Westen & Morrison, 2001; Westen et al., 2004a).

Figure 4.1 presents data on the percentage of patients screened for inclusion who actually receive treatment in the average RCT for six disorders (from Westen & Bradley, in press). As can be seen, the average patient screened for inclusion does not begin and complete treatment in most RCTs. These data likely underestimate exclusion rates in RCTs because researchers rarely report on patients excluded during telephone prescreening prior to a structured interview. For clinicians trying to apply the results of RCTs to a given patient, the high exclusion rates and variable exclusion criteria used across studies are problematic, requiring them to guess without empirical guidance whether the results of a body of evidence will likely apply to their patient. The situation is even more discouraging for clinicians who treat racial or ethnic minority patients, for whom data on generalizability from RCTs are almost entirely lacking (Zane, Hall, Sue, Young, & Nunez, 2004). I do not mean to imply that all patients in all RCTs are "clean;" many are not. The problem is that the inclusion and exclusion criteria used in RCTs render them unrepresentative.

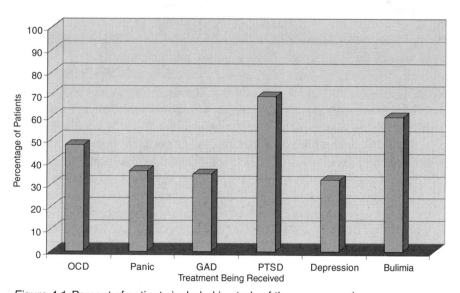

Figure 4.1 Percent of patients included in study of those screened.

ARE TREATMENTS IN RCTS REPRESENTATIVE OF TREATMENTS IN PRACTICE?

We now briefly consider the extent to which treatments tested in the laboratory are representative of treatments or treatment circumstances in the community. As noted previously, the requisites of research will always produce some differences between patients and procedures in the laboratory and those in the clinic or private practice. For example, patients in RCTs know that they have been randomly assigned to one of several possible conditions, and unless they are in treatment for a persistent coma they will surely have hypotheses about which treatment they are receiving. Researchers cannot do anything about this, other than to try to avoid giving patients any hints that one condition is intended as the "good" condition (or, preferably, to compare different treatments championed by different members of the research team).

We focus here on two issues that bear on the generalizability of research treatments to everyday practice: the representativeness of treatments selected and the representativeness of treatment length.

Representativeness of Treatments Selected for Testing

The first question is how researchers select which treatments to test. Most psychotherapy researchers share the viewpoint of the philosopher of science Karl Popper (1959), who equated scientific methods with hypothesis testing. From this vantage point, where we get our hypotheses is our own business, as long as we test them appropriately. I would argue, however, that the question of how we choose which hypotheses to test is of central scientific significance, and that treatments tested should be sampled from treatments widely practiced in the community as well as promising treatments developed in the laboratory. The reasons are multifold.

From a scientific standpoint, the current situation, in which researchers primarily test variants of CBT (and occasionally interpersonal psychotherapy [IPT]) and then draw conclusions about treatment of choice, is intellectually untenable, akin to the ethnocentric practice of holding a "World Series" of baseball in which only U.S. teams compete. Suppose, for example, psychiatrists had been using Selective Serotonin Reuptake Inhibitors (SSRIs) to treat depression for decades without any evidence other than the clinical observation that they are helpful to many patients. Then suppose pharmaceutical researchers discovered St. John's Wort and proceeded to test it in study after study without ever comparing it to the (unpatentable) SSRIs. They would likely have found that St. John's Wort outperforms placebo and begun exhorting clinicians to stop their scientifically invalid practice of treating depression with SSRIs. The problem in psychotherapy research is heightened by the fact that most treatments for most disorders tend to work when tested by investigators and conducted by therapists who believe in them (Luborsky et al., 1999; Wampold, 2001). We cannot make determinations of treatment of choice unless we compare laboratory-generated treatments to treatments in widespread use in the community.

The normative research practice of comparing laboratory treatments to everything but the longer-term eclectic, integrative, and psychodynamic treatments that evolved over the last century is not only scientifically problematic but is pragmatically inadvisable. The journals today are filled with hand-wringing about why clinicians will not wake up and smell the empirically supported coffee (i.e., why they will not give up their practices and prejudices and make way for scientifically supported treatments). Although clinician hubris, ignorance, and resistance all likely play some part, researcher hubris, ignorance, and resistance probably account for at least as much variance. If researchers want clinicians to test-drive their manuals, they need to show that their treatments outperform what good clinicians in the community can expect to accomplish with similar patients, not that they can outperform placebos, waitlists, obviously inert or technically limited intent-to-fail conditions, or treatment-as-usual (TAU) conditions with overworked masters-level clinicians in community mental health settings (unless their goal is only to show that their treatment should be implemented in such settings, rather than in broader clinical practice). The failure to test treatments that have evolved over a century of clinical work is not only unfortunate for clinicians who would genuinely like to learn from RCTs but it also betrays a devaluation of clinicians and what they might have learned through years of training and experience (and can only increase their resistance to ESTs).

Consider again the TADS. In the CBT condition, 1 of 5 patients who had gone through multiple screening steps (and hence could be presumed to be highly motivated) dropped out of treatment, and of those who completed treatment, the average patient no-showed 1 out of every 4 sessions. Even putting aside the modest outcomes obtained in the CBT-alone condition, as a practicing clinician, if my patients were to vote with their feet in such high numbers, I would seek supervision. Except for a handful of studies on specific anxiety disorders (see Roth & Fonagy, 1996) and on parasuicidal behaviors in BPD patients (Linehan, 1993), I cannot remember the last time I read the results of an RCT and was impressed that the average patient was better off than the average patient in my practice.

How do researchers currently select treatments to test? In my experience as a reviewer of grant proposals and manuscripts, researchers tend to select treatments to test on the basis of the answer to one or more of the following questions: What have we used before? What have we used in related disorders, for which we already have a manual? What is readily manualized? What won't take too long? What is likely to be funded? And finally what might make sense theoretically or in light of relevant findings from basic science? One more question might be worth considering: Which clinicians in the community are getting the best outcomes, and what are they doing (Westen et al., 2004a, 2004b)?

Representativeness of Treatment Length in Clinical Trials

Aside from the question of which treatments to test is the question of how long to test them. The average RCT for adult disorders is between 8 and 20 weeks (Westen et al., 2004a). For child and adolescent disorders, the average is 9 weeks (Weisz et al., 2005). To the experienced clinician, these statistics reflect a profound misunderstanding of the complexity and tenacity of psychopathology. And empirically the experienced clinician is right: Except for a handful of treatments for a handful of disorders, most brief treatments tested in RCTs for most disorders leave most patients, including those described as "responders," symptomatic at termination and vulnerable to relapse within 2 years (Westen & Morrison, 2001; Westen et al., 2004a). In contrast, the average treatment in practice lasts roughly 2 years, and even the average CBT treatment in the community tends to take about a year (Morrison, Bradley, & Westen, 2003; Thompson-Brenner & Westen, in press). Whether these longer treatments yield better outcomes than brief treatments in RCTs is largely unknown, although many naturalistic studies suggest that longer-term treatments would be worth testing in RCTs.

It is unfortunate that, with a few exceptions, researchers have considered treatment length to be the prerogative of researchers constructing manuals rather than a variable that should be tested extensively to identify optimal parameters. Researchers have recently begun to test longer-term versions of short-term therapies for depression because of the finding that brief psychotherapy trials did not produce comparable outcomes to long-term medication maintenance trials (Hollon, Thase, & Markowitz, 2002). Unfortunately, they have not yet considered comparing long-term extensions of CBT or IPT to long-term therapies that were intended from the start to be long-term therapies. Absent such comparisons, we do not know whether clinicians should practice long-term versions of short-term therapies or whether they should continue to practice treatments that reflect the clinically derived hypothesis, now proven accurate, that depression is not readily treated in 16 weeks.

CONCLUSIONS

The EBP movement (and the variant of it that emphasizes ESTs) has led to dramatic changes in practice and training, and has dominated the psychotherapy agenda since the mid-1990s. There is no doubt that we have made many steps forward in the development of effective treatments, particularly for anxiety disorders. What we do not know is how many steps we have taken backward in psychotherapy practice and training for the myriad patients who present for treatment of multiple, often less focal concerns.

If researchers want clinicians to take their research seriously, they will need to take clinicians seriously. That is, they will need to compare their treatments to treatments as practiced by experienced, well-paid professionals in private practice, not to no treatment, waitlist controls, worst-practice labeled TAU (i.e., treatment by overworked, often undereducated therapists in underfunded settings), or intent-to-fail conditions (e.g., "supportive" therapy with no theoretical goals carried out by graduate students who know they are in the non-bona fide treatment condition; Wampold, 2001). They will also need to study patients who resemble patients treated in the community, using the same exclusion criteria used by competent clinicians in private practice. At this point, if the goal is to generalize to everyday practice, there is no excuse for continuing to exclude patients from RCTs for mood, anxiety, eating, or substance use disorders for virtually anything other than psychosis, mania, or closed head injury. Nor is there any excuse for comparing experimental treatments to anything but what the best clinicians in private practice do.

We have learned enough about internal validity. Now let's learn something about psychotherapy.

Research Patients and Clinical Trials Are Frequently Representative of Clinical Practice

Shannon Wiltsey Stirman and Robert J. DeRubeis

The differences between research and practice are not substantial enough to warrant a dismissal of the applications of RCT results to clinical practice. Although differences certainly exist between some aspects of RCTs and routine clinical practice, some of these differences have been overstated. We draw this conclusion in part on the basis of the findings of recent studies that suggest patients who participate in psychotherapy outcome research are more representative of patients who receive treatment in clinical practice than previously assumed. To support these positions, we will review some recent data on comorbidity among research participants, as well as the results of studies that compare treatment-seeking outpatients to patients in RCTs. We will then consider other issues related to the external validity of clinical trials.

PATIENT CHARACTERISTICS

Concerns regarding the differences between patients who participate in research and those who receive treatments in clinics or private practice have been based primarily on the fact, well documented by Westen and Morrison (2001), that during the intake process the typical RCT screens out about two-thirds of the patients referred to it. Critics of RCTs have inferred from such findings that (a) the typical treatment-seeking patient is unlikely to fit the profiles necessary for participation in RCTs, and (b) the typical patient who is excluded from an RCT presents with problems, symptoms, or diagnoses that would make him or her more difficult to treat than the typical included patient. On the basis of these inferences, the claim is made that the improvement rates reported in RCTs are overestimates of what clinicians could expect if they were to use the tested treatments in their own practices or clinics (Westen & Morrison).

These conclusions are worthy of consideration, but the data they are based on (exclusion rates) are consistent with a host of other possibilities as well. A patient can be excluded from an RCT for at least five other kinds of reasons, aside from presenting with symptom constellations that would prove too difficult for the manualized, relatively brief treatments typically tested in RCTs:

(1) *The excluded patient presented with symptoms that did not meet the study criteria for symptom severity.* The research literature does not tell us whether this excluded patient is likely to respond to the treatments offered in the RCT better or worse than the typical included patient, but a reasonable hypothesis is that such patients will respond at least as well as the typical included patient.

(2) *The excluded patient is deemed to have a disorder generally considered to be milder or less chronic than what is being studied in the RCT, and for which there are currently no empirically supported treatments (ESTs).* An example of this type of exclusion is the patient who presents for a treatment study for major depression but is diagnosed not with MDD but with an adjustment disorder or a minor depression. In a recently completed RCT for MDD, nearly half of those excluded from the study were excluded for one of these first two reasons (DeRubeis, Amsterdam, O'Reardon, & Young, 2004).

(3) *The excluded patient warrants a diagnosis that would make him or her eligible for other RCTs but not the one to which he or she was referred.* A typical example is the patient who is referred for a treatment study of social phobia; at intake it is discovered that he or she meets the criteria for MDD but does not meet the criteria for social phobia. Had this patient been screened for a typical RCT of treatments for MDD, he or she may indeed have been screened into it.

(4) *The excluded patient met criteria for the disorder under study, but it was deemed at intake that another disorder is primary.* A patient with MDD self-

refs, or is referred by a health professional, to a study of treatments for depression. The study diagnostician discovers that the patient has a primary diagnosis of substance dependence. The substance dependence interferes with functioning more than the depressive symptoms, and the judgment is made that treatment of the substance dependence will likely lead to an alleviation of the symptoms of the depressive episode, but not vice versa. This patient, with comorbid depression, may have been screened into a typical RCT of treatments for substance dependence. Not knowing anything more about this patient, we can expect that he will respond to an EST for substance dependence at a level typically found in those studies.

(5) *The excluded patient is given a diagnosis for which little, if any, individual, manualized psychotherapy research exists.* Examples of such diagnoses include an adjustment disorder, bipolar disorder, and dysthymia.

On the basis of exclusion rates alone, it has been impossible to differentiate between the reasons for exclusion listed previously. Different kinds of empirical data are required to decide between the set of possibilities posed by Westen and Morrison (2001), which, if correct, render the findings of RCTs relatively uninformative vis-à-vis clinical practice, or the other possibilities, which lead to more differentiated, and more optimistic, conclusions about the applicability of the RCTs' findings. A further problem is that, although high overall screen-out rates have been documented in published studies, and the exclusion criteria are spelled out in the reports of RCTs, very often the number of potential subjects in each screen-out category has not been listed. Thus, until recently, the specific reasons why most potential patients from the community were not included in research have been the subject of speculation rather than empirical inquiry.

In a recent study, Stirman, DeRubeis, Crits-Christoph, and Brody (2003) mapped information from the charts of patients who had coverage under a managed behavioral health care network to the inclusion and exclusion criteria of nearly 100 RCTs for individual therapies for common adult mental health diagnoses. The largest group in this sample (47% of the patients) had been given an adjustment disorder diagnosis, with no other Axis I diagnosis. No EST exists for adjustment disorders, so these patients presumably would not have fit into any of the published RCTs. Among those who had diagnoses represented in the literature, however, raters (who were uninformed as to the purpose of the study) determined that 80% would have been eligible for at least one study for their primary diagnosis, and 70% would have been eligible for two or more studies. Many of the patients who did not have an adjustment disorder but were nonetheless ineligible to participate in research were determined to be ineligible because they had levels of severity that were too low to meet the criteria for the otherwise relevant studies. Thus, the majority of patients in our managed-care sample did not have more complex diagnostic profiles than the patients who participated in psychotherapy outcome research. In fact, the opposite appeared to be true.

Although these results suggested that the RCTs' findings might generalize reasonably well to at least some kinds of clinical practice, the limitations of the study indicated that further research was necessary before such conclusions could confidently be drawn. The diagnostic information used in the Stirman et al. (2003) study was obtained through unstructured interviews, and the reliability of the diagnoses was therefore questionable. Moreover, the facts that nearly half the patients were diagnosed with an adjustment disorder as well as that a very low rate of diagnosed Axis II comorbidity was observed suggested that the sample may not have represented a typical outpatient clinic. We therefore replicated the methodology of our study, this time with a sample of patients who sought and were denied participation in one of several RCTs at the University of Pennsylvania. Unlike the patients in the previous sample, these patients were diagnosed using reliable, structured diagnostic interviews. An Axis I or II comorbid diagnosis was present in 59% of the patients, and the patients were also of greater ethnic diversity than was true of the earlier sample (Stirman, DeRubeis, Crits-Christoph, & Rothman, 2005).

Of the 220 patients in this sample, 165 (73%) had a primary diagnosis that is represented in the RCT literature. Among those patients, 95% were judged to be eligible for at least one study for the primary diagnosis, and 74% were judged to be eligible for at least two studies. The rates of eligibility for patients with any occurrence of each studied diagnosis (rather than just a primary diagnosis of a particular disorder) were also calculated. The majority of patients with depression (94%), panic disorder (100%), and generalized anxiety disorder (100%) were determined to be eligible for participation in at least one study that targeted these diagnoses. Inclusion rates were high among patients with obsessive–compulsive disorder and social anxiety disorder as well, although fewer patients in our sample were given these diagnoses. The most striking exception to this pattern among all the disorders considered in the study was our findings in the subsample of substance dependent patients. The rates of eligibility were lowest among the studies that tested individual treatments for substance-dependent patients, often because the studies tested treatments for the use of a single substance, whereas most substance-dependent patients use multiple substances. Because group treatments, which are more common in the treatment of (and in RCTs of treatments for) substance dependence, were not included in our study, we could not report on whether the substance abuse literature as a whole is more inclusive.

The results of the Stirman et al. (2005) study suggest that when the entire RCT literature is considered, with the exception of the substance-dependent patients, most treatment-seeking individuals would be eligible for an RCT for their primary diagnosis and frequently for their secondary diagnoses as well. Of those not eligible, many would have been excluded because they were in partial remission or had levels of severity that were lower than the minimum severity criteria for the studies. Thus, it appears that treatment-seeking outpatients, whether they present in a clinic or are excluded from a research trial, do not have more complex diagnostic profiles than patients who participate in research.

Of course, inclusion in an RCT does not guarantee successful treatment. Success rates of RCTs, depending on a range of factors, including the criteria chosen to determine "success," typically range from 50% to 75%. It is therefore possible that outpatients who might meet inclusion criteria for an RCT despite complex diagnostic profiles might be less likely to be successfully treated using a therapy studied in an RCT. As Newman, Moffitt, Caspi, and Silva (1998) pointed out, if comorbid cases are under- or over-represented in such studies relative to the general outpatient population, the extent to which findings can be generalized to the population of people with the disorder may be limited.

For example, Axis I comorbidity has been associated with differential outcomes in studies for MDD (DeRubeis et al., 2004; Goodyer, Herbert, Secher, & Pearson, 1997). Axis II comorbidity has been associated with poorer outcomes in studies of MDD and other Axis I disorders (Chambless, Renneberg, Gracely, Goldstein, & Fydrich, 2000; Crits-Christoph & Barber, 2002; Ezquiaga, Garcia, Pallares, & Bravo, 1999; Reich & Vasile, 1993; Shea et al., 1990). Thus, if RCT participants have lower levels of severity, or lower rates of diagnostic characteristics that are predictors of poor outcome, than nonrandomized outpatients, the RCT results might not be expected to generalize to an outpatient population.

In fact, many psychotherapy RCTs have reported relatively high rates of comorbidity among participants. Shea and associates (1990) reported that 74% of patients who participated in the Treatment of Depression Collaborative Research Project (Elkin et al., 1989) had personality disorders. In a recently completed RCT comparing CBT and antidepressants for MDD (DeRubeis et al., 2004), 69% of the patients were diagnosed with an Axis I comorbidity and 49% were diagnosed with an Axis II comorbidity. In addition, Miranda and colleagues (2003) reported that in an RCT comparing treatments for depression among low-income minority women, 47% carried an additional diagnosis of PTSD. Stangier and colleagues (2003) reported a 75% rate of Axis I comorbidity and a 35% rate of Axis II comorbidity among patients in their study comparing treatments for social anxiety disorder. Also, Cottraux and colleagues (2000) reported a 72% rate of avoidant personality disorder among participants in an RCT for social anxiety. It appears that, perhaps especially in more recent research, RCT participants have relatively complex diagnostic patterns.

Direct comparisons of patients who participate in research and those who do not can also provide information regarding their similarities and differences. Pham, Tang, and Elkin (2004) compared the diagnostic profiles of depressed patients who were receiving treatment in outpatient settings to the profiles of participants in two RCTs for depression (Elkin et al., 1989;

DeRubeis et al., 2004). Participants in the Elkin study had similar rates of Axis II diagnoses and somewhat lower rates of Axis I comorbidity than the outpatient sample, but patients in the DeRubeis study had very similar rates of Axis I and II comorbidity to those of the outpatient sample. These results provide further evidence that both research and nonresearch patients have more similar diagnostic profiles than previously assumed.

In fact, in our experience, it is at least as common for patients in research studies to present with comorbidities as it is for patients in clinical practice to do so. Many patients who present in research clinics are uninsured, underemployed as a result of their psychiatric condition, and cannot afford to pay for treatment. Others have received psychotherapy or medications elsewhere with little success and therefore seek out a research clinic because they want to try a "cutting-edge" treatment. Indeed, if a comprehensive comparison of "research" and "clinic" patients were undertaken, a reasonable prediction is that research patients would be found to have more features associated with poor responses than would clinic patients. Fortunately, treatments and studies are emerging that specifically target patients with comorbidities (Barrowclaugh et al., 2001; Brady, Dansky, Back, Foa, & Carroll, 2001; Linehan et al., 1991; Zlotnick, Najavits, Rohsenow, & Johnson, 2003), as well as those who present with Axis II diagnoses (Svartberg, Stiles, & Seltzer, 2004) or substance dependence comorbid with an Axis I or II diagnosis (Linehan et al., 2002).

ASSESSMENT AND TREATMENT

Just how different are the clinical procedures in research settings when compared to nonresearch environments? In this section, we will address some issues related to assessment and treatment in research and nonresearch settings. We will also consider the likely impact of the differences that exist between research and practice on the patients' treatment experiences and on treatment outcomes.

In a typical RCT, a patient is first screened for the symptoms that are the focus of the study. If patients do endorse these symptoms, a diagnostician gives the patient a diagnosis in person after completing a structured clinical interview and will not subsequently provide treatment if the patient is entered into the study. This is a notable difference between research and practice. Although some larger mental health care clinics do ask potential patients to come in for a more formal assessment before assigning their case to a therapist, this policy is the exception rather than the rule in outpatient settings. Background and diagnostic information on the patient is generally not available to a clinician in private practice before the therapist's first meeting unless the patient is referred to him or her by another clinician who knows the patient well. A therapist in a first meeting typically diagnoses patients, and the diagnosis can be revised in subsequent meetings, typically via unstructured interviews. In contrast, only after a patient is entered into a clinical trial does he or she meet the study therapist, who by that time either has watched a tape of the evaluation meeting or has been briefed by study personnel. Thus, a therapist in an RCT may have more reliable and more comprehensive diagnostic information at the beginning of treatment than a typical therapist in clinical practice. The availability of more complete diagnostic information at the outset may allow research therapists to anticipate obstacles that may arise even before their first meeting with the patient and enable them to choose the most efficient and appropriate methods of addressing these obstacles.

Researchers do exclude some potential participants from clinical trials, but therapists in clinical practice do not have "the luxury of screening out patients they do not believe will respond" (Westen & Morrison, 2001, p. 876). However, like researchers, therapists in a clinical practice do have a responsibility to make sure that their patients receive the most appropriate and competent treatment available. Consider a therapist who has not had experience treating patients with eating disorders, who discovers that his or her new patient requires treatment for bulimia. The therapist would have two choices: to seek supervision in the treatment of bulimia and continue to work with that patient or to refer the patient to a therapist who has experience treating patients with eating disorders. The latter choice is analogous to the choice made by researchers after discovering that a potential participant has a diagnosis that is not the subject of study but requires another kind of treatment before the patient could expect to experience the alleviation of the symptoms that are the subject of the study.

Despite differences in assessment, early meetings between the therapist and patient, whether in a research setting or in a clinical practice, share some common features. In both settings, the therapist works to build a rapport with the patient as they discuss the patient's history and goals. The patient learns what he or she can expect during the course of therapy, and the patient has an opportunity to ask questions. In a typical RCT, the therapist works with the patient for a prescribed number of sessions. The patient is then either referred if he or she is still symptomatic or is followed for a given number of months, sometimes with an allotment of "booster sessions." This time-limited nature of treatment may distinguish research from clinical practice, although in clinical practice many patients engage in time-limited psychotherapy, if for no other reason than that they cannot afford long-term treatment.

The use of time-limited, manual-based treatments is perhaps the greatest difference between treatment in private practice and research. In a national survey of practicing therapists, 47% of the psychologists who responded reported that they never use treatment manuals in their practices, and only 6% of the therapists surveyed reported using manuals in almost all cases (Addis & Krasnow, 2000). Thus, psychotherapy in clinical practice most likely does not resemble the psychotherapy practiced in clinical trials. Whether it will in the future depends in part on whether manual-based therapies can be used effectively in clinical settings. The relation of adherence to a treatment manual and treatment outcome has been debated extensively (see chap. 3 of this volume) and will therefore not be discussed here. Of note, however, are findings that indicate that the outcomes of benchmarking and effectiveness studies (e.g., Merrill, Tolbert, & Wade, 2003; Persons, Bostrom, & Bertagnolli, 1999; Wade, Treat, & Stuart, 1998) show that the treatments studied in RCTs can be successfully transported to clinical practice without a loss of treatment integrity. In addition, some evidence suggests that therapists who are cognitive–behavioral in orientation have a favorable view of treatment manuals and make extensive use of them (Najavits, Weiss, Shaw, & Dierberger, 2000). These findings run counter to the assumption that in order for manual-based treatments to be effective in clinical settings, they need to be modified to such a degree that they no longer resemble the treatments that were conducted in clinical trials. From what we have seen in many clinics and practices that specialize in cognitive–behavioral treatments, therapists frequently use manuals flexibly yet in a manner that is consistent with cognitive–behavioral principles, even as they integrate cognitive–behavioral techniques to treat patients who present with multiple diagnoses.

Whether in private practice or a research setting, there comes a point in time at which the therapist must decide whether continued treatment is indicated and, if so, whether a different approach should be pursued. Some evidence suggests that patients seen in private practice require a greater number of sessions to benefit from treatment, and it has been suggested that the primary reason for this difference is the presence of co-occurring conditions (Morrison, Bradley, & Westen, 2003; Persons et al., 1999). It is expected that patients who present with multiple diagnoses will, on average, require longer-term treatments to address all their symptoms sufficiently. But we suggest that other factors may contribute to the difference in average treatment length between research and practice. Some evidence indicates that patients and therapists work harder when the number of psychotherapy sessions is limited from the outset (Reynolds, Stiles, & Barkham, 1996). This is one feature of treatment in the typical RCT that may serve to increase the effectiveness of therapy. Evidence also shows that clinicians in private practice overestimate, on average, the number of sessions that their patients will require (Cohen & Cohen, 1984; Vessey et al., 1994), which may influence the pace at which therapy proceeds. Certainly, some patients will need more than the typical number of sessions allotted in RCTs to benefit fully from treatment because of the presence of comorbid conditions, a higher than average vulnerability to relapse, or a lack of progress. However, whether or not competent TAU would provide more relief to patients in fewer sessions is unknown at this point because of a dearth of studies that compare EBPs to competent usual care.

Another highly relevant question with regard to the types of patients and treatments seen in research versus those seen in clinical practice is, can the treatments tested in psychotherapy outcome research be effective with the patients seen in practice? Several findings suggest that these treatments are effective when conducted in real-world circumstances. Franklin and colleagues (2000) treated patients who were excluded from a study comparing treatments for obsessive–compulsive disorder (OCD), using exposure and response prevention. Non-RCT patients achieved substantial and clinically meaningful reductions in their OCD and depressive symptoms, which were comparable with those reported in the RCTs. Warren and Thomas (2001) reported similar findings with a sample of clinic patients with OCD. Additionally, Wade, Treat, and Stuart (1998) compared the results of CBT for panic disorder among CMHC patients to the results of several efficacy studies. The magnitude of change from pretreatment to follow-up and the maintenance of change from post-treatment to follow-up in the CMHC sample were comparable with what has been reported in efficacy studies. At follow-up, 89% of the CMHC clients were panic free, and a substantial proportion of the sample had successfully discontinued benzodiazepine use. Merrill, Tolbert, and Wade (2003) also found that CBT was as effective for clinic patients as it had been for patients in two RCTs for depression, although patients in clinical practice received more sessions than patients in the RCTs. Persons, Bostrom, and Bertagnolli (1999) demonstrated that depressed clinic patients treated with CBT experienced a statistically and clinically significant symptom reduction that was comparable to that of the research samples, despite a more complex symptom profile among the clinic patients. These results suggest that the types of patients who are treated in nonresearch settings can, in fact, benefit from the treatments studied in RCTs.

CONCLUSIONS

In summary, the differences that exist between patients in research settings and those in clinical practice are still not well characterized, but the data thus far suggest that they are not nearly as great as some have assumed (see Seligman, 1995), particularly as RCTs have evolved to address the shortcomings of earlier studies. The nascent research and our own experience led us to the conclusion that research patients and clinical trials are frequently representative of clinical practice. Further, research is becoming ever more relevant to clinical practice. Clinical researchers and practicing clinicians should continue to work together to bridge all the gaps between research and practice, an aim that requires persistence and adjustment to current methods, not the abandonment of the scientific methods that have contributed greatly to practical knowledge thus far.

Dialogue: Convergence and Contention

Drew I. Westen

I am in general agreement with the broad message of Stirman and DeRubeis's position paper that "The differences between research and practice are not substantial enough to warrant a dismissal of . . . RCTs . . . ." My argument has never been that we should exclude the results of RCTs from EBP any more than we would exclude results of RCTs for treatments of heart disease. What I have argued is that we should make better use of RCTs, of scientific methods other than RCTs, and of clinicians as collaborators. In this response, I will address two broad issues: (a) Why do researchers exclude patients from RCTs? and (b) Why do researchers exclude the knowledge they might derive from genuine collaboration with practicing clinicians?

Stirman and DeRubeis present an impressive body of evidence from recent studies designed to demonstrate that patients in RCTs are not very different from patients in clinical practice. The question, then, is why researchers have spent the last two decades excluding patients whose inclusion would have had no impact. I suspect the answer has to do with an assumption about psychopathology that has turned out to be wrong and an assumption about the goals of treatment research that is equally problematic.

A central assumption of the EST movement (but not of RCT methodology in general; Westen, Novotny, & Thompson-Brenner, 2004a, 2004b) is that specific disorders require specific treatments. The primary criticism of a prior era of psychotherapy research, which led the Division 12 Task Force to minimize the contributions of the vast majority of RCTs conducted from the 1950s through the 1980s, was that specific problems required specific interventions, and hence that relatively little can be learned from diagnostically heterogeneous samples treated using a general approach (e.g., CBT or psychodynamic). This assumption reflected a number of converging trends: the imbalance toward medications in psychiatric practice guidelines, the emergence of the *DSM–IV* as the taxonomic basis for all research on psychopathology and treatment, and the congeniality of this assumption to CBT researchers, who constitute the vast majority of EST advocates. Combined with the goal of developing treatment *packages* that can be "transported" to clinical practice and "delivered" in the community, this assumption has necessarily led researchers to apply wide exclusion criteria.

Why? If one is developing a specific treatment for depression, the presence of cooccurring conditions is likely to require additional interventions, create within-condition variance in the experimental condition, and lead to increased, and variable, treatment duration (because if specific problems require specific interventions, the presence of two problems necessarily requires more time than one). The problem is compounded if one does not assume that comorbidity is additive (e.g., that patients with depression and substance abuse just happen to have the misfortune of having two problems instead of one) and is independent of personality. Stirman and DeRubeis repeatedly make these assumptions when they suggest that a patient with multiple conditions excluded from one study can simply enter one for a different disorder, that clinicians can readily prioritize problems as "primary" and "secondary" without considering shared diatheses, that comorbid patients can be treated sequentially with manuals designed for each disorder considered separately, and that a clinician might evaluate a patient and decide that the "most appropriate treatment" is one for bulimia (rather than, for example, a treatment that focuses on the bulimic symptoms as well as broader problems of impulse regulation of which they may be an indicator; Thompson-Brenner & Westen, in press).

The problem is that we now know that comorbidity is not random or additive, and that much of it reflects diatheses rooted in personality variables such as negative affect (Kendler, Prescott, Myers, & Neale, 2003; Krueger, 1999). This recognition has led some prominent EST researchers to begin developing pan-disorder treatments (e.g., Barlow, Allen, & Choate, 2004; Fairburn, Cooper, & Shafran, 2003), which we consider a welcome development, moving away from the focus on treatment packages rather than treatment processes.

A second question is why researchers consistently exclude from psychotherapy research the knowledge they might derive from genuine collaboration with practicing clinicians. As colleagues and I argue elsewhere (Westen, Novotny, & Thompson-Brenner, in press), the model of researcher–clinician collaboration associated with the EST movement—reflected in terms such as transportation and dissemination, and in the tendency to equate TAU or "treatment in the community" with treatment provided by underfunded bachelors- or masters-level clinicians in CMHCs—is not one of equal partnership. Despite the many limitations of "clinical data," these data led decades ago to treatments predicated on two hypotheses: that most mental processes are encoded on associational networks to which people lack access, and that most psychological symptoms are moored in enduring personality dispositions. A century later, these two hypotheses are well documented empirically and suggest substantial limits to many of the brief treatments that have been the near-exclusive focus of the EST movement (see Westen, 1998; Westen et al., 2004a). This historical fact might give us pause before relegating clinicians primarily to the role of beta testers for manuals (Westen & Weinberger, in press).

From a strictly scientific standpoint, if researchers want to argue for the generalizability of their studies to everyday clinical practice, they need to use samples drawn from the same population as patients in everyday practice. They also need to compare experimental treatments to treatments sampled from the population of comparison treatments to which they hope to generalize when they claim that their therapies are the treatment of choice. That is, they need to compare them to treatments as practiced by experienced private practitioners.

In the meantime, the data from RCTs provide one compelling source of interventions for clinicians to incorporate into their practices, but the superiority of ESTs can be generalized only to no-treatment, waitlist, and intent-to-fail conditions with patients who may be healthier or sicker than patients treated in private practice in one study or another but who are decidedly different. Rather than suggesting that we abandon science, I am suggesting quite the opposite: that we limit ourselves to scientifically valid generalizations from our studies, alter our experimental designs so that they are more generalizable and clinically useful, and integrate the findings of experimental studies with all available data if our goal is best practice.

Shannon Wiltsey Stirman and Robert J. DeRubeis

Psychotherapy outcome research continues to evolve, with enhancements in both the internal and external validity of its studies. The result is that today policy makers, clinicians, and patients can place more confidence than ever before in the body of knowledge that has emerged from the vast psychotherapy research literature. The principle contributors to this literature, experienced, dedicated clinicians by and large, have of course not addressed all the questions to which they or their fellow clinicians would like answers. They have made choices, as have the peer reviewers and funding agencies that control support in this labor-intensive research area. For a very long time, we suspect, it will be true, and not tritely so, that more research will be needed if we are to continue to use science to inform practice.

Professor Westen has again provided a service to the field by pointing to some limitations in the psychotherapy research literature, relative to a reasonable set of priorities that focus more on longer-term treatments than has been the norm in the literature to date. We interpret some of the existing data differently than does Westen, especially data that speak to the match, or mismatch, between the kinds of patients who have participated in research, and the kinds of patients who are treated in private practices, CMHCs, and managed care consortia. Westen and Morrison's article from 2001, in which they focused on the high screen-out rates typical of RCTs, was a wake-up call for those who, like us, see that the external validity of treatment research is essential if we are to apply the findings in the clinic. Thus, it has been reassuring to discover, as we have in our nascent research program on this problem, that the exclusions of patients by and large are for sensible, clinically relevant reasons and do not appear to undermine appreciably the practical value of findings from the RCT literature. Indeed, the rates of screen-outs from individual studies are very high in some studies, a good example being the unusually high rate (85%) reported in the TADS cited by Westen. But even high screen-out rates should not necessarily undermine the clinical utility of a study's findings, as we have argued (in this chapter) and shown (Stirman et al., 2003, 2005).

There are times, however, when the screen-out policies of a single study raise serious questions, such as the one raised by Westen about suicidality and the TADS. Indeed, researchers face a difficult ethical–practical–scientific decision when defining the level of suicidality that will lead to a referral outside the study. In our own research on treatments for severe, chronic, and recurrent depression, we have found that some patients who participate in the screening process are so acutely suicidal that the most appropriate course of action is to escort them to the hospital. After a hospital stay, if outpatient pharmacotherapy or psychotherapy is deemed to be a safe option, such a patient may then be admitted to our research protocol. Responsible practitioners repeat this sequence in an analogous fashion throughout the country every day. That is, outpatient treatment often follows a hospital stay for patients who present to a clinician in a suicidal crisis. No study, then, of the effects of once- or twice-weekly outpatient sessions should include patients who require more intensive treatment than can be offered through the study. That said, research targeting suicidal and parasuicidal behaviors is encouraging (Bruce et al., 2004; Evans et al., 1999; Linehan et al., 1991; MacLeod et al., 1998; Tyrer et al., 2003), as such treatments may be more beneficial for some patients, at least initially, than a depression treatment protocol.

We would also like to highlight research progress on the concern, raised by Westen, that racial and ethnic minorities are underrepresented in clinical trials. Although no consistent pattern has emerged indicating that minority status predicts either better or poorer outcome, researchers are beginning to adapt and test treatments for underrepresented populations, such as minorities (Carter, Sbrocco, Gore, Marin, & Lewis, 2003; Ginsburg & Drake, 2002; Kohn, Oden, Muñoz, Robinson, & Leavitt, 2002; Miranda et al., 2003) and unemployed patients (Creed, Machin, & Hicks, 1999), with promising results. The positive findings from these trials provide reason for optimism about the potential for modifying treatments to suit specific needs or populations.

We agree with Westen about the need to compare the treatments studied in RCTs against competent TAU. The dearth of informative studies of this type may be largely due to the difficulty of funding such endeavors, but we agree with Westen that funding priorities should change. We will briefly describe a research approach that would address many of the questions that still remain about the alleged value of ESTs. A large population of (willing-to-participate) therapists in a variety of clinics would be randomly assigned either to continue their practice as usual or to learn and follow a treatment protocol, or a set of treatment protocols, with either a single, disorder-defined population (e.g., patients with panic disorders) or a set of populations (e.g., patients with nonpsychotic affective or anxiety disorders). Care would be taken to ensure that the "experimental" group of therapists received no more support than the control therapists, so, for example, patient loads would be equated, as would meeting time. Whereas the experimental therapists meet for ongoing supervision, the control therapists would likewise meet to discuss cases. Research of this type would be necessary to determine which patient populations, if any, would be best served by the time, money, and effort required to train clinicians in new treatments.

Along with thousands of clinician–scientists and clinicians who engage in EBPs, we have been energized and edified by the findings in the psychotherapy research literature as they have emerged over the last half-century. We are proud to contribute to this literature, and we believe it is vital that clinical scientists continue to pursue research that will ultimately improve the day-to-day delivery of mental health care.

REFERENCES

Addis, M., & Krasnow, A. (2000). A national survey of practicing psychologists' attitudes toward psychotherapy treatment manuals. *Journal of Consulting and Clinical Psychology, 68*, 331–339.

American Psychiatric Association. (1994). *Diagnostic and statistical manual of mental disorders* (4th ed.). Washington, DC: Author.

Barlow, D. (2002). *Anxiety and its disorders* (2nd ed.). New York: Guilford Press.

Barlow, D. H., Allen, L. B., & Choate, M. L. (2004). Toward a unified treatment for emotional disorders. *Behavior Therapy, 35*, 205–230.

Barrowclough, C., Haddock, G., Tarrier, N., Lewis, S., Moring, J., O'Brien, R., et al. (2001). Randomized controlled trial of motivational interviewing, cognitive behavior therapy, and family intervention for patients with comorbid schizophrenia and substance use disorders. *American Journal of Psychiatry, 158*, 1706–1713.

Bradley, R., Greene, J., Russ, E., Dutra, L., & Westen, D. (in press). A multidimensional meta-analysis of psychotherapy for PTSD. *American Journal of Psychiatry.*

Brady, K., Dansky, B., Back, S., Foa, E., & Carroll, K. (2001). Exposure therapy in the treatment of PTSD among cocaine-dependent individuals: Preliminary findings. *Journal of Substance Abuse Treatment, 21*, 47–54.

Brown, T. A., Chorpita, B. F., & Barlow, D. H. (1998). Structural relationships among dimensions of the *DSM-IV* anxiety and mood disorders and dimensions of negative affect, positive affect, and autonomic arousal. *Journal of Abnormal Psychology, 107*, 179–192.

Bruce, M., Ten Have, T., Reynolds, C., Katz, I., Schulberg, H., Mulsant, B., et al. (2004). Reducing suicidal ideation and depressive symptoms in depressed older primary care patients: A randomized controlled trial. *Journal of the American Medical Association, 29,* 1081–1091.

Carter, M. M., Sbrocco, T., Gore, K. L., Marin, N. W., & Lewis, E. L. (2003). Cognitive–behavioral group therapy versus a wait-list control in the treatment of African American women with panic disorder. *Cognitive Therapy and Research, 27,* 505–518.

Chambless, D., Renneberg, B., Gracely, E., Goldstein, A., & Fydrich, T. (2000). Axis I and II comorbidity in agoraphobia: Prediction of psychotherapy outcome in a clinical setting. *Psychotherapy Research, 10,* 279–295.

Cohen, P., & Cohen, J. (1984). The clinician's illusion. *Archives of General Psychiatry, 41,* 1178–1182.

Cottraux, J., Note, I., Albuisson, E., Yao, S., Note, B., Mollard, E., et al. (2000). Cognitive behavior therapy versus supportive therapy in social phobia: A randomized controlled trial. *Psychotherapy and Psychosomatics, 3,* 137–146.

Creed, P. A., Machin, M. A., & Hicks, R. E. (1999). Improving mental health status and coping abilities for long-term unemployed youth using cognitive–behaviour therapy-based training interventions. *Journal of Organizational Behavior, 20,* 963–978.

Crits-Christoph, P., & Barber, J. P. (2002). Psychosocial treatments for personality disorders. In P. Nathan & J. Gorman (Eds.), *A guide to treatments that work* (pp. 611–624). New York: Oxford University Press.

DeRubeis, R. J., Amsterdam, J. D., O'Reardon, J. P., & Young, P. R. (2004, July). Cognitive therapy versus medications: Acute treatment of severe depression. In S. D. Hollon (Chair), *Cognitive therapy versus medications: Treatment and prevention of severe depression.* Symposium conducted at the annual meeting of the American Psychological Association, Honolulu, Hawaii.

Elkin, I., Shea, M. T., Watkins, J. T., Imber, S. D., Sotsky, S. M., Collins, J. F., et al. (1989). National Institute of Mental Health Treatment of Depression Collaborative Research Program: General effectiveness of treatments. *Archives of General Psychiatry, 46,* 971–982.

Evans, K., Tyrer, P., Catalan, J., Schmidt, U., Davidson, K., Dent, J., et al. (1999). Manual-assisted cognitive–behaviour therapy (MACT): A randomised controlled trial of a brief intervention with bibliotherapy in the treatment of recurrent deliberate self-harm. *Psychological Medicine, 29,* 19–25.

Ezquiaga, E., Garcia, A., Pallares, T., & Bravo, M. (1999). Psychosocial predictors of outcome in major depression: A prospective 12-month study. *Journal of Affective Disorders, 52,* 209–216.

Fairburn, C., Cooper, Z., & Shafran, R. (2003). Cognitive behaviour therapy for eating disorders: A "transdiagnostic" theory and treatment. *Behavior and Research Therapy, 41,* 509–528.

Fava, G. A., & Mangelli, L. (2001). Assessment of subclinical symptoms and psychological well-being in depression. *European Archive of Psychiatry and Clinical Neuroscience, 251,* 47–52.

Franklin, M. E., Abramowitz, J. S., Kozak, M. J, Levitt, J. T., & Foa, E. B. (2000). Effectiveness of exposure and ritual prevention for obsessive–compulsive disorder: Randomized compared with nonrandomized samples. *Journal of Consulting and Clinical Psychology, 68,* 594–602.

Ginsburg, G. S., & Drake, K. L. (2002). School-based treatment for anxious African-American adolescents: A controlled pilot study. *Journal of the American Academy of Child & Adolescent Psychiatry, 41,* 768–775.

Goodyer, I., Herbert, J., Secher, S., & Pearson, J. (1997). Short-term outcome of major depression: I. Comorbidity and severity at presentation as predictors of persistent disorder. *Journal of the American Academy of Child and Adolescent Psychiatry, 36,* 179–187.

Hollon, S. D., Thase, M. E., & Markowitz, J. C. (2002). Treatment and prevention of depression. *Psychological Science in the Public Interest, 3,* 39–77.

Kendler, K. S., Prescott, C. A., Myers, J., & Neale, M. C. (2003). The structure of genetic and environmental risk factors for common psychiatric and substance use disorders in men and women. *Archives of General Psychiatry, 60,* 929–937.

Kohn, L. P., Oden, T., Muñoz, R. F., Robinson, A., & Leavitt, D. (2002). Adapted cognitive behavioral group therapy for depressed low-income African American women. *Community Mental Health Journal, 38,* 497–504.

Krueger, R. F. (1999). The structure of common mental disorders. *Archives of General Psychiatry, 56,* 921–926.

Krueger, R. F., & Piasecki, T. M. (2002). Toward a dimensional and psychometrically-informed approach to conceptualizing psychopathology. *Behaviour Research and Therapy, 40,* 485–499.

Linehan, M., Dimeff, L., Reynolds, S., Comtois, K., Welch, S., Heagerty, P., et al. (2002). Dialectal behavior therapy versus comprehensive validation therapy plus 12-step for the treatment of opioid dependent women meeting criteria for borderline personality disorder. *Drug and Alcohol Dependence, 67,* 13–26.

Linehan, M. M. (1993). *Cognitive–behavioral treatment of borderline personality disorder.* New York: Guilford Press.

Linehan, M. M., Armstrong, H., Suarez, A., Allmon, D., et al. (1991). Cognitive–behavioral treatment of chronically parasuicidal borderline patients. *Archives of General Psychiatry, 48,* 1060–1064.

Luborsky, L., Diguer, L., Seligman, D. A., Rosenthal, R., Krause, E. D., Johnson, S., et al. (1999). The researcher's own therapy allegiances: A "wild card" in comparisons of treatment efficacy. *Clinical Psychology: Science and Practice, 6,* 95–106.

MacLeod, A., Tata, P., Evans, K., Tyrer, P., Schmidt, U., Davidson, K., et al. (1998). Recovery of positive future thinking within a high-risk parasuicide group: Results from a pilot randomized controlled trial. *British Journal of Clinical Psychology, 37,* 371–379.

March, J. S., Silva, S., Petrycki, S., Curry, J., Wells, K., Fairbank, J., et al. (2004). Fluoxetine, cognitive–behavioral therapy, and their combination for adolescents with depression: Treatment for adolescents with depression study (TADS) randomized controlled trial. *Journal of the American Medical Association, 292,* 807–820.

Merrill, K. A., Tolbert, V. E., & Wade, W. A. (2003). Effectiveness of cognitive therapy for depression in a community mental health center: A benchmarking study. *Journal of Consulting and Clinical Psychology*, 404–409.

Miranda, J., Chung, J., Green, B., Krupnick, J., Siddique, J., Revicki, D., et al. (2003). Treating depression in predominantly low-income young minority women: A randomized controlled trial. *Journal of the American Medical Association*, 290, 57–65.

Morrison, K., Bradley, R., & Westen, D. (2003). The external validity of controlled clinical trials of psychotherapy for depression and anxiety: A naturalistic study. *Psychology and Psychotherapy: Theory, Research and Practice*, 76, 109–132.

Najavits, L. M., Weiss, R. D., Shaw, S. R., & Dierberger, A. E. (2000). Psychotherapists' views of treatment manuals. *Professional Psychology: Research and Practice*, 31, 404–408.

Newman, D., Moffitt, T., Caspi, A., & Silva, P. (1998). Comorbid mental disorders: Implications for treatment and sample selection. *Journal of Abnormal Psychology*, 107, 305–311.

Persons, J. B., Bostrom, A., & Bertagnolli, A. (1999). Results of randomized controlled trials of cognitive therapy for depression generalize to private practice. *Cognitive Therapy and Research*, 23, 243–248.

Pham, T., Tang, T., & Elkin, I. (2004). *Real world patients versus research patients: How big is the gap?* Unpublished manuscript, Northwestern University.

Popper, K. (1959). *The logic of scientific discovery*. London: Hutchinson.

Reich, J., & Vasile, R. (1993). Effect of personality disorders on treatment outcome of Axis I disorders: An update. *Journal of Nervous Mental Disease*, 182, 475–484.

Reynolds, S., Stiles, W. B., & Barkham, M. (1996). Acceleration of changes in session impact during contrasting time-limited psychotherapies. *Journal of Consulting and Clinical Psychology*, 64, 577–586.

Roth, A., & Fonagy, P. (1996). *What works for whom? A critical review of psychotherapy research*. New York: Guilford Press.

Seligman, M. E. P. (1995). The effectiveness of psychotherapy: The *Consumer Reports* study. *American Psychologist*, 50, 965–974.

Shea, M. T., Pilkonis, P., Beckham, E., Collins, J., Elkin, I., Sotsky, S., et al. (1990). Personality disorders and treatment outcome in the NIMH Treatment of Depression Collaborative Research Program. *American Journal of Psychiatry*, 147, 711–718.

Stangier, U., Heindreich, T., Peitz, M., Lauterback, W., & Clark, D. (2003). Cognitive therapy for social phobia: Individual versus group treatment. *Behaviour Research and Therapy*, 41, 991–1007.

Stirman, S. W., DeRubeis, R. J., Crits-Christoph, P., & Brody, P. E. (2003). Are samples in randomized controlled trials of psychotherapy representative of community outpatients? A new methodology and initial findings. *Journal of Consulting and Clinical Psychology*, 71, 963–972.

Stirman, S. W., DeRubeis, R. J., Crits-Christoph, P., & Rothman, A. (2005). Can the randomized controlled trial literature generalize to non-randomized patients? *Journal of Consulting and Clinical Psychology, 73*, 127–135.

Svartberg, M., Stiles, T., & Seltzer, M. (2004). Randomized controlled trial of the effectiveness of short-term dynamic psychotherapy and cognitive therapy for cluster C personality disorders. *American Journal of Psychiatry, 161*, 810–817.

Thompson-Brenner, H., & Westen, D. (in press). A naturalistic study of psychotherapy for bulimia nervosa, Part 1: Comorbidity and therapeutic outcome. *Journal of Nervous and Mental Disorders.*

Tyrer, P., Thompson, S. Schmidt, U., Jones, V., Knapp, M., Davidson, K., et al. (2003). Randomized controlled trial of brief cognitive behaviour therapy versus treatment as usual in recurrent deliberate self-harm: The POPMACT study. *Psychological Medicine, 33*, 969–976.

Vessey, J. T., Howard, K. I., Lueger, R., Kächele, H., & Mergenthaler, E. (1994). The clinician's illusion and the psychotherapy practice: An application of stochastic modeling. *Journal of Consulting and Clinical Psychology, 62*, 679–685.

Wade, W. A., Treat, T. A., & Stuart, G. L. (1998). Transporting an empirically supported treatment for panic disorder to a service clinic setting: A benchmarking strategy. *Journal of Consulting and Clinical Psychology, 66*, 231–239.

Wampold, B. E. (2001). *The great psychotherapy debate: Models, methods, and findings.* Mahwah, NJ: Erlbaum.

Warren, R., & Thomas, J. (2001). Cognitive–behavior therapy of obsessive–compulsive disorder in private practice: An effectiveness study. *Journal of Anxiety Disorders, 15*, 277–285.

Weisz, J. R., Jensen Doss, A., & Hawley, K. M. (2005). Youth psychotherapy outcome research: A review and critique of the evidence base. *Annual Review of Psychology, 56*, 337–363.

Westen, D. (1998). The scientific legacy of Sigmund Freud: Toward a psychodynamically informed psychological science. *Psychological Bulletin, 124*, 333–371.

Westen, D., & Arkowitz-Westen, L. (1998). Limitations of Axis II in diagnosing personality pathology in clinical practice. *American Journal of Psychiatry, 155*, 1767–1771.

Westen, D., & Bradley, R. (in press). Empirically supported complexity: Avoiding dichotomous thinking in the evaluation of psychotherapies. *Current Directions in Psychological Science.*

Westen, D., & Morrison, K. (2001). A multidimensional meta-analysis of treatments for depression, panic, and generalized anxiety disorder: An empirical examination of the status of empirically supported therapies. *Journal of Consulting and Clinical Psychology, 69*, 875–899.

Westen, D., Novotny, C., & Thompson-Brenner, H. (2004a). The empirical status of empirically supported therapies: Assumptions, methods, and findings. *Psychological Bulletin, 130*, 631–663.

Westen, D., Novotny, C., & Thompson-Brenner, H. (2004b). The next generation of psychotherapy research. *Psychological Bulletin, 130*, 677–683.

Westen, D., Novotny, C., & Thompson-Brenner, H. (in press). EBP–EST: Reply to Crits-Christoph, Wilson, and Hollon (2005) and Weisz, Weersing, and Henggeler (2005). *Psychological Bulletin.*

Westen, D., & Weinberger, J. (in press). In praise of clinical judgment: Meehl's forgotten legacy. *Journal of Clinical Psychology.*

Wixom, J., Ludolph, P., & Westen, D. (1993). Quality of depression in borderline adolescents. *Journal of the American Academy of Child and Adolescent Psychiatry, 32,* 1172–1177.

Zane, N., Hall, G. N., Sue, S., Young, K., & Nunez, J. (2004). Research on psychotherapy with culturally diverse populations. In M. J. Lambert (Ed.), *Bergin and Garfield's Handbook of Psychotherapy* (5th ed., pp. 767–804). New York: Wiley.

Zlotnick, C., Najavits, L., Rohsenow, D., & Johnson, D. (2003). A cognitive–behavioral treatment for incarcerated women with substance abuse disorder and posttraumatic stress disorder: Findings from a pilot study. *Journal of Substance Abuse Treatment, 25,* 99–105.

5

WHAT SHOULD BE VALIDATED?

The Treatment Method

Dianne L. Chambless and Paul Crits-Christoph

Psychotherapy is a complex endeavor. Whether it is successful depends on many variables, only one of which is the treatment method the therapist follows. That the treatment method is not the only factor in treatment outcome does not diminish its importance. Consistent with the thrust of the evidence-based medicine approach (Sackett, Richardson, Rosenberg, & Haynes, 1997), we hold that examination of the empirical basis of the treatment method is essential to the improvement of treatment outcomes. Moreover, knowledge of the evidence for our treatment method versus other potential methods is required by the ethical principle that psychologists' work be based on scientific knowledge (American Psychological Association, 2002).

WHAT IS A TREATMENT METHOD?

We begin by defining what we mean by a treatment method. A treatment consists of therapists' behaviors designed to foster therapeutic benefit. The treatment may be highly complex, involving many different components, such as dialectical behavior therapy (Linehan, 1993), or the treatment may be one quite specific intervention, such as empty chair work for unresolved conflicts with an important other (Paivio & Greenberg, 1995), one intervention of many used in Gestalt therapy. What is critical is that the treatment can be detailed and taught. From a public health perspective, it doesn't help us to know that some gifted psychotherapists can achieve demonstrably good outcomes if they cannot also articulate to others the principles behind their successes. The tacit knowledge of such individuals benefits only their patients and cannot be passed on to students and colleagues. For a treatment method to be of public health significance, someone must be able to identify its principles and procedures. Only then can the treatment be disseminated to students and other professionals and tested in any meaningful way.

Suppose that someone has been successful in developing a treatment that is successful for all kinds of clients with all kinds of problems, from an autistic child to a martially dissatisfied couple, and the treatment is relatively inexpensive and easy for therapists to learn to administer. Our task as psychotherapy researchers would be over once we determined that this treatment did indeed work for all kinds of problems, and our training as clinicians could stop as soon as we learned to administer this treatment. It is improbable to us that such a treatment exists or ever will. Given that this is the case, ethical therapists are left with choosing which treatment method to use with a given client or with selecting their clients to be compatible with the sort of treatment they are prepared to offer.

On what basis does the therapist choose? In reviewing the literature on clinical decision-making for this position paper, we were struck by the dearth of research on therapists' choices about treatment. This stands in contrast to the large body of research on clinicians' decision-making regarding psychological assessments (e.g., Garb, 1998). We argue here, as we have elsewhere (Task Force on Promotion and Dissemination of Psychological Procedures, 1995), that treatment decisions should be made, whenever possible, on the basis of the results of empirical research that tests what treatment works for what problems experienced by clients with what important characteristics that might moderate the treatment outcome. Only such an approach fulfills the commitment of psychologists to blend science and practice. Thus, for example, the research literature tells us that relaxation training is a poor treatment for obsessive–compulsive disorder (see Chambless & Ollendick, 2001), whereas exposure plus response prevention is a good one. Our responsibility seems clear: to use exposure and response prevention rather than relaxation training if we are competent to do so, or to refer to someone who is.

Empirically Supported Versus Nonsupported Treatments

On what basis, other than research, would psychotherapists choose a treatment? Would they provide the type of treatment they enjoy delivering? Or would they provide the simplest treatment regardless of its benefits? Surely, the compassionate, ethical clinician would not. We suspect that therapists who do not value the empirical literature base their treatment decisions on clinical lore passed on by the people who taught them, by workshop leaders, or by influential writers, or they base their decisions on their own prior experience. Indeed, in the only study we found on the selection of treatment methods, clinicians treating patients with psychosomatic disorders were open to considering the empirical evidence the investigators provided them, but only if that evidence did not contradict their own clinical experience (Raine et al., 2004). We do not wish to be critical of clinical lore. Such lore is often the first step in developing a new efficacious treatment. Rather, we argue that clinical lore is not sufficient and that, whenever possible, we need to subject it to a rigorous empirical test. Historical examples such as the use of clitoridectomy, cocaine, bloodletting, and trephining to treat mental illness remind us that clinical lore can be disastrously wrong. More recently, we have the less drastic but sad example of facilitated communication for people with developmental disabilities, an intervention about which there was great excitement until controlled research repeatedly demonstrated that the positive results reported either did not occur or were due to unintended direction from the facilitator (e.g., Hirshoren & Gregory, 1995).

Currently, many problems do not have corresponding empirically supported treatments (ESTs), and in many cases the available EST fails. Even when a therapist uses an empirically supported method, for a given case hundreds of minidecisions must be made, and there will never be data to guide all of them. Thus, it is impossible for the therapist's every action to be driven by hard data. However, we should aspire to test as many treatments and aspects of treatments as possible, realizing that we will also need to generalize from the available empirical literature or draw on clinical lore, failing all else. Thus, in the face of evidence that Treatment A works, it is not sufficient for the practitioner who prefers Treatment B to rest on the fact that no one has shown that Treatment B is ineffective. Treatment A remains the ethical choice until the success of Treatment B is documented, unless in the process of informed consent the practitioner describes the alternatives and evidence for each, permitting the client to make an educated decision. Meeting this ethical demand is not a death knell for the clinician's practice. Clients may be as satisfied with suggestions based on the therapist's clinical experience as with research data (O'Donohue, Fisher, Plaud, & Link, 1989).

If many consumers are satisfied with clinical experience as the basis for their treatment, why are we less sanguine? As psychologists, we know more than consumers about the limitations of humans as information processors.

Can clinicians reliably assess and remember accurately what the causal factors were in their clients' improvement? Without systematic research, it is unlikely that, amid all the variability and uncontrolled factors in treatment outcome, clinicians can be confident about which of their many behaviors are consistently related to the results of treatment for a particular type of client or problem. A simpler piece of information, how long clients in one's practice remain in treatment, is far less subject to memory's distortion than factors involved in treatment outcome. Nonetheless, practitioners consistently overestimate the percentage of their clients who remain in their practice for long-term therapy (Vessey, Howard, Lueger, Kachele, & Mergenthaler, 1994).

Space does not permit a review of the entire catalogue of errors in information processing that seem pertinent to psychotherapy (for comprehensive reviews, see Baron, 2000; Turk & Salovey, 1988; see also the Hollon paper in this volume). We will limit ourselves to a consideration of a few. When therapists draw on their memory banks for what treatment approach has worked with similar clients in the past, they are in danger of having their decisions biased by the availability heuristic. That is, the ease of thinking of examples about the intervention's success or failure will affect estimations of how likely it is the treatment will help. One or two salient successful cases may be sufficient to override one's memory of the cases when this approach did not work. For example, no doubt blinded by initial dramatic successes, one of us (DLC) was an early advocate of paradoxical intention as an addition to exposure instructions for people with panic disorder with agoraphobia. Alas, later controlled research showed no benefit for this approach over exposure alone (Michelson, Mavissakalian, & Marchione, 1985), and it also showed that most clients quietly ignored the instruction to try to initiate a panic attack when in the phobic situation (Edelman & Chambless, 1993).

The effects of a confirmation bias may be such that the therapist sees success where it is expected and overlooks any evidence of failure. After all, therapists are human beings and need to protect their confidence and self-esteem in a stressful profession that carries a great deal of responsibility. It is hardly surprising then that Kendall, Kipnis, and Otto-Salaj (1992) found evidence of a self-serving bias in therapists' assessment of their cases: When psychologists described a treatment failure, they were most likely to attribute the reason for that failure to client attributes, whereas Kipnis, Hansen, and Fallon (1989, as cited by Kendall et al., 1992) found therapists were most likely to attribute successes in treatment to themselves and their skills.

Depending on the kind of clients a therapist sees, perhaps one third will improve over the passage of time or from environmental influences apart from the therapy (Smith, Glass, & Miller, 1980). This so-called spontaneous remission sets the stage for the development of illusory correlations, wherein the therapist attributes improvement to the treatment when this conclusion is not warranted. Therapists in specialty clinics who see the same kind of case over and over may well accurately discern patterns in improvement over time. It is much more difficult for a general practitioner who sees a wide variety of cases to develop a clear view of cause–effect relationships in a clinical practice. Why then do clinicians have more confidence in clinical experience, their own and that of others, than in data? Two factors seem likely to come into play. First, in general, people tend to be overconfident that their judgments are right (Baron, 2000). Second, direct experience is much more vivid and more likely to affect subsequent behavior than indirect experience, such as reading dry statistics (Snyder & Thomsen, 1988). Accordingly, a colorful case study described by a supervisor or a striking case in one's own practice is likely to override the latest meta-analysis.

Given the crush of these biases, how can we encourage clinicians to be more skeptical about untested treatments and more enthusiastic about evidence-based treatments? Part of the answer lies in graduate training. Exposure to the evidence of cognitive biases and the integration of an empirical approach to treatment in students' practices should strengthen the likelihood that students will continue to draw on science once they are in practice. Presenting case studies treated with ESTs to graduate students and professional audiences should also be helpful. Moreover, the growth of evidence that ESTs work in practice settings in the community should help allay clinicians' concerns that cases treated in research programs are too different from their own to benefit from ESTs (Chambless & Ollendick, 2001). Finally, the increasing practice in many clinics of monitoring treatment outcomes with standardized assessment instruments will provide clinicians with the feedback on all their cases that is necessary to encourage a more objective look at what works for whom in their own practice. Such an assessment may stimulate the appetite for ESTs.

TREATMENT METHODS VERSUS OTHER VARIABLES

A common point of confusion among critics of the EST approach is the belief that those of us who advocate the identification and use of ESTs believe the treatment method is the only important contributor to psychotherapy outcome. This is certainly not the case, as we hope we have and will make clear in this position paper. In addition, these critics often suggest that other features of psychotherapy should trump any focus on treatment methods. These features include aspects of the patient, the therapist, and the therapist–patient relationship. We will consider a number of these arguments in this section.

Treatments Versus Patient Variables

Critics of ESTs have argued that patient variables affect treatment outcome and therefore that creating a list of ESTs ignores the fact that some outcome variance is attributed to patient variables (Garfield, 1998). A more sophisticated version of this argument calls attention to possible interactions between patient variables and treatments; that is, some treatments work well for certain types of patients but not others. The concern inherent in these arguments is that studies of treatment methods might tell us that a given treatment is, on average, superior to a control condition or other treatment, but this information does not guarantee that the treatment will work with a particular patient currently in a therapist's office (because that patient has characteristics that might lead to a relatively poorer outcome).

Neither of these arguments is a reason to abandon studying treatments or compiling a listing of the treatments that have been shown to be efficacious. The fallacy in these arguments is the assumption that treatment research is designed to guarantee a certain outcome with every patient with the given problem. The purpose of disseminating ESTs is to do the most good, that is, to help as many patients as possible. Thus, treatment research is conducted with a public health view: How much suffering, illness, or disability can be diminished across the population if a new treatment is empirically supported (and then disseminated)? Further, we fail to see the logic in the argument that it is better that therapists fly by the seat of their pants than to try an EST that might not help each and every patient but has a good chance of doing so.

With any treatment it is likely that patient variables account for some outcome variance (perhaps even more than the treatment versus control difference). It would certainly be ideal to disseminate a treatment with highly specific qualifications on its use (e.g., this treatment works with younger men with a moderate severity of the disorder, but it does not work with the elderly), but much can still be gained when treatments are disseminated even without such qualifications. Once additional research clarifies the types of patients for whom the treatment should not be used, this information can be immediately disseminated to enhance population average outcomes further. Given that few patient variables have consistently, and robustly, predicted treatment outcome (Luborsky, Crits-Christoph, Mintz, & Auerbach, 1988), and that response rates to most psychological interventions are fairly high (in the range of 50%–80%), the rate of treatment failures, while a concern, needs to be balanced against the importance of the treatment successes that result in the population from the use of ESTs. If, before we disseminate a treatment, we wait the decades it would take for research to nail down all the patient variables that may or may not predict outcome or that interact with treatment types, we run the risk of allowing enormous amounts of patient suffering to continue over those decades when much of that suffering could have been reduced. It is not uncommon, for example, for patients with obsessive–compulsive disorder (OCD) to have reported essentially no improvement over the course of 20 or more years of treatment with various nonempirically tested psychotherapies. Many of these patients would achieve substantial symptom relief and improvement in quality of life if exposed to an EST, even though not all would improve.

The question of patient variables that might affect treatment outcome reduces again to an issue of, what are the alternatives for choosing a treatment? Without research evidence that a particular EST (e.g., exposure and response prevention for OCD) is not effective (or relatively less effective than another treatment) with a certain type of patient (e.g., patients with OCD and comorbid depression), we argue that the EST remains the best available choice for such patients. If a patient fails to improve in an EST, then clinical options (alternative treatment or longer-term treatment) can always be considered. In summary, we have to act on the best empirical knowledge we have at the moment and continue to add to, and refine, such knowledge over time.

Relationship Variables Versus Treatments

Another spurious argument is that the heart of change is in the therapeutic relationship, not the treatment method, and therefore any effort to focus attention on the treatment method is misguided. First of all, although the therapeutic alliance has shown to be a consistent predictor of treatment outcome, the size of the statistical relationship is actually relatively small. On the basis of meta-analytic evidence across a wide range of psychotherapies, only about 5% of the outcome variance is attributed to the therapeutic alliance (Martin, Garske, & Davis, 2000). Moreover, only a few studies have ruled out a third-variable interpretation of the alliance–outcome relationship, namely that the alliance is in part a function of early improvement in therapy (patients have a better relationship with their therapist when they have achieved early gains). Although it appears as though some component of the alliance–outcome relationship is independent of this third variable (e.g., Klein et al., 2003), the direct causal contribution of the alliance to the outcome is likely to be of a magnitude somewhat less than the 5% figure currently documented.

Having said this, we should make clear that we also view the therapeutic relationship as a key element of most treatment methods. In fact, many ESTs (e.g., Beck, Rush, Shaw, & Emery, 1979) include the therapy relationship as one component of an overall treatment package. Thus, it is inaccurate to view these ESTs as ignoring the therapy relationship. However, it is also inaccurate to generalize from existing psychotherapy studies showing that the alliance is related to outcome to a claim that it is central to all treatments for all disorders. It may be that the alliance is not an important causal factor for some treatments. For example, a number of studies indicate that cognitive–behavior therapy (CBT) for a panic disorder delivered by bibliotherapy and web-based programs is efficacious (see review by Chambless &

Peterman, 2004). Obviously, in such treatments there is no therapist with whom to have an alliance.

Assuming the therapeutic alliance is indeed important to the outcome for most treatments, the relevant question is, can therapists influence the quality of alliance? If so, then therapist behaviors designed to improve the alliance are part of the treatment that should be specified. If the alliance is a function of what the patient brings to therapy, we still need to focus on what the therapist can also do to enhance outcome above and beyond the impact of the alliance. Only when patient contributions to the alliance predict 100% of the outcome variance would focusing on treatment techniques be futile.

If the quality of the alliance is something that can be improved by certain therapist behaviors (techniques that can be taught), then the alliance is not an alternative to an emphasis on treatment techniques; it is fully within the domain of research that attempts to validate treatment techniques. Along these lines, one of us (PCC) has created a treatment manual for fostering the alliance and conducted a pilot study evaluating whether therapists can improve their alliance when they are taught techniques designed to improve the alliance or repair ruptures in the alliance (Crits-Christoph, Connolly Gibbons, Narducci, Schamberger, & Gallop, in press). Further research is needed to determine whether techniques that enhance the alliance are sufficient to achieve maximum patient outcomes or need to be combined with other types of techniques. Additional research is also needed to establish what proportion of therapists can effectively learn to use such alliance-fostering techniques.

Treatments Versus the Therapist

Related to the argument about alliance is the position that a focus on a treatment method ignores the therapist's contribution to the outcome. The inherent qualities of the therapist (e.g., warmth and genuineness) may be more important than treatment techniques. As with patient characteristics, the existence of the therapist's personal characteristics that influence the outcome is not antithetical to the testing and dissemination of treatment models. Unless 100% of the outcome variance is due to therapist variables (or patient plus therapist variables), we can still enhance the outcome by teaching therapists behaviors that improve the outcome.

Therapists of course need to be appropriately selected, trained, and certified to do therapy. Unless we restrict the practice of psychotherapy to gifted therapists who, with little formal training, are able to achieve good outcomes (and this scenario is very distant from the current processes that allow people to conduct psychotherapy), teaching therapists how best to help their patients will play an important role.

Treatments Versus Principles

An additional criticism of the movement to direct attention to ESTs is that treatment manuals are cookbooks that focus too much on specific techniques rather than on general principles. A better approach, according to this argument, is to teach general empirically supported principles that would allow clinical flexibility in their application. This argument contains multiple fallacies. The first is equating ESTs with cookbooks. Many existing treatment manuals that have considerable empirical support (e.g., cognitive therapy for depression) are not cookbooks at all. Therapists are taught general principles and have considerable flexibility in implementing the treatment model, although a prototypical course of treatment is often outlined to assist the therapist in training, and some treatment manuals (Luborsky, 1984) are explicitly based on principles.

Thus, assuming that principles can be taught, there is no reason why a principle-based psychotherapy manual cannot be created and the treatment evaluated. Care would need to be taken to ensure that the manual is not so flexible that the implementation of the treatment could not be replicated. If other therapists cannot replicate the implementation, such principles of treatment cannot be empirically supported in a way that is useful to other therapists. Thus, a call for a greater emphasis on the principles of treatment reduces to a preference for a certain type of treatment manual. We fully support the pursuit of such research, provided that the treatment principles can be consistently learned and implemented. Such treatment models (principles), appropriately validated, would be added to the growing list of ESTs.

WHY THE TREATMENT METHOD?

In sum, we believe that treatment principles, treatment techniques, and therapist behaviors designed to increase the alliance with the patient are all part of treatment methods. It may be of interest to know, if it were true, that a particular kind of client will benefit from therapy no matter what the method or that a psychotherapist of a particular personality will have positive outcomes no matter what method he or she uses. Nonetheless, unless we are prepared to only offer psychotherapy to those select patients or to only allow those fortunate psychotherapists to practice, these facts would be of little import to the actual practice of psychotherapy.

What are we left with that does matter if we are to improve patient care? The treatment method. Why is this so? Of all the aspects of psychotherapy that influence outcomes, the treatment method is the only aspect in which psychotherapists can be trained, it is the only aspect that can be

WHAT SHOULD BE VALIDATED?   199

manipulated in a clinical experiment to test its worth, and, if proven valuable, it is the only aspect that can be disseminated to other psychotherapists. As clinical psychologists and psychotherapy researchers, the process of psychotherapy itself fascinates us. However, our primary concern is that psychotherapy be used to improve patients' lives. If psychotherapists are to help patients decrease their suffering and increase their functioning, they must be informed about and trained in effective treatment methods. This is what drives our work on empirically supported therapies.

SUMMARY

Our view is that patient, therapist, relationship, and technique variables all contribute to treatment outcome. Validating treatments is simply an effort to improve the care of patients in ways that can be modified. Knowledge about treatments is in a constant state of flux, with new information about modifiers of existing ESTs and new treatment methods accumulating over time. Other ways of improving the care of patients (e.g., the most clinically relevant ways of selecting people to become therapists) should also be pursued. But any approach to psychotherapy research that does not focus on what we can reliably teach therapists to improve their outcomes runs the risk of ignoring avenues to reduce patient suffering and disability. Treatment methods are not where all the action is in relation to outcome, but they are the logical place to intervene to improve care.

The Psychotherapist

Bruce E. Wampold

The fundamental question is, what is the purpose of validating any aspect of psychotherapy? The answer, from my perspective, is that ultimately the validation process will benefit patients. Nevertheless, the validation process exists in a context that involves other factors, such as professional and personal considerations (Wampold & Bhati, 2004). For example, the EST movement explicitly stated that one of the goals was to promote clinical psychology: "if clinical psychology is to survive in this heyday of biological psychiatry, APA must act to emphasize the strength of what we have to offer—a variety of psychotherapies of proven efficacy" (Task Force, 1995, p. 3). Moreover, the EST movement privileges some treatments (i.e., those that are designed as an EST) and disadvantages others.

Independent of the motivations behind ESTs and evidence-based practices (EBPs), the question about the benefits to patients must be answered: Does the validation of a certain aspect of psychotherapy demonstrably benefit patients? This position paper will focus most directly on this question, although the implications of answering the question will be addressed later.

SOURCES OF VARIABILITY IN OUTCOMES

The validation of a certain aspect of psychotherapy involves establishing that the aspect is related to the outcome. Some aspects of therapy are by necessity present (viz., the common factors); validation in this instance would involve associating benefits (i.e., outcomes) with the degree to which a common factor is present (e.g., the frequency of empathic responses) or the quality of the factor (e.g., client-rated alliance; Horvath & Bedi, 2002). In other instances, validation involves comparing the presence to the absence of some aspect of therapy, as is the case when a treatment is compared to no treatment or to another treatment. In either case, the critical determination of the choice of an aspect of therapy to be validated is that it must be shown to be reliably related to outcomes.

A source of variability in outcomes that has not been prominently considered as an object of validation is the psychotherapist (Wampold, 2001a; Wampold & Bhati, 2004), despite evidence that suggests it is an important, if not the most important, source of variability in outcomes. In this position paper, the research that has examined psychotherapist effects will be summarized and compared to other sources. However, before summarizing the literature, some critical methodological considerations relating to the treatment of psychotherapists in research needs to be discussed.

Methodological Considerations

Typically, in the primary analysis of clinical trials psychotherapists are ignored as a factor, which raises two important issues (Crits-Christoph & Mintz, 1991; Crits-Christoph et al., 1991; Kim, Wampold, & Bolt, in press; Wampold & Bhati, 2004). First, if psychotherapists are not considered in the design and analysis, it is impossible to determine how much of the variability in outcomes is because of the psychotherapist. Second, ignoring psychotherapist effects results in an overestimation of treatment effects (Wampold & Serlin, 2000).

When determining psychotherapist effects, it is necessary to treat the psychotherapists as a random factor or as a fixed factor (Crits-Christoph & Mintz, 1991; Serlin, Wampold, & Levin, 2003; Siemer & Joormann, 2003; Wampold & Serlin, 2000). If psychotherapists are treated as fixed, the results are conditioned on the particular psychotherapists included in the clinical trial. Although restricting the generality of the results yields an increase in power to test the main effects, conclusions about a particular small set of psychotherapists would appear to be an unreasonable restriction (see Serlin, Wampold, & Levin, 2003; Siemer & Joormann, 2003). More informative results are obtained when psychotherapists are considered as being randomly selected from a population of psychotherapists so that conclusions can be made about psychotherapists in general (or at least to psychotherapists similar to the ones used in the trial).

Having decided to treat psychotherapists as a random factor necessitates that the appropriate statistical model be used. Variations among psychotherapists creates observed variations among treatments that are not because of true treatment differences. Thus, in clinical trials, a mixed model (treatments fixed, psychotherapists random) must be used in either an analysis of a variance model (Wampold & Serlin, 2000) or in a multilevel model (Moerbeek, 2004).

Variability in Outcomes Due to Psychotherapists

Here I review the literature to estimate the proportion of variability in outcomes that are due to psychotherapists. One must consider several points as the studies are reviewed. First, psychotherapist effects are estimated by examining the ratio of the variability among psychotherapists to the total variation in outcomes; the resulting intraclass correlation coefficient is an estimate of the proportion of variability due to psychotherapists (see Wampold & Serlin, 2000). According to this conception, it is not necessary, nor is it desirable, to designate some psychotherapists as competent either through expert ratings or from various categorizations of outcomes (e.g., using median splits). The estimates to be cited rely solely on the outcomes produced by the psychotherapists; in this sense, competence is defined empirically.

A second point is that the studies to be cited involve, for the most part, reanalyses of data obtained from clinical trials using a variety of methods. Nevertheless, the studies seem to be sufficient to determine a robust estimate of psychotherapist effects (Kim, Wampold, & Bolt, in press).

A third point is that the estimates obtained for psychotherapist effects will need to be compared to the effects for other psychotherapy factors. Expressed as a percentage of variability in outcomes accounted for by the factor, we have summarized or obtained the following estimates (Baskin, Tierney, Minami, & Wampold, 2003; Wampold, 2001b): treatment versus no treatment, 13%; differences among treatments, 0% to 1%; EST versus the psychotherapy placebo, 0% to 4%; working alliance, 5%. The evaluation of the importance of psychotherapist effects will be judged by placing the estimate within the range of 0% (difference among treatments) to 13%, which serves as an upper limit of the percentage of variability due to psychotherapy itself (Wampold, 2001b).

In the early 1990s, researchers began to analyze data from clinical trials to estimate psychotherapist effects. Crits-Christoph and Mintz (1991) reanalyzed data from 10 clinical trials and found that the proportion of variance due to psychotherapists ranged from 0% to 13.5% on the basis of the mean of variables within studies. On the basis of 27 treatment groups, Crits-Christoph et al. (1991) found overall that 8.6% of the variance in outcomes was attributable to psychotherapists.

Kim and colleagues (in press), in a reanalysis of the National Institute of Mental Health (NIMH) Treatment of Depression Collaborative Research Program (TDCRP) data, used various multilevel modeling methods and found that about 8% of the variance in the outcomes of psychotherapy within each treatment was due to psychotherapists. This percentage varied by the outcome measure analyzed and the manner in which the psychotherapist variance was modeled. The proportion of variance due to psychotherapists, within CBT and interpersonal therapy (IPT), was compared to the proportion of variance due to differences between the two treatments, as shown in Table 5.1 for the patients who completed the treatments. For this sample, the estimated percentage of variance accounted for by the differences among psychotherapists within treatments ranged from 5% to 10% for the four outcome measures. For all four outcome measures, the estimated proportion of variance due to differences between the treatments was zero.

Recently, Huppert and colleagues (2001), in a reanalysis of cognitive–behavioral treatments in a multicenter trial for panic disorder, reported psychotherapist effect sizes for the various measures used in the study as ranging

TABLE 5.1
Multilevel Analysis of Treatment (Fixed) and Therapists'
(Random Intercept, Fixed Slopes) Effects for Completers

	Treatment (fixed)					Therapists (random effect)			Error variance σ^2
Variable	coefficient $\hat{\gamma}_{01}$	SE	t	p	$\hat{\omega}^2$	Variance component τ_o^2	p	$\hat{\rho}_I$	
HRSD	−.903	1.432	−.631	.537	.000	2.44	.211	.069	33.03
GAS	1.50	2.93	.513	.615	.000	16.67	.062	.097	114.01
BDI	−3.197	1.99	−1.606	.129	.000	4.10	.293	.050	78.56
HSCL	−.048	.107	−.449	.659	.000	.018	.143	.090	.181

Note. $\hat{\omega}^2$ is the estimator of the population proportion of variance because of differences between CBT and IPT; $\hat{\rho}_I$ is the estimator of the population proportion of variance because of therapists; HRSD is the Hamilton Rating Scale for Depression; GAS is the Global Assessment Scale; BDI is the Beck Depression Inventory; HSCL is the Hopkins Symptom Checklist. From "Therapist Effects in Psychotherapy: A Random Effects Modeling of the NIMH TDCRP Data," by D. M. Kim, B. E. Wampold, and D. M. Bolt, in press, *Psycotherapy Research.* Copyright by Taylor and Francis, www.tandf.co.uk. Adapted by permission.

from 1% to 18%. Accounting for assignments to the different cognitive–behavioral treatments did not alter materially the psychotherapist effects.

Taking all the reanalyses of clinical trials into account, it appears that about 8% of the variability in outcomes is because of differences among psychotherapists (Wampold & Brown, in press). This estimate is generalizable to psychotherapists similar to those used in clinical trials, a context in which psychotherapists typically are selected for their skill, are specially trained, receive supervision, and are guided by a manual (Elkin, 1999; Wampold & Serlin, 2000; Westen, Novotny, & Thompson-Brenner, 2004). Additionally, psychotherapist effects determined in clinical trials are restricted by other contextual variables, such as the homogeneity of the patients enrolled in clinical trials (Westen et al., 2004). Nevertheless, in clinical trials, the variability of outcomes due to therapists (8%–9%) is larger than the variability among treatments (0%–1%), the alliance (5%), and the superiority of an EST to a placebo treatment (0%–4%), making it the most robust predictor of outcomes of any factor studied, with the exception of the initial level of severity.

Somewhat surprisingly, the variability in outcomes among psychotherapists in practice is somewhat smaller than the 8% found in clinical trials. Wampold and Brown (in press), in a study of 6,146 patients seen by 581 psychotherapists in private practices, found that about 5% of the variability in outcomes (taking into account the initial severity) was attributable to psychotherapists. Initially, this appears confusing, as one would expect psychotherapists in private practices to be less homogenous than psychotherapists in clinical trials; however, the patients in private practices are similarly less homogenous, increasing the error variance (Wampold & Brown). Although 5% seems modest, Wampold and Brown illustrated the size of these effects by identifying the best (top quartile) and worst (bottom quartile) psychotherapists in one time period, on the basis of residualized gain scores, and then examined their outcomes in a second time period.

Table 5.2 presents the results of this analysis for psychotherapists who saw at least 6 patients (3 in the predictor and 3 in the criterion subsamples) and 18 patients (9 in the predictor and 9 in the criterion subsamples) in terms of residual gain scores, the proportion of patients who reliably changed (i.e., improved more than two standard errors of the differences from the initial outcome measure to the final outcome measure; Jacobson & Truax, 1991), and the effect size for the patients (pretest minus posttest, divided by the standard deviation of the outcome measure in the norming sample). Clearly, those identified as effective psychotherapists (the top quartile in the predictor sample) had better outcomes with their successive patients. The patients of the "best" psychotherapists, in this cross-validated sample, had negative residualized gain scores (patients did better than expected), had a higher probability of displaying a reliable change than did the "worst" psychotherapists (7%–13% greater, depending on the sample used), and produced pre-post

Variable	Quartile 1 (best)	Quartile 4 (worst)
3 cases (k = 483 therapists)		
Residualized change	−1.30	1.90
Proportion reliably changed	.32	.25
Effect size	.43	.23
9 Cases (k = 73 therapists)		
Residualized change	−1.81	2.30
Proportion reliably changed	.35	.22
Effect size	.47	.20

Note. Therapists were placed in quartiles on the basis of the residualized gain scores of the predictor sample. The results in this table are the means derived from the criterion sample.

effect sizes approximately twice as large as the "worst" psychotherapists. In other words, the 5% of variability in the treatment outcome attributable to psychotherapists in private practices makes significant differences, statistically and clinically, to patient benefits.

The relatively large proportion of variability in outcomes due to psychotherapists infers that some psychotherapists consistently produce better outcomes than others; consequently, psychotherapists are a worthy locus of validation.

VALIDATING PSYCHOTHERAPISTS

In this section, I discuss several issues in validating psychotherapists. First, it is important to understand that many variables may be confounded with therapists, creating some difficulty in making statements about whether the therapist, rather than some other variable associated with the therapist, is the cause of the observed variability. Second, it also important to identify the characteristics and actions of the therapists who consistently produce superior outcomes. Finally, using outcomes in practice raises issues that must be resolved.

Confounding Variables

One threat to validating psychotherapists is the potential variables that are confounded with the psychotherapists. If patients are not randomly assigned to therapists, then there exist the possibility that some therapists produce better outcomes not because of any variable related to the therapists but because of differences between the patients they treat and the patients other therapists treat. For example, patients of psychotherapists producing "poorer" outcomes may be more resistant, have more intractable diagnoses (e.g., Axis II diagnoses), and may be more severely disordered. However, this does not appear to be the case. In the reanalyzed clinical-trials data, patients were typically randomly assigned to psychotherapists; even when they were not randomly assigned, they were homogeneous in terms of diagnosis and in the absence of comorbidity, concurrent medication, and suicidality (see Westen et al., 2004). In the Wampold and Brown (in press) study of psychotherapists in private practice, variables such as psychotherapist degree, psychotherapist experience, psychotherapist and patient sex and age, patient medication status, and patient diagnosis accounted for none or very little of the psychotherapist variability.

Psychotherapists Versus Psychotherapist Characteristics and Actions

Validating particular therapists also raises questions of whether therapist characteristics are common to those who produce better outcomes or whether psychotherapist actions are common to psychotherapists who produce better outcomes. If either case, it would be the psychotherapist characteristics or the psychotherapeutic actions that should be validated, rather than the particular psychotherapists.

Although psychotherapist variables have been studied for decades, few variables have been reliably shown to be related to treatment outcomes (Beutler et al., 2004). Perhaps of greater interest are the psychotherapist variables that have not been associated with outcomes. Blatt, Sanislow, Zuroff, and Pilkonis (1996), in the reanalysis of the three active treatments (viz., imipramine plus clinical management, CBT, and IPT) of the NIMH TDCRP, found that psychotherapist age, sex, race, religion, marital status, general clinical experience, and clinical experience with specific therapies were not related to psychotherapist effectiveness. However, psychotherapist effectiveness was positively related to the use of psychological interventions (as opposed to biological interventions), psychological mindedness, and the expected length of treatment. Huppert and colleagues (2001), in the analysis of CBT psychotherapists treating panic disorders, found that psychotherapist effectiveness was not related to the psychotherapist's age, gender, gender match, and experience with CBT, although on some variables psychotherapist effectiveness was related to overall experience in conducting psychotherapy. It also appears that adherence to and expert-rated competence in the EST protocols are not related to psychotherapist variability (Huppert et al., 2001; Shaw et al., 1999).

Of course, certain aspects of psychotherapy have consistently been shown to be related to outcomes, such as the therapeutic alliance, empathy, goal consensus, and customizing therapy to the patient (Norcross, 2002). However, it has not been shown that such variables can account for the psychotherapist variability that has been consistently detected in clinical trials and private practice, although Vocisano and colleagues (2004) recently found that more effective therapists emphasized the relationship more than less effective therapists. Disentangling therapists from therapist characteristics or actions is complicated by the data structures because therapist characteristics and actions cannot be randomly assigned. Attempts to partition therapist variability to other variables involves complicated statistical methods, and future research needs to address this important question. Moreover, with the exception of a few naturalistic studies (e.g., Wampold & Brown, in press), therapist variability has been estimated using data from clinical trials using homogeneous samples of patients, particularly with regard to diagnosis, as well as with similar treatments. It may well be that much of the variability in outcomes in naturalistic settings involves other considerations, such as greater heterogeneity of treatments administered and treatment–patient matching (e.g., Beutler, Moleiro, & Talebi, 2002a, 2002b). Therapist flexibility to match treatment to patients is something that is precluded in clinical trials but likely occurs frequently in practice. Nevertheless, until such time as therapist and therapist–patient matching variables can be shown to account for the variability due to psychotherapists, it is the psychotherapist per se that should be validated.

Use of Outcome Data

Validating psychotherapists raises issues related to the management of psychotherapeutic services. The astute observer will notice the parallels with high-stakes testing in education and the No Child Left Behind legislation. In the education context, low-performing schools are first given the opportunity to improve (with some but very limited additional resources); if they do not, they are penalized (e.g., students may transfer to another school; administrative duties might be assumed by the state). Identifying and validating psychotherapists may lead to actions by managers of care such as behavioral health-managed care organizations and clinic directors.

It is beyond the scope of this paper to provide a comprehensive discussion of this complicated issue (Miller, Duncan, & Hubble, in press), but several points need to be made. First, knowledge of psychotherapist effectiveness is important in making informed decisions. Although care must taken in the use of such data, it should be uncontroversial that it can be useful. On what basis could it be argued that information about psychotherapist effectiveness should be suppressed? Second, psychotherapist effectiveness data can be used to improve systems of care (Miller et al., in press). Indeed, Lambert and his colleagues (e.g., Lambert, Hansen, & Finch, 2001) have shown that simple feedback to psychotherapists with regard to how their patients are progressing results in more effective and efficient service provision.

CONCLUSIONS

The argument presented here that psychotherapists should be validated should not be construed to indicate that some psychotherapists should be punished because they are "invalidated" (and shame on anyone who cites this article to make that case). Rather, we need, as Lambert and colleagues have done, to research ways in which data about psychotherapist effectiveness can be used to increase the benefits to patients. Of course, certain psychotherapists may be impaired or, even with intervention, may consistently fail to provide benefits to patients, and it may be that these psychotherapists should be enjoined from providing services. Using outcomes to make that determination is superior to reprimanding psychotherapists for actions unrelated to outcomes, such as failing to acquire the necessary continuing education credits.

We are at the origin of a revolution for using outcomes to inform practice and guide management of services. Care must be taken to use this precious data to benefit patients rather than curtail costs. In the end, we (practitioners, researchers, and third parties) should be united in our desire to optimize the benefits that psychotherapy can provide to patients. To do so, we must emphasize those aspects of psychotherapy that account for the variability in outcomes. At this point, the evidence indicates that the psychotherapist is critical.

The Therapy Relationship

John C. Norcross and Michael J. Lambert

Health care policy makers around the globe are promulgating practice guidelines and privileging evidence-based treatments in mental health. These are noble efforts to distill scientific research into clinical applications and to direct graduate training. Such efforts wisely demonstrate that, in a climate of accountability, psychotherapy stands up to empirical scrutiny with the best of health care interventions. The substantial body of empirical research on the effects of psychotherapy provides an impressive base by which to guide psychotherapy practice.

At the same time, as with any initial effort, the evidence-based movement is incomplete and potentially misleading, on at least three counts. First, the evidence favoring specific treatments for specific disorders has been overstated (Wampold et al., 1997). Those who advocate specific interventions for specific disorders do so without acknowledging the complexity of psychotherapy, patients, therapists, and the human side of research (Lambert &

Ogles, 2004; Wampold, 2001b). Psychotherapy is far more than delivering manualized techniques to patients with Axis I disorders. Second, the emphasis on evidence-based treatment largely neglects the evidence for the importance of the therapy relationship, an interpersonal quality that makes substantial and consistent contributions to the psychotherapy outcome (Norcross, 2002). Third, the initial efforts at distilling empirically supported treatments (ESTs) typically ignore the complexity of patients and their individual circumstances. Therapists treat patients in all their complexity, matching therapeutic activities and relational stances to the individual patient beyond his or her diagnosis.

In this position paper, we review the robust research and clinical evidence for the curative power of the therapy relationship and argue that it, in addition to the treatment method, the therapist, and the patient, should routinely be emphasized in EBPs in psychotherapy. Much of the research reviewed here was compiled by an APA Division of Psychotherapy Task Force (Norcross, 2001, 2002), which identified, operationalized, and disseminated information on empirically supported (therapy) relationships or ESRs.

SOURCES OF PSYCHOTHERAPY OUTCOME

Psychotherapy outcome studies generally account for or explain only 40% to 50% of the total outcome variance. This fact reminds us of how much we still need to learn about conceptualizing and measuring the complex sources of treatment success (Roberts, Kewman, Mercier, & Hovell, 1993).

Averaging across hundreds of psychotherapy outcome studies and many meta-analyses, we estimate that the patient (including the severity of his or her distress) accounts for approximately 25% to 30% of the total variance, the therapy relationship for 10%, the therapist for 8% (when not confounded with treatment effects), and the specific treatment method for 5% to 8%. The interactions among patient, treatment, and relationship may or may not account for an additional 5%. These are, of course, crude attempts to divide the indivisible clinical reality. Of the dozens of variables that contribute to patient outcome, only a few can be included in any given study. This complexity limits the degree to which we can accurately estimate the relative importance of all the variables that influence successful treatment.

Still, without question, the largest determinant of psychotherapy outcome is the patient. Research makes clear that the degree of patient disturbance, however measured (Garfield, 1994), is the most important patient variable affecting treatment outcome. Those who begin treatment near the normal range of functioning show only small gains, whereas those who are most disturbed show large gains during treatment but often fail to return to normal functioning (particularly if they suffer from comorbid disorders or incapacitating chronic disorders, such as schizophrenia). The most promising patients are neither too healthy nor too disturbed. They show large treatment gains and are likely to terminate therapy in the normal range of functioning. In addition to severity, the client brings a variety of other characteristics to treatment. These include positive expectations, a readiness for change, and the like. We estimate that the patient, including the severity of his or her distress, accounts for approximately 25% to 30% of the total variance.

Beyond the patient, the therapeutic relationship and the therapist contribute most to patient change, but the individual therapist's contribution has been rarely studied. Although both client and therapist determine the quality of the therapy relationship, clients attribute the success of treatment directly to therapists and the degree to which they provide an empathic, supportive, and respectful encounter. The importance of the relationship is also supported by the fact that paraprofessionals and trainees are often found to be as effective as fully trained professionals, by the limited evidence for the differential value of specific school-based treatments, and by improvements in therapy that occur well before the methods of school-based treatments have been used (Haas, Hill, Lambert, & Morrell, 2002). The quality of the relationship accounts for approximately 10% of the total outcome variance, with therapist effects adding another 8%. By contrast, the specific treatment method accounts for only 5% to 8% of the total outcome variance.

The magnitude of these percentages differs depending on the design, measures, and context of each study. Estimates of outcome variance are quite different when comparing, for example, psychotherapy to no treatment, treatment A to treatment B, or any treatment to a placebo. In the latter case, placebos are quite powerful, typically demonstrating one half or more of the success of formal treatment (Baskin, Tierney, Minami, & Wampold, 2003; Fisher & Greenberg, 1997; Kirsch, 2002). We interpret the ambiguous "placebo effect" as a combination of several factors but primarily the active efforts, positive expectancies, and therapeutic contributions of the patient (see Bohart, this volume).

THE EVIDENCE FOR THE POWER OF THE RELATIONSHIP

Here we canvass the large base of evidence on the therapeutic relationship by reviewing, in turn, meta-analyses, individual outcome studies, and client self-reports.

Meta-Analyses

The therapeutic alliance refers to the quality and strength of the collaborative relationship between client and therapist, typically measured as agreement on therapeutic goals, consensus on treatment tasks, and a relationship bond. Across 89 studies, the mean correlation between the therapeutic alliance and therapy outcome among adults was .21, a modest but very robust association (Horvath & Bedi, 2002). An independent meta-analysis of 23 studies of child and adolescent therapy found similar results. The weighted mean correlation between alliance and outcome was .20 (Shirk & Karver, 2003). These correlations correspond to a d of .45, a medium-size effect.

Cohesion in group therapy, a parallel of the therapeutic alliance in individual therapy, also demonstrates consistent relations to patient benefit. Approximately 80% of the studies support positive relationships between cohesion (mostly member to member) and therapy outcome (Burlingame, Fuhriman, & Johnson, 2002).

Quantitative reviews and meta-analyses of specific relational behaviors on the part of the psychotherapist also predict salutatory client outcomes. Empathy, to take one prominent example, refers to the therapist's sensitive ability and willingness to understand clients' thoughts, feelings, and struggles from their point of view (Rogers, 1957). A meta-analysis of 47 studies (encompassing 190 tests of the empathy–outcome association) revealed a median r of .20 for effect-level analyses and .26 for study-level analyses (Bohart, Elliott, Greenberg, & Watson, 2002). Goal consensus and collaboration, to take two additional examples related to the therapeutic alliance, refer to therapist–patient agreement on treatment goals and mutual involvement of the participants in the helping relationship, respectively. Fully 68% of the studies found a positive association between goal consensus and outcome, and 88% of the studies reported the same for collaboration and outcome (Tryon & Winograd, 2002).

The Division of Psychotherapy Task Force reviewed the extensive body of empirical research and generated a list of empirically supported relationship (ESR) elements. For each, we judged whether the element was demonstrably effective, promising and probably effective, or insufficient research to judge. The evidentiary criteria for making these judgments were the number of supportive studies, the consistency of the research results, the magnitude of the positive relationship between the element and outcome, the directness of the link between the element and outcome, the experimental rigor of the studies, and the external validity of the research base. The preceding five elements—alliance, cohesion in group therapy, empathy, goal consensus, and collaboration—were judged to be demonstrably effective elements. We also determined that seven additional therapist relational elements were promising and probably effective: positive regard, congruence, feedback, repairing alliance ruptures, self-disclosure, management of countertransference, and the quality (but not quantity) of relational interpretations (see Norcross, 2002, for details).

Individual Outcome Studies

A brief discussion of a few individual studies will provide examples of the typical connection between the therapeutic relationship (frequently measured as the alliance) and client outcome. Safran and Wallner (1991) studied a sample of 22 outpatients who received time-limited cognitive therapy. The alliance was measured using the Working Alliance Inventory and the California Psychotherapy Alliance Scale. Results indicated that both alliance measures were predictive of outcome when administered after the third session of treatment. These findings underscored the importance of the alliance in cognitive therapy, not only in person-centered and psychodynamic therapy, and were consistent with research indicating that therapy outcome can be predicted by ratings of the relationship in the early stages of treatment (Horvath & Luborsky, 1993).

In a classic study of alcohol abusers, Miller, Taylor, and West (1980) examined the comparative effectiveness of several behavioral approaches in reducing alcohol consumption. The authors also collected data on the contribution of therapist empathy to patient outcome. At the 6- to 8-month follow-up interviews, client ratings of therapist empathy correlated significantly ($r = .82$) with client outcome, thus accounting for 67% of the variance on the criteria. These results argue for the importance of therapist empathy, even within behavioral and other technique-centered treatments.

In another study, Gaston, Marmar, Thompson, and Gallagher (in press) used hierarchical regression analysis to examine the alliance in elderly depressed patients who participated in dynamic, cognitive, or behavioral therapy. Symptomatic improvement up to the time of the alliance measurement and the patient and therapist alliance scores were used to predict symptoms at termination. The alliance assessed near termination accounted for 36% to 57% of the outcome variance in the study.

Castonguay and colleagues (1996) compared the impact of a treatment variable unique to cognitive therapy (the therapist's focus on distorted cognitions) and two variables common to other forms of treatment (the therapeutic alliance and client emotional involvement) on the psychotherapy outcomes of 30 clients experiencing major depression. Results revealed that the two common variables, the therapeutic alliance and the clients' emotional experiencing, were both found to be positively related to client improvement. To the contrary, the variable deemed to be distinctive to cognitive therapy, connecting distorted thoughts to unwanted emotions, was positively correlated to depressive symptoms following therapy.

In the NIMH Collaborative Study, Krupnick and colleagues (1996) examined the impact of the therapeutic alliance on the treatment of depressed individuals. The therapeutic alliance in both psychotherapy and pharmacotherapy emerged as the leading force in reducing a patient's depression. In summarizing the results of this study, the authors stated, "these results are most consistent with the view that the therapeutic alliance is a common factor across modalities of treatment for depression that is distinguishable from specific technical or pharmacological factors within the treatments" (p. 538).

Client Reports of What's Effective

Apart from sophisticated statistical analyses on the reliable association between the therapy relationship and treatment outcomes, a robust body of clinical experience and client reports attests to the palliative, if not curative, nature of the therapy relationship. When clinicians ask patients what was helpful in their psychotherapy, patients routinely identify the therapeutic relationship (Sloane, Staples, Cristol, Yorkston, & Whipple, 1975). At least a hundred such studies have appeared in the literature with similar conclusions. Clients do not emphasize the effectiveness of particular techniques or methods; instead, they primarily attribute the effectiveness of their treatment to the relationship with their therapists (Elliott & James, 1989).

In an illustrative study, Murphy, Cramer, and Lillie (1984) asked outpatients to list the curative factors they believed were associated with their successful CBT. The factors endorsed by a significant portion of patients were advice (79%), talking to someone interested in my problems (75%), encouragement and reassurance (67%), talking to someone who understands (58%), and the instillation of hope (58%). The clients in this study were mainly from the lower socioeconomic class, whom past research has suggested expect more expert advice in therapy (Goin, Yamamoto, & Silverman, 1965).

In an investigation by Najavits and Strupp (1994), 16 therapists were assigned clients with similar difficulty levels. After 25 sessions, therapists were evaluated according to outcome, the client's length of stay, and therapist in-session behavior. Therapists whose clients evidenced better outcomes used more positive behaviors and fewer negative behaviors than the less effective therapists, with the largest differences occurring in relationship behaviors rather than technical skills. Warmth, understanding, and affirmation were considered positive, whereas subtle forms of belittling, blaming, ignoring, neglecting, attacking, and rejecting were considered negative behaviors. From these results, the authors concluded, "Thus, basic capacities of human relating—warmth, affirmation, and a minimum of attack and blame—may be at the center of effective psychotherapeutic intervention. Theoretically based technical interventions were not nearly as often significant in this study" (Najavits & Strupp, 1994, p. 121).

Clients' perspectives on the helpful aspects of their psychotherapy experiences were also examined in the NIMH Collaborative Treatment Study (Elkin et al., 1989). The findings revealed that, even among patients receiving manualized treatments in a large research study, the most common responses fell into the categories of My Therapist Helped (41%) and Learned Something New (36%). At posttreatment, fully 32% of the patients receiving a placebo plus clinical management wrote that the most helpful part of their "treatment" were their therapists (Gershefski, Arnkoff, Glass, & Elkin, 1996).

As a final illustration, we would point to studies on the most informed consumers of psychotherapy: psychotherapists themselves. In two studies, U.S. ($N = 380$) and British ($N = 710$) psychotherapists were asked to reflect on their own psychotherapy experiences and to nominate any lasting lessons they acquired concerning the practice of psychotherapy (Norcross, Dryden, & DeMichele, 1992; Norcross, Strausser-Kirtland, & Missar, 1988). The most frequent responses all concerned the interpersonal relationships and dynamics of psychotherapy: the centrality of warmth, empathy, and the personal relationship; the importance of transference and countertransference; the inevitable humanness of the therapist; and the need for more patience in psychotherapy. Conversely, a review of five published studies that identified covariates of harmful therapies received by mental health professionals concluded that the harm was typically attributed to distant and rigid therapists, emotionally seductive therapists, and poor patient–therapist matches (Orlinsky & Norcross, 2005).

THE EVIDENCE FOR RELATIONAL MATCHMAKING

The first aim of the Division 29 Task Force was to identify those relationship behaviors, primarily provided by the psychotherapist, that are effective. That is, what works in general. The second aim of the Task Force was to identify those patient behaviors or qualities that served as reliable markers for customizing the therapy relationship. That is, what works for particular patients.

Clinicians strive to offer or select a therapy that is responsive to the patient's characteristics, proclivities, and worldviews in addition to diagnosis. In this section we review the research evidence for adapting the therapy relationship to two such patient characteristics that, in the judgment of the Task Force, serve as demonstrably effective (resistance) and probably effective (stages of change) means of customizing the relationship to the individual patient.

Client resistance refers to being easily provoked by external demands. Research confirms that high patient resistance is consistently associated with poorer therapy outcomes (in 82% of studies). But, in 80% of studies, matching therapist directiveness to client level of resistance improves therapy efficiency and outcome (Beutler, Moleiro, & Talebi, 2002b). Specifically, clients presenting with high resistance benefit more from self-control methods, minimal therapist directiveness, and paradoxical interventions. By contrast, clients with low resistance benefit more from therapist directiveness and explicit guidance. The clinical implication is to match the therapist's level of directiveness to the patient's level of resistance.

People progress through a series of stages—precontemplation, contemplation, preparation, action, and maintenance—in both psychotherapy and self-change. A meta-analysis of 47 studies (Rosen, 2000) found effect sizes of .70 and .80 for the use of different change processes in the stages. Specifically, cognitive–affective processes are used most frequently by clients in the precontemplation and contemplation stages, and behavioral processes most frequently by those in the action and maintenance stages. The therapist's optimal stance also varies depending on the patient's stage of change: a nurturing parent with patients in the precontemplation stage, a Socratic teacher with patients in the contemplation stage, an experienced coach in the action stage, and a consultant during the maintenance stage (Prochaska & Norcross, 2002). The clinical implications are to assess the patient's stage of change, match the therapeutic relationship and the treatment method to that stage, and systematically adjust tactics as the patient moves through the stages.

Different folks do indeed need different strokes, and the preceding two client characteristics illustrate the success of relational matchmaking supported by the research. The Task Force determined that, in addition to client resistance, the client's functional impairment was also demonstrably effective as a means of customizing the relationship. And, in addition to stages of change, the client's coping style, anaclitic–sociotropic versus introjective–autonomous styles, expectations, and assimilation of problematic experiences were all promising and probably effective means of customizing therapy. The current research was insufficient for the Task Force to make a clear judgment on whether customizing the therapy relationship to the following patient characteristics improves treatment outcomes: attachment style, gender, ethnicity, religion and spirituality, preferences, and personality disorders.

CHALLENGES IN VALIDATING THE THERAPY RELATIONSHIP

Practitioners and researchers who trumpet the positive association between the therapy relationship and treatment outcome frequently encounter a number of challenges. We will briefly consider three of these here.

The first and immediate concern is typically the correlational, as opposed to the causal, connection between the relationship element and treatment outcome. Causal inferences are always difficult to make concerning process variables such as the therapy relationship (see Feeley, DeRubeis, & Gelfand, 1999). Does the relationship cause improvement or simply reflect it? Is the relationship produced by something the therapist does or is it a quality brought to therapy by patients? However, several unconfounded regression, structural equation, and growth curve studies persuasively demonstrate that the therapy relationship causally contributes to treatment outcome. Barber and colleagues (2000), for example, demonstrated that alliance at all sessions significantly predicted subsequent change in depression when prior change in depression was partialled out. The alliance remained a potent and causal predictor of further improvement. Using growth-curve analyses, Klein and colleagues (2003), for another example, found that the early alliance significantly predicted subsequent treatment improvement in 367 chronically depressed patients after controlling for prior improvement and eight prognostically relevant patient characteristics. Further, experimental designs and aptitude-by-treatment interaction studies have also demonstrating the cause–effect nature of several client dimensions in relational matching (e.g., Beutler et al., 2003). Thus, although we need to continue to parse out the causal linkages, the therapy relationship has already been shown to exercise a causal association to outcome.

A second and prevalent challenge is that the therapy relationship may be powerful for some treatments and disorders but not for others. In other words, perhaps we are not sufficiently attending to the treatment-specific and disorder-specific nature of the therapy relationship. With regard to the former, some have argued that the alliance-outcome and empathy-outcome associations might be larger in those therapies in which empathy is held to be a key change process. However, meta-analyses on the effects of the therapy alliance (Horvath & Bedi, 2002) and empathy (Bohart et al., 2002) turn up little evidence for differential effect sizes as a function of theoretical orientation. On the contrary, "there is a hint that empathy might be more important to outcome in cognitive–behavioral therapies than in others" (Bohart et al., 2002, p. 96).

With regard to the latter, that the therapy relationship might be less powerful in the treatment of some disorders than others, we agree that little systematic evidence exists and thus it is too early to aggregate the research. But we concur that the patient's primary disorder might differentially impact the therapy relationship. It is more likely that the importance of the relationship varies as a function of the degree of patient disturbance rather than the diagnosis per se. The alliance is harder to establish with clients who are more impaired, delinquent, homeless, drug abusing, fearful–anxious, and dismissive (Horvath & Bedi, 2002). In the treatment of severe anxiety disorders, such as panic and OCD, there are early suggestions that specific treatments seem to exhibit a greater effect size than the therapy relationship, but in depression the relationship appears more powerful (Krupnick et al., 1996; Stevens, Hynan, & Allen, 2000). As with research on specific treatments, it may no longer suffice to ask "Does the relationship work?" but "How does the relationship work for this disorder and this patient?"

A third challenge in arguing for the potency of the therapy relationship is the tendency to underestimate the contributions of the client and the treatment method to therapy effectiveness. It is true that, across hundreds of psychotherapy outcome studies, preexisting client characteristics account for the single greatest portion of outcome variance. We should be careful not to be "therapist-centric" in minimizing the client's relational contribution and self-healing processes.

From the other side, we are occasionally criticized for neglecting the material effect of the specific treatment method. Our response is crystal clear: The empirical research shows that both the therapy relationship and the treatment method make contributions to treatment outcome. It remains a matter of judgment and methodology on how much each contributes, but there is virtual unanimity that both the relationship and the method (insofar as we can separate them) "work." Looking at treatment interventions or therapy relationships (or client contributions) alone is incomplete.

CONCLUSIONS AND RECOMMENDATIONS

Two crucial omissions have detracted from the first-generation compilations of evidence-based treatments: the therapy relationship and relational matchmaking. We share the view of many that the advocacy of specific treatments for specific disorders can lead to an overemphasis on the least curative aspects of the therapeutic endeavor. The promotion of evidence-based treatments (as opposed to evidence-based practices) may inadvertently lead to neglecting the human relationship (Bergin, 1997).

The therapy relationship makes substantial and consistent contributions to psychotherapy outcome for all types of treatments, including pharmacotherapy. Efforts to promulgate lists of evidence-based treatments without including the therapy relationship are thus seriously incomplete on both clinical and empirical grounds. Correspondingly, EBPs should explicitly address therapist behaviors and qualities that promote a facilitative therapy relationship.

At the same time, the therapy relationship probably acts in concert with discrete interventions, patient characteristics, and clinician qualities in determining treatment effectiveness. A comprehensive understanding of effective (and ineffective) psychotherapy will consider all of these determinants and their optimal combinations.

Adapting or tailoring the therapy relationship to specific patient characteristics (in addition to diagnosis) enhances the effectiveness of treatment. Although the research indicates that certain psychotherapies make better marriages for certain disorders, psychological therapies will be increasingly matched to people, not only diagnoses.

The Division of Psychotherapy Task Force reports (Norcross, 2001, 2002) close with a series of general, practice, training, research, and policy recommendations. Here we conclude by echoing several of those recommendations for establishing comprehensive and balanced EBPs:

- Practitioners are encouraged to make the creation and cultivation of the therapy relationship, characterized by the elements found to be demonstrably and probably effective, a primary aim of their treatment.
- Practitioners are encouraged to adapt the therapy relationship to patient characteristics in the ways shown to enhance treatment outcome.
- Practitioners are encouraged to routinely monitor patients' responses to the therapy relationship and ongoing treatment. Such monitoring leads to increased opportunities to repair alliance ruptures, improve the relationship, modify technical strategies, and avoid premature termination (see Lambert, 2005, for a review).
- The concurrent use of ESRs and ESTs tailored to the patient's disorder and characteristics is likely to generate the best outcomes.

The Active Client

Arthur C. Bohart

Psychotherapy works primarily as a collaborative dialogue between two (or more) intelligent, thinking beings who bend their common effort to help one of them overcome obstacles to living a more productive life. Through their own efforts to self-right, clients are able to use the learning structures, modalities, and ideas of many different psychotherapy approaches to accomplish this. Their self-healing ability to do this overwhelms outcome differences attributable to techniques and procedures.

In this position paper, I argue that clients' active self-healing abilities are primary determinants of psychotherapy outcome and, further, that the EST approach in advancing the notion that different treatments are needed for different disorders restricts our view of alternative models of effective therapy. It privileges treatment packages over the potential of client resourcefulness, a privilege not supported by my interpretation of the research evidence.

THE CLIENT AS ACTIVE SELF-HEALER

Psychotherapy can be viewed as a process of facilitating or releasing clients' natural self-healing tendencies. Miller and Rollnick (1991, p. 62) observed, "We believe that each person possesses a powerful potential for change. Your task as a therapist is to release that potential, to facilitate the natural change processes already inherent in the individual. In this approach, the client is treated with great respect, and as an ally." Orlinsky, Grawe, and Parks (1994, p. 278) said, "we view psychotherapy as 'the activation through the process of interpersonal communication of a powerful endogenous therapeutic system that is part of the psychophysiology of all individuals and the sociophysiology of relationships'" (Kleinman, 1988, p. 112).

Despite these sentiments, theoretical and research writings on psychotherapy still largely portray it as a process in which therapists' interventions cure clients' pathology. In general, therapists recognize that clients must play an active role in therapy, but typically this role is restricted to their willingness to participate. The idea that clients can be generative forces of their own growth, unless therapists "treat clients" with potent interventions, has been given little recognition. In the medical model, the central power to correct behavior lies in the therapist's hands. Views such as these leave little room for the possibility that clients are capable of their own generative thinking and that therapy works by providing a supportive, dialogical relationship where such thinking and problem-solving can occur. Put another way, although virtually all psychotherapists agree that client activity and resilience play a role in positive outcomes, a careful analysis of their positions reveals a therapist-centric bias. They give passing acknowledgement to the client's contribution but devote far more attention to the power of treatment rendered by an expert.

The client as active self-healer has at least two different meanings. The first, emphasized by most therapists, is that clients must be active in participating in the treatment. Accompanying this is what many therapists mean by collaboration, which is that clients must comply with the treatment. However, another, stronger meaning places the client in a more central and genuinely collaborative role in terms of dialoging with the therapist, having a say in which treatment he or she receives, and cogenerating ideas about what will be helpful. That second meaning is based on the idea that all clients have the capacity to be actively involved in generatively learning about their lives and making changes. They may enter therapy demoralized or discouraged and so not take initiative. However, in their everyday lives they have generally been at least partially successful as active problem solvers (Cantor, 2003). To be an active self-healer in this sense in psychotherapy means to (a) actively involve oneself in the process; (b) actively try on, learn from, or "inhabit" whatever interventions or interactions constitute the therapy process; (c) actively contribute through one's generative capacity to think dialectically, make inferences, and extract meaning; (d) use one's capacities for logical thinking; (e) creatively misinterpret therapists' interventions; (f) use therapists' interventions as tools in one's own way; (g) learn through an iterative process of trying ideas from therapy out and then shaping them on the basis of feedback from life; (h) experience the interventions and draw inferences from that experience; and (i) apply what is being learned in everyday life. In other words, therapists are not the only "local clinical scientists"(Trierweiler & Stricker, 1998) or "reflective practitioners" (Schön, 1983) in therapy. As the personality psychologist Cantor (2003, p. 53) has observed, "One of the signature features of individuals' proclivity for constructive cognition is its creativity . . . . In fact, a great deal of what people think about themselves and others is adaptive precisely to the extent that it plays creatively with 'reality.'"

THE MEDICAL MODEL OF PSYCHOTHERAPY

This view of the client as active self-healer contrasts to the dominant metaphor of psychotherapy as treatment (Orlinsky, 1989) or the medical model. In the medical model, therapy is analogous to a medical operation: Interventions operate on clients to change dysfunctional behaviors, cognitions, affects, and personality structures. This is the metaphor favored by the EST movement. A diagram of the medical model of therapy is as follows:

Therapists' interventions → operate on clients → to produce effects

The client is the "dependent variable" on which the independent variables of the therapist's interventions operate. Research following this paradigm tends to minimize the client's contribution (Angus, 1992; Dreier, 2000).

The medical metaphor has several implications. First, it has led to the belief that the power of psychotherapy rests primarily on techniques, tailored to specific disorders. Second, the therapy relationship is hierarchically structured: The therapist is the expert who determines the problem, sets the agenda, and chooses and applies the healing balms. The client's role is to comply and participate. Third, as in medicine, the relationship is secondary to "real treatment;" a good doctor–patient relationship plays a supportive role, increasing the chances the patient will comply. Fourth, placebo effects are things to be ruled out by appropriate research strategies so that the potency of "real" interventions can be demonstrated, rather than thought of as legitimate components of therapy (Snyder, Michael, & Cheavens, 1999).

On the basis of the medical metaphor we would expect therapists' interventions to be powerful and to account for most of therapeutic outcome, the relationship to be less important than interventions, the therapist's expertise to be a powerful correlate of effectiveness, the therapist's implementation of procedures to be a virtually necessary part of the change process, and clients to see interventions as the primary healing components. However, the evidence does not generally support this view, as is reviewed elsewhere in this volume (see also Bohart & Tallman, 1999).

Instead, the evidence suggests that most therapies work approximately equally well for most disorders, that interventions do not have the specific effects on the outcome postulated by various theories, that change happens in therapy before the supposed effective ingredients have "kicked in," and that self-help procedures produce effects as or almost as strong as those produced by the supposed expert-applied interventions of therapists.

None of this makes sense if psychotherapy is a business of an expert applying specific interventions to specific problems. However, as I have argued (Bohart & Tallman, 1999), it does make sense if one postulates an active client who is able to use useful structures offered by different therapies to create change. I suggest this is the most parsimonious explanation for these findings.

EVIDENCE FOR THE CLIENT AS THE MAJOR HEALING FORCE IN THERAPY

Here I consider evidence supporting the idea that the client is the major healing force in therapy. On the basis of his research on family therapy, Dreier (2000, p. 241) concluded,

> Treatment does not progress as an effect therapists make on their clients. It progresses primarily because of the clients' changing pattern of interrelating different modes of experiencing and dealing with their problems in their diverse social contexts. It is not the therapists but the clients who are the primary agents of therapy . . . . (p. 241)

Lambert (1992) estimated that client factors account for the lion's share of outcome, followed by therapeutic common factors, of which the most significant is the therapeutic relationship. In this paper I argue that this is primarily the client's use of the relationship. Healing due to the placebo effect is client generated, and if clients make a substantial contribution to the usefulness of the relationship, then more outcome variance can be attributed to the client than to the therapist.

Researchers have concluded that the client's active effort and involvement is key to the therapeutic outcome. Orlinsky (2000, p. 4) advised therapists, "To judge your patient's treatment progress, pay attention to the qualities of the patient's on-going interpersonal and emotional–psychological involvement in the process, and if those are positive then your patient is most likely progressing towards a positive outcome."

The alliance between therapist and client is a more important component of outcome than techniques (Bachelor & Horvath, 1999). The alliance provides a platform for client involvement and effort. The client's point of view on the alliance correlates more highly with outcome than do therapists' perceptions (Bachelor & Horvath, 1999; Busseri & Tyler, 2004). That has to do with how much the client agrees with what the therapist is doing (Horvath & Greenberg, 1986). If clients don't agree with the therapist's agenda, they are less likely to actively invest effort in the process and nothing will happen.

Evidence also supports the role of client hope, expectation, and optimism (Snyder et al., 1999). Factors that enhance hope and optimism can be healing only through the mobilization of clients' self-healing capacities.

These streams of evidence are all consistent with the idea that humans in general have a capacity for self-healing and personal growth (Deci & Ryan, 1991; Prochaska, Norcross, & DiClemente, 1994). Evidence supporting this can be found in studies of self-change and human resilience. Masten, Best, and Garmazy (1990, p. 438) have concluded that "studies of psychosocial resilience support the view that human psychological development is highly buffered and self-righting." Other studies have found that between 40% to 60% of individuals who experience major trauma grow from the experience (Tedeschi, Park, & Calhoun, 1998), many alcoholics recover on their own (Miller & Rollnick, 1991), many individuals exhibiting antisocial behavior mature out of it by age 40 (Pulkkinen, 2001), and many schizophrenics achieve at least a reasonable level of adjustment as they grow older without drugs (Harding et al., 1987). A Gallup poll of 1,000 Americans revealed that 90% had successfully overcome a significant health, emotional, addiction, or lifestyle problem in their recent past on their own (Gurin, 1990). Finally, Miller (2004) and colleagues documented the frequent phenomenon of "quantum change," cases where individuals experienced sudden and significant life-altering change without the aid of mental health services.

In my view, clients are primarily responsible for therapy's effectiveness by drawing on the general human capacities for resilience and personal growth. In therapy, it is clients' agreement with what is going on, the investment of effort, and hope and optimism that drive the change process. As we shall see in the next section, clients make further active contributions in the form of their intelligent capacities for drawing inferences, creatively generating ideas, and applying what they learn to their everyday lives.

HOW CLIENTS MAKE THERAPY WORK

Individuals who come to therapy have come because they have been unable to solve their problems with the resources available in their natural life spaces. They need assistance. However, if clients are actively involved in therapy they may, in many cases, make use of a wide variety of different therapies. This is because therapies and their techniques are not really treatments that operate on clients to change them but rather tools used by clients in their self-healing and problem-solving efforts. Techniques do not operate on clients so much as clients operate on techniques, which is one reason clients can use many different techniques to arrive at the same outcome. From the standpoint of the client as active self-healer, therapy looks like the following:

Clients → operate on techniques and therapists' inputs → to produce outcomes

Because of therapist-centrism in clinical research, evidence is limited on how clients contribute to change. The following conclusions are drawn from suggestions in quantitative, qualitative, and case history studies:

- Clients creatively operate on and interpret the input they receive from therapists. They actively work to get what they want (Rennie, 2000); sift through what is useful to them from what is not useful (Elliott, 1984); interpret, fabricate, or misinterpret therapists' inputs to get what they need (Bohart & Boyd, 1997); and work with and around therapists (Rennie, 1994). Talmon's (1990) interview findings with ex-clients are illustrative. Talmon discovered that

  > I had taken my interventions and my words much too seriously. Patients reported following suggestions that I could not remember having made. They created their own interpretations, which were sometimes quite different from what I recollected and sometimes more creative and suitable versions of my suggestions . . . . (p. 60).

  Kühnlein (1999), in another example, found from interviews with 49 inpatients who had CBT that participants did not blindly adopt what was presented in therapy. They took what they found useful and combined it with their own previously existing schemas.
- Clients use the therapeutic environment as a kind of "workspace" in which they can talk out their problems and gain some perspective on them (Phillips, 1984). Clients feel freer to talk out things with their therapists because the therapists are strangers who are not involved in their lives (Dreier, 2000).
- Clients use therapy as an opportunity to reflect on their problems (Rennie, 1992; Watson & Rennie, 1994). Clients may get insights from this self-generated activity and not report them to therapists. Rennie (1990) found that clients are continually thinking during therapy. This is done covertly and much of it is not reported to therapists because of the effort of reifying

thinking into words. Clients also make their own interpretations (Angus, 1992).

- Clients work outside of therapy. Several studies have found that it is common for clients to show improvement even before their first therapy session (McKeel, 1996). Therapy does not take place primarily in the therapist's office. Clients do not merely transfer what they have learned to life situations but rather actively transform and apply it. "Clients configure the meaning of therapy within the structure of their ongoing social practice" (Dreier, 2000, p. 253). Clients may also increase the utilization of resources outside of therapy; for instance, clients increase their use of other people to talk to (Cross, Sheehan, & Kahn, 1980).

- Clients may use the same procedures outside of therapy that therapists use in therapy (Prochaska et al., 1994). For instance, a common procedure used by behavior therapists is exposure, yet the idea of exposure is part of everyday wisdom (Efran & Blumberg, 1994). Silverman and colleagues (1999) found, contrary to their expectations, that education support control groups for parents and children worked as well as exposure-based treatments for childhood phobias. They suspect that the education support conditions might have led to self-initiated exposure by clients.

- At least some clients operate as their own integrative therapists (Gold, 1994). They may purposefully see therapists of different orientations sequentially, or they may use the devices of one type of therapy to get the insights of another type.

In sum, clients are not operated on by treatments but instead are the ones who do the operating. They do not merely make treatments work by complying and investing effort in them; they actively invest thought and intelligence in them also. They listen to the therapist, evaluate what he or she says, and understand it from their own frames of reference. Patients sometimes creatively misinterpret it, derive implications from it (not always the ones we think), and then use what they have learned to solve problems in their life spaces. Because clients are active transformers of what they get, no simple, one-to-one relationship exists between the intervention and outcome.

CONCLUSIONS

Within EBPs in mental health, the client as an active self-healer is presented in either a weak version or a strong version. In the weak version, the idea of the client as active self-healer is not incompatible with ESTs. In fact, many cognitive–behavioral treatment packages encourage clients to be their own therapists in the sense of applying techniques outside of therapy between sessions and after therapy has ended. In this version, the client is primarily active by following the prescriptions of the therapist, not through his or her own generative capacity. In fact, approaches that rely on common factors to promote client self-healing are distrusted by some who write as if they believe that unless clients are taught specific skills by expert therapists that any changes generated by clients in "nonspecific" treatment will be ephemeral (e.g., Karoly & Anderson, 2000). Therefore, in the weak version of the client as active self-healer, the client can and must be an active contributor to therapy in order for it to work, but it is still the expert therapist applying treatment that is primarily responsible for change.

The stronger version suggests an alternative paradigm for psychotherapy. In this view, the client's self-healing capacity is primary and the treatment package is less important. Treatments are helpful primarily in that they provide a useful structure for clients' generative capacities. Psychotherapy is a dialogue between two intelligent beings rather than an application of specific treatments for specific disorders. The optimal role of the therapist is more along the lines of a collaborative problem-solver than an expert who applies specific interventions. The idea of the therapist coming into the session with a preset treatment plan (Suinn, 1999) or choosing a treatment on the basis of manuals is not compatible with this strong version. Therapists and clients may still use ESTs, but decisions would not be based on applying an EST template or formula to the client's problem on the basis of a preset formula. Rather, the client and the therapist would engage in mutual dialogue and the specific techniques, if any, to be used would emerge from that dialogue.

Given this stronger version of the client as active self-healer, the EST paradigm becomes inappropriate for conducting psychotherapy research. As Westen and colleagues (2004) have said, referring to the manualization requirement of ESTs,

> The scientific utility of treatment manuals is maximized in treatments in which the therapist sets the agenda for each session. Where patients have a substantial degree of control over the content or structure of treatment hours, therapists by definition have less control . . . . Modeled after dosing in medication trials . . . manualization commits researchers to an assumption that is only appropriate for a limited range of treatments, namely that therapy is something done to a patient—a process in which the therapist applies interventions—rather than a transactional process in which patient and therapist collaborate. (p. 11)

The EST paradigm therefore should not dominate either how therapy is practiced or how it is researched. Alternate research strategies would place an emphasis on understanding how therapy works in terms of clients' active self-healing efforts, aided and abetted by a collaborative, dialogical relationship. This would include a study of how a facilitative therapy relationship supports clients being productive, reflective practitioners, why clients seem to place so much value on being listened to and understood, and how they productively use that. A greater research focus on clients would also explore individual differences in clients' motivational and information-processing styles. There would also be a focus on how therapy is contextually embedded in clients' lives, as well as an emphasis on how this affects clients' understanding of what happens in therapy and how they use it (Dreier, 2000).

Given an actively involved client who is persistent and invests effort in the process, whatever particular approach the therapist uses has a good chance of being helpful in many cases. In this respect, psychotherapy is akin to other learning environments, such as school, where factors that promote student effort and involvement are more important than different classroom styles and environments (Murphy, 1999; Shaffer, 2000).

Alternatives to ESTs exist as ways of construing EBPs that are more compatible with the stronger version of the client as an active self-healer. These rely more on a convergence of evidence from a variety of sources than on manualized forms of treatments for specific disorders in randomized clinical (or controlled) trials (RCTs; Bohart, 2005; Orlinsky, Rønnestad, & Willutzki, 2004; Rozin, 2001). Evidence for common factors in general, and the client as active self-healer in particular, comes from a variety of converging sources (including RCTs). Considerable converging evidence serves to "validate" the client as an active self-healer and to establish client-centric EBPs in mental health. It is important that we take a broader view of EBPs and embrace alternative paradigms. As Ogles and colleagues (1999, p. 218) observed, "Models are essential to the advancement of psychotherapy research and practice. Importantly, however, these models need not necessarily include techniques . . . . Rather, such a model might emphasize the development of a warm and compassionate client–therapist relationship." I would add "an emphasis on the client as an active self-healer."

Principles of Change

Larry E. Beutler and Brynne E. Johannsen

The field of psychology is currently engrossed in a debate regarding whether treatment procedures or relationship variables and therapist qualities are preeminent in determining positive treatment outcomes. Some scholars (e.g., Lambert, 1992; Wampold, 2001b) cite the importance of relationship and contextual factors where desired change in the patient arises as a function of the therapeutic alliance formed between the patient and the therapist. To these authors, patient and therapist factors, rather than techniques, are the major contributors (see Norcross, 2002). To other scholars (e.g., Chambless & Hollon, 1998; Chambless & Ollendick, 2001; Nathan & Gorman, 1998, 2002), the influence of common factors is incidental and the power of treatments is based on the procedures that underlie and guide what the therapist does. To these authors, effective treatment is realized through the identification of treatments that are most effective with patients that share a common diagnosis, and the treatment itself is described and guided via manuals.

This is a debate in which scientifically both sides are right. Both common variables embodied in the relationship and in the therapists' skill, as well as specific procedures within the theoretical model and treatment manual, can and do elicit changes in patients' feelings and behaviors (Castonguay & Beutler, in press). However, the either-or debate has prevented a rapprochement between both partially correct perspectives. Although select variables representing the patient, therapist, context, relationship, and treatment model are all related to improvement, it has been clearly shown that any one of these variables in isolation does not account for a very large share of the total therapeutic change.

More than 150 different treatment manuals have met research criteria of "efficacy" and have been deemed effective (Chambless & Ollendick, 2001), but negligible differences exist among the actual effects of these ESTs. Most psychotherapies account for less than 10% of the total variance among outcomes (Luborsky et al., 2001). The belief that one must focus on either relationship and context or the treatment model is lacking in efficiency and effectiveness for planning treatments and predicting outcomes on an individual level.

A different perspective is necessary to represent accurately the complexity of psychological treatments and to guide effective practice. This new approach must consider the ways in which all relevant variables work individually and interact with one another to optimally affect a patient's problems. One effective way of integrating participant, context, relationship, and treatment variables is through the establishment of research-informed principles of change. Principles, when established firmly in the cumulative body of psychotherapy research, can serve as effective guidelines for planning and implementing treatment. Such research-based principles describe direct and indirect relationships among variables and different outcomes. Principles of treatment that are empirically derived in this way are not wedded to any particular treatment model; rather, they are extracted from research evidence and are prioritized with respect to variables (patient, therapist, context, relationship, and procedural) that can both alert the clinician to the patient's prognosis and help the clinician adjust the environment and treatment.

DEFINING CURATIVE FACTORS

In this section we briefly review the relationship, participant, and treatment factors identified in the research literature. These factors form the basis of the principles of change summarized in the next section of this position paper.

Relationship Factors

Scholars who view the benefits of psychotherapy as being dependent on the signal importance of a therapeutic relationship place great stock in the empirical demonstrations that (a) head-to-head comparisons of different treatments usually demonstrate their relative equivalence, and (b) patients frequently improve regardless of the particular techniques used. Because the strength of the therapeutic bond is frequently associated with good outcomes (e.g., Martin, Garske & Davis, 2000; Norcross, 2002), it is easy to conclude that change must be causally related to this relationship between therapist and patient. Although this conclusion is persuasive, it is important to observe that the relationship between the therapeutic alliance and outcome only accounts for about 10% of the change variance (Beutler et al., 2003; Horvath & Symonds, 1991). Further, research has not convincingly demonstrated that a causal connection exists between relationship quality and outcome. The correlation between these domains could arise from extraneous factors (e.g., patient or therapist variables, the nature of the treatment) or these variables may interact differentially as a function of the treatment provided.

Participant Factors

Participant factors are enduring and relatively stable traits that are brought into treatment by the patient or therapist involved in the process. Patient factors exert two kinds of effects on treatment outcomes. The first is a general and direct effect on treatment prognosis. Relatively stronger effects than these direct ones are observed, however, when one adds the influence of the treatments being provided. The pattern of findings supports the role of patient factors as mediators of treatment outcome. That is, patient qualities differentially affect how well different treatments will work (Castonguay & Beutler, in press; Norcross, 2002). In many cases, it is only when treatment procedures are considered in conjunction with patient qualities that specific effects of treatment emerge. Different folks need different strokes; that is, certain patient dispositions respond differentially to the application of specific models or procedures of psychotherapy (Barber & Muenz, 1996; Beutler et al., 1991; Calvert, Beutler, & Crago, 1988; Cooney et al., 1991). Conventional models of inspecting either common or specific interventions fail to identify the impact of these patient–treatment interactions. Research-informed principles of change, by contrast, can capture the direct and complex interactive effects of patient, therapist, contextual, relationship, and treatment variables.

Treatment Factors

Most clinical practice relies on treatments whose benefits are assumed by virtue of strong opinion and theory, rather than relying directly on the results of scientific evidence (Beutler, 2000). Yet practitioners who want to use scientific evidence to guide their practices are confronted with several major problems. First, they are confronted with the reality that not many models demonstrate how to apply ESTs in contemporary practice. Second, they are faced with a large number of treatments described in research-based manuals and that require long hours of training. Such a time commitment is often not possible, and even if it is available, it is unclear which specific manuals and how many different treatments one needs to learn to treat patients effectively.

Thus, research-minded practitioners are virtually forced to pick a single model of treatment, in which they seek training, and hope it is flexible enough and broad enough to meet the needs of the particular mix of patients in their own practices. However, selecting a given model of therapy and hoping it fits all problems is a bit more hazardous than one might think. Even manuals of treatment that derive from the same theory are dramatically different in how they are applied and in their profile of interventions (Malik, Beutler, Gallagher-Thompson, Thompson, & Alimohamed, 2003). The lack of successful generalization from one manual to another and from one patient to another provides ample reason to invest efforts in developing a set of research-informed principles of change to guide a practice. Principles, better than techniques, manuals, or models of treatment, can cut across different occasions and conditions to provide a clear and consistent way of keeping one's practice grounded in science.

Integration of Factors

Intuitively, most clinicians know that all patients are unique and that treatments will be more or less effective with any given person, depending on the patient fit with the specific demands of that treatment. Further, we understand that therapists differ in their abilities to deliver various methods and that all therapists work better with some patients than with others. Several studies have found that patient factors, treatment types, the therapeutic relationship, and the fit among patient and treatment variables all contribute uniquely to the prediction of treatment outcome (e.g., Beutler et al., 2003).

Collectively, the prediction of treatment outcome approaches 90% efficiency when all these factors are considered and treatment is planned to optimize the fit of patient and treatment characteristics.

PRINCIPLES OF CHANGE

Research-guided principles of change allow clinicians to select, create, and modify the procedures from which psychotherapy is drawn, on the basis of the unique variation of each patient. This process does not require the clinician to learn new theories and a host of specific techniques to apply to various combinations of diagnostic groups (Beutler, Clarkin, & Bongar, 2000). Two major efforts, and several more limited ones, have been made to develop a reasonably comprehensive list of principles that specify the conditions of therapeutic change and that can be used specifically to guide the development of a treatment plan and the implementation of effective psychotherapy. Beutler, Clarkin, and Bongar developed the first of these under the title of Systematic Treatment Selection (STS). This effort focused largely on the predictors of change in patients whose problems included depression. It led to a second and more comprehensive effort by two professional societies to derive an extensive list of principles that can be applied to a wide range of problems. Here we will provide a brief introduction to the first of these efforts but will focus largely and more specifically on the second effort because of its broad applicability and because it represents the work of a large and representative group of scientists who have devoted effort to defining the generalizable principles of change.

Systematic Treatment Selection (STS)

STS (Beutler, Clarkin, & Bongar, 2000) represents an effort to identify empirically established principles of treatment that cut across models and disciplines. The development of this approach took place in several steps. First, an extensive review of research literature on psychotherapy outcomes resulted in the extraction of six patient characteristics that have been shown to be related either directly to patient prognosis or indirectly to outcome as mediators of treatment effects. These six characteristics were the patient's level of functional impairment, problem complexity or comorbidity, the patient's level of probable resistance, the patient's coping styles, the level of social support, and the patient's level of subjective distress.

Beutler et al. (2000) concluded that each of these six patient dimensions was advantageously matched with one or more patient dimensions in an optimally planned treatment. Thus, the patient's level of impairment served as an apparent indicator for the level of treatment intensity needed to induce an effect—the greater the impairment, the greater the intensity (length, frequency, modality, etc.) of the treatment used.

Likewise, the literature review concluded that patient problem complexity was a likely indicator for the use of treatment combinations, including medication and the intensity of treatment. The level of resistance was an indicator of the level of directiveness to be used, and the coping style, along with problem complexity, served to indicate the probable value of insight or symptom-focused interventions. The available social support indicated the relative need for a multiperson involvement in treatment (e.g., group or family treatment), and the level of subjective distress might serve as an indicator for the use of supportive and confrontive treatments.

Research on this model of treatment planning provided a good deal of support for most of the principles and led to a refinement of the treatment-planning dimensions, reducing them to six basic patient and treatment dimensions (Beutler et al., 2000). It also resulted in the development of a specific manual to guide the application of the principles for the individual treatment of patients with depression and chemical abuse (Beutler & Harwood, 2000). The manual came with a subsequent demonstration showing that the patient–treatment-matching dimensions enhanced the effective treatment of these groups (Beutler et al., 2003; Karno, Beutler, & Harwood, 2002).

Principles of Therapeutic Change

Drawing from the foregoing work to identify the general principles of treatment-induced change, a joint task force of the Society for Clinical Psychology (APA Division 12) and the North American Society for Psychotherapy Research (NASPR; Castonguay & Beutler, in press) was formed with the mission of identifying, clarifying, and extending the list of principles that can be applied to the planning and prediction of treatment responses. This task force specifically selected a large group of investigators to look at a broad range of literature, extending to four problem areas (depression, anxiety, personality disorder, and chemical use disorders) and three variable domains (relationships, participant factors, and treatments), to bring together and integrate the diverse and sometimes disparate recommendations of the previous task forces formed to look, respectively, at "Treatments That Work" (Nathan & Gorman, 1998) and "Therapy Relationships That Work" (Norcross, 2002).

The questions posed by this latter task force included (a) What is known about the nature of participants, relationships, and procedures within treatment that induce positive effects across theoretical models and methods? and (b) How do the factors related to participants, relationships, and treatments work with, against, *and* within one another to enhance change?

The goals of answering these questions were to generate guidelines that would identify how therapists could select efficient and optimal interventions for each patient's presenting problem while still maintaining allegiance to their overriding theoretical orientation.

The task force was comprised of senior investigators representing expertise in different treatment variables and patient populations. They were divided into pairs to ensure that a diversity of perspectives was represented, and subsequently additional authors and task force members were added to expand the generalizability and expertise represented. In total, nearly 50 participants worked together to define what is known and not known about principles that govern therapeutic change within the four problem areas. The task force defined principles of change as

> general statements that identify the conditions, therapist behaviors, and classes of interventions that produce change under identified circumstances and for particular kinds of patients. Principles are more general statements than those constituting mere description of techniques and they are more specific statements than those comprising theoretical formulations. (Castonguay & Beutler, in press)

By leaving the confines of a particular theoretical orientation, practitioners are able to serve a wider range of patients and optimize their effectiveness. Task force members worked in groups to address the roles of relationship factors, participant factors, and treatment factors within the four large problem areas.

Principles of Change Related to Relationships

These principles take into account both patient and therapist factors such that the therapist can tailor his or her treatment decisions based on what will optimize the treatment outcome while still maintaining the favored theoretical orientation. Some principles stress the importance of certain therapist characteristics that will facilitate the development of a therapeutic alliance, such as flexibility and empathy. Other principles highlight the fit between the patient and the therapist on factors relating to background and culture, emphasizing the value of matching within this dimension. Still others emphasize the importance of a good therapeutic alliance to the effective use of different psychotherapy techniques.

Principles of Change Related to Participants

These change principles relate to identifying those patients who have a good and poor prognosis and estimating the likelihood that a patient will benefit from treatment. Other principles identify factors that do not appear to contribute to therapeutic change, even though some theory and logic tend to believe that they do. For example, the beliefs that a clinician must have had an addictive disorder to effectively treat it or that certain problems must be treated in a particular context are not supported in the available research to incorporate into practice. Still other principles identify the types of procedures best suited for certain patient and therapist factors, emphasizing the fit of such things as therapist directives and patient resistance, or between the behavioral or insight focus of treatment and the patient's coping strengths.

Principles of Change Related to Treatment Models

These treatment principles covered a wide range of therapeutic models. We strived specifically to define treatments without reference to their theories of origin. Thus, the principles apply to both the structure of therapy (early versus late sessions, multiperson versus individual format, directive versus nondirective, the use of homework, etc.) and the content (cognitive versus insight and emotional focus, behavior change and skill development versus awareness, etc.) but without reference to conventional brand names. Some principles were found to be specific to certain types of problems, whereas others were found to be quite general across problem areas. Moreover, principles at this level reflected those at other levels. For example, one principle of treatment emphasizes that all treatment procedures should be implemented within the context of a stable and supportive therapeutic alliance. Another emphasized that adding interventions from different models was indicated when problems were quite severe and impairing, and still another emphasized that the relative value of direct symptom change and the facilitation of self-understanding were moderated by the patient's usual method of dealing with change and stress.

CONCLUDING COMMENTS

The research literature is increasingly supporting the integration of treatment methods with aspects of the patient's characteristics and situation beyond diagnosis. We have reviewed two efforts to define the nature of effective principles and their effects on enhancing therapeutic outcomes. The identified principles of change attempt to assimilate and integrate the variety of factors that often compete for attention within different models of psychotherapy. Yet the principles currently identified have not yet reached the status where they can be used as guidelines for which treatment procedures should be implemented per se but rather are research-based suggestions for structuring therapy sessions and intervention as a function of patient presentation, problems, goals, and situations.

When properly applied, principles of change will allow clinicians to operate research-informed practices, enhance their ability to serve a wider range of patients, and use an eclectic array of empirically supported clinical methods. The systematic use of the foregoing principles of change to customize the psychotherapy procedures used to fit the patient's proclivities will also improve the rate and magnitude of outcome. At this point, it is not precisely known to what extent the participant, relationship, and treatment factors will contribute to the therapeutic outcome or which of these should take priority. However, to exclude any one of these factors or to consider them in isolation is to provide incomplete care to the consumers of mental health services. Conducting psychotherapy is a multifaceted practice that requires a systematic incorporation of all the factors contributing to behavior change.

Dialogue: Convergence and Contention

Dianne L. Chambless and Paul Crits-Christoph

We welcome the opportunity to address a number of misconceptions about the importance of identifying ESTs that are apparent in the position papers here as well as in other critiques of ESTs.

MISCONCEPTION 1: EST ADVOCATES IGNORE CONTRIBUTIONS OF THE PSYCHOTHERAPIST

We would hope it is clear from our position paper that we do not and have never suggested that no meaningful differences exist among psychotherapists in their efficacy. Surely, anyone who seeks to make a referral knows that often one is more eager to refer to certain therapists than others. But what are we to do with the findings, such as those discussed by Wampold, showing some therapists are more effective than others? Unless psychology licensing boards are prepared to weed out those therapists who are less effective than others (as opposed to those who are clearly incompetent or unethical), then a demonstration of such effects is interesting but merely a first step in using psychotherapy research to benefit the public.

One thing that can be done is to standardize treatments in such a way as to include the important known components of a treatment approach to raise the poorer therapists' level of performance. Indeed, the degree to which therapists differ in outcome is reduced by the use of treatment manuals (Crits-Christoph et al., 1991). Another step that can be taken is to study the more effective therapists in an attempt to distill what makes them more effective and incorporate these behaviors in the treatment such that other therapists can learn to adopt them too.

As Wampold's review makes clear, we know precious little to date about what makes one therapist better than another. It is premature to dismiss an adherence to treatment techniques and competence as potential factors, as little research has been conducted to test whether these factors account for therapist differences. Wampold cites two studies suggesting these factors are irrelevant, but one of these (Shaw et al., 1999) did not address this question, and the other (Huppert et al., 2001) did find a relationship between competence and therapist outcomes, albeit a curvilinear one. A number of studies have found that adherence to or competence in specific procedures of treatments predicts a better treatment outcome (e.g., Barber, Crits-Christoph, & Luborsky, 1996; DeRubeis & Feeley, 1990; Feeley, DeRubeis, & Gelfand, 1999). Thus, it seems reasonable to hypothesize that such differences would be related to therapist effects. However, clinical trials that attempt to standardize the treatment variable through therapist selection, training, certification, supervision, and adherence–competence monitoring are not well suited to test such questions. We know of no study that adequately addresses this issue by including a large number of therapists and a full range of adherence–competence. Accordingly, these remain obvious possibilities but certainly not the only ones.

MISCONCEPTION 2: EST ADVOCATES HOLD THAT THE THERAPEUTIC RELATIONSHIP IS NOT IMPORTANT

As psychotherapy researchers who have conducted research demonstrating the importance of the treatment alliance in behavioral and psychodynamic therapies, as psychotherapists, and as sometime clients ourselves, we are certainly aware of the importance of the relationship between the therapist and client. We are astonished to learn that anyone would think that our suggesting the importance of disseminating evidence-based treatments means that we think only techniques matter. So let us say it clearly here: The therapeutic relationship is important too! We are not alone among EST researchers. We have never seen a treatment manual for ESTs that suggests that the therapist should be indifferent to the relationship, and many manuals explicitly describe the importance of the relationship and even prescribe its nature (e.g., the collaborative relationship in cognitive therapy). Thus, we would agree with Norcross and Lambert that in all practice guidelines and summaries of the literature on empirically supported psychotherapies, the importance of a positive therapeutic relationship be mentioned as well.

However, the therapy relationship is but a piece of therapy outcome. We seek to identify teachable treatment methods that are also related to better outcome, and we argue that these clearly exist (e.g., Chambless & Ollendick, 2001; Crits-Christoph, 1997). For example, Borkovec and Costello (1993) compared nondirective therapy to CBT in the treatment of generalized anxiety disorder (GAD). The quality of the therapeutic relationship did not differ between treatment conditions, and the same therapists delivered both treatments. Nonetheless, clients who received CBT were significantly more likely to be treatment responders (58%) than were nondirective therapy clients (22%). This and other studies led us to designate CBT for GAD as empirically supported.

Furthermore, we argue that research on the relationship must move beyond correlational research to be useful (no matter how fancy the statistics, correlational research does not establish causality). We need to know what effective therapists do to foster good relationships with their clients, to train other therapists in these behaviors, and to test whether this makes a difference in outcome. Only then will we be able to make use of research on the therapeutic relationship to improve rather than simply describe treatment outcomes and thus benefit the public.

MISCONCEPTION 3: EST ADVOCATES HOLD THAT CLIENTS ARE PASSIVE RECIPIENTS OF TREATMENTS

Bohart offers an important message in saying that clients' contribution to their own healing is of immense importance. This is true not only in psychotherapy but also in medical treatments. However, clients come to us because they expect us to have some expertise, and we should have information to offer them about which treatments are likely to help them achieve the changes they want to make. They, of course, make the final decision about which treatments are acceptable to them. Finally, we propose that part of our job as therapists is to figure out how to help more clients engage fully in treatment and to improve the quality of their lives. That is, the buck stops with us.

Bruce E. Wampold

No one would question that each of the loci of validation discussed in this chapter is important to the process and outcome of psychotherapy. Indeed, a *treatment*, on the basis of *principles of change*, conducted by a *psychotherapist* with a *client* in the context of a *relationship*, constitutes the essential ingredients of what we know as psychotherapy. However, it is the relative emphases placed on these aspects and the inferences drawn from the evidence that are important for the delivery of optimal services to clients.

One reading of the chapter appears to contrast treatment versus the other factors as loci of validation. Chambless and Crits-Christoph make the claim that failure to use a treatment other than an empirically validated treatment is unethical, whereas the other authors address the complex interplay of aspects involved in the process of psychotherapy. Underlying the Chambless and Crits-Christoph claim is an implicit adoption of a medical model, in which treatment is royal and other aspects of the endeavor are subservient. The history of modern medicine is a story of establishing the specificity of the chemical ingredients of the treatment so that the medical profession could escape the shadows of pharmacopoeias containing myriad substances and practitioners administering legions of procedures. The emphasis on treatment ingredients, however, ignores all other aspects that might be important to producing benefits (Wampold & Bhati, 2004). Although the emphasis on the specificity of treatments might be appropriate in medicine, it contradicts the evidence in psychotherapy, in which the variability in outcomes because of therapists, relationships, clients, and strategies of change is significant and, indeed, is much greater than the variability due to treatments, as discussed in this chapter.

Research demonstrating that treatment A produces better outcomes than no treatment or placebo-type treatment (e.g., supportive counseling) does not logically establish that the specific ingredients of treatment A are responsible for the change, nor does it indicate that treatment A is superior to another treatment. Privileging treatment A elevates that status of treatment over all other factors and ignores the evidence supporting the other aspects of treatment. It is a false dichotomy to suggest that the alternative to providing treatment A is to base the delivery of services on clinical lore. This chapter contains a great deal of research cited on nontreatment aspects of psychotherapy that a clinician could and should use to ensure that beneficial services are being delivered.

A useful way to view validation is from the three perspectives of the client, the therapist, and the payer or manager of services. What decisions will maximize the benefits for the client from these perspectives? The client must select a therapist and a treatment, two aspects that, for practical purposes, are confounded in that the therapist selected typically will deliver a particular treatment. The research indicates that the variability due to therapists is at least an order of magnitude greater than the variability due to the particular treatment, and thus the client should choose the most effective therapist above all else. Researchers who design clinical trials know as well as anyone that the choice of therapist is vital; they will attempt to use the most effective therapists available to increase the effect of the treatment. Furthermore, because research indicates that the relationship (Horvath & Bedi, 2002) and expectations (Arnkoff, Glass, & Shapiro, 2002) are related to the outcome, the client would be well served to ensure that he or she has formed a good relationship with the therapist and that he or she believes the treatment will be effective. Bohart would suggest to the client that he or she actively make use of the therapist and the therapy, regardless of the particular treatment delivered. With regard to the therapist, it would be prudent for each therapist to ensure that he or she is obtaining appropriate outcomes. Adopting a particular treatment, whether designated empirically validated or not, does not guarantee that the client will benefit, and it is important that each therapist have some evidence that his or her services are effective (Miller et al., in press). Furthermore, research that indicates that customizing the treatment and relationship to the individual patient (e.g., Beutler, Harwood, Alimohamed, & Malik, 2002; Beutler, Moleiro, & Talebi, 2002a, 2002b) would suggest that therapist flexibility is more important than the adoption of a particular treatment.

Finally, payers and managers of care who wish to efficiently spend limited resources should act to attain maximum benefits to their covered lives. In the managed care environment, little evidence shows that the resources spent mandating and monitoring treatments, requiring treatment plans, and otherwise managing the nature of the treatments delivered result in better outcomes. Because the provider explains most of the variability in treatment outcomes in managed care (Wampold & Brown, in press), managers of care should spend resources to assist poorer-performing therapists (Miller et al., in press). A promising way to assist therapists is to provide them with feedback (e.g., Lambert, Hansen, & Finch, 2001), a strategy successfully used by Pacificare Behavioral Health (Matumoto, Jones, & Brown, 2003).

The various aspects of psychotherapy that have been claimed to be validated in this chapter are indispensable to the psychotherapy endeavor. An adoption of a medical model would place the emphasis, above all else, on the choice of treatment. However, the evidence does not support such a position. A more appropriate approach would be to consider psychotherapy as a complex endeavor in which the various aspects interact to produce benefits.

John C. Norcross and Michael J. Lambert

We find ourselves in fundamental agreement with most of the positions taken by the authors contributing to this chapter. We agree that the treatment method, the individual therapist, the therapy relationship, and the patient are vital contributors to the success of psychotherapy, and all must be studied. Comprehensive EBPs will consider all these determinants and their optimal combinations. We, like the other authors, are firmly committed to using research to enhance patient outcomes, believing that patients are best served when empirical methods are combined with clinical wisdom.

Each author approaches the proverbial elephant of effective psychological practice from a different angle. One finds the elephant's trunk, another the elephant's leg, and so on. What we find and prize, however, is not due to mere caprice and perceptual handicap. Rather, our interpretation of the evidence is deeply anchored in our philosophical worldviews and probably our personality dispositions.

Our strongest disagreement is the degree to which school-based therapies should be regarded as the essential aspect of clinical training and service delivery. Chambless and Crits-Christoph properly note the importance of variables other than the treatment method; nonetheless, in our view, they continue to minimize the salience of relationship variables and undermine the strength of evidence indicating a causal link between treatment outcome and the therapeutic relationship. We also believe they overstate the evidentiary value favoring specific techniques for specific problems. They take this to an extreme when they assert an ethical responsibility of providing services based largely on the results of RCTs.

Our position is not that "any effort to focus attention on treatment method is misguided." To the contrary, we explicitly argue in our position paper that

> The empirical research shows that *both* the therapy relationship and the treatment method make contributions to treatment outcome. It remains a matter of judgment and methodology on how much each contributes, but there is virtual unanimity that both the relationship and the method (insofar as we can separate them) "work."

The tendency to perceive the world in a dichotomous, black and white manner is a central barrier to reaching a consensus on EBPs. So let us be clear: We argue for the centrality, not the exclusivity, of the therapeutic relationship. Of course, as we note in our position paper, the client him- or herself actually accounts for more of the treatment outcome than either the relationship or method.

The relationship should be emphasized as a fundamental aspect of treatment delivery, therapist selection, and clinical training. As evidence of the primacy of relationship variables, consider the fact that researchers do not hesitate to control and manipulate treatment methods, but rarely consider conducting experiments in which relationship variables are similarly manipulated. Clinical trials in which therapists are intentionally tepid, rejecting, disrespectful, distracted, phony, and defensive will never be conducted. Practitioners, researchers, and human participant committees all understand how damaging such behaviors can be. The lack of experimental research on such variables is not attributable to shortcomings in the research base but because of the obvious power that such variables exert, especially on the vulnerable.

Chambless and Crits-Christoph argue that a lack of causality between relationship and outcome is apparent because "cognitive–behavior therapy (CBT) for a panic disorder delivered by bibliotherapy and web-based programs is efficacious" (p. 197). They fail to note, however, that those who create such resources go out of their way to express their understanding of client concerns and symptoms in their self-help resources. Self-help authors provide considerable hope, warmth, acceptance, and respect in their materials. We are avid supporters of self-help resources (e.g., Finch, Lambert, & Brown, 2000; Norcross et al., 2003), but these materials hardly show an absence of relational factors. In fact, they illustrate the opposite: the importance of the human "encounter" even when the "therapist" is embodied in a self-help book, computer program, or Internet site.

We largely agree with the positions of Wampold on the impact of the psychotherapist and with Bohart on the centrality of the active client, but would offer a few small twists. In Wampold's case, we would not rely as heavily on meta-analysis to determine the estimates of the impact of treatments. We collegially believe that treatments exercise somewhat more impact than he does, particularly for severe and chronic disorders. In Bohart's case, we would amplify his arguments by reference to patients' early dramatic response and outcomes. Haas and colleagues (2002) followed clients' progress on a weekly basis and found a subset of clients who made early dramatic responses to treatment. These clients responded prior to the introduction of "active technical ingredients" of psychotherapy. Significantly, these patients showed a dramatic response not only early in treatment but also at follow-up (an average of 1-year post-termination). The authors suggested that client characteristics, such as resourcefulness, were the most likely explanation.

As for Bohart's paper itself, we were impressed with his passion for the patient's contribution and agree that much of the literature is indeed "therapist-centric" (p. 219). At the same time, he occasionally blended personal passion and the empirical evidence without adequate distinction.

Beutler and Johannsen make the valuable point that principles of change might represent a more parsimonious, efficient, and consensual focus. We concur—to a point. We believe that they exaggerate both the EST position and the relational or common factors position, making them appear more oppositional or incompatible than they are. Further, we are not as optimistic about the empirical base for matching treatment methods to client characteristics. Little research has been conducted, many of the results are preliminary, and replication of results has not occurred (see reviews in Norcross, 2002). We look forward to additional research on not only matching patients to treatments but also to the principles of change advocated by Beutler and Johannsen.

Lest our recitation of small differences obscure our larger agreements, let us conclude with two take-home messages from reading the position papers in this chapter. First, comprehensive EBPs in mental health will embrace the treatment method, the individual therapist, the therapy relationship, the patient, and their optimal combinations. That's good practice and good research. Second, let us all avoid the ubiquitous pull toward dichotomous and polarizing characterizations of the evidence and each other's positions. That's good science and good relationships.

Arthur C. Bohart

The position papers of Wampold and Norcross and Lambert converge with mine to empirically support a relational paradigm of psychotherapy. Empirically supported principles (Beutler & Johannsen) are also compatible with that paradigm. On the other hand, a "strong" view of the client as an active self-healer is incompatible with the ESTs paradigm (Chambless & Crits-Christoph).

When I was in my twenties, I suffered from generalized anxiety disorder. I saw a psychodynamic therapist who related to me in Rogerian ways. He supported me as I followed my nose in treating my problem as an existential crisis in meaning. Over the course of 5 months I gradually improved and have not suffered a recurrence. My therapist practiced in an ethical, empirically supported way, although he did not use an EST. Why? First, he did not impose treatment but rather worked collegially with my worldview to establish a therapeutic direction, supporting a collaborative, discovery-oriented process in which I was ultimately the "therapist" (Bohart). Second, he facilitated an empathic relational base from which I could do my own work (Norcross and Lambert). Third, various aspects of his personal presence as a therapist were facilitative (Wampold). Overall, his work was based on (now) established scientific and professional knowledge of the discipline. Therefore, his practice was in accord with section 2.04 of the APA ethics code, which says, "Psychologists' work is based upon established scientific and professional knowledge of the discipline" (p. 1064).

The question raised by Chambless and Crits-Christoph's position paper on treatment methods is, if these authors had their way: Would I have a choice if I were to have a recurrence and want the same kind of therapist, or would I be forced to "be treated" with an EST because they claim it is the "ethical" way to proceed? Although I respect EST advocates as scholars, I am disturbed by the hegemonic tendencies I have found in some of their writing. They seem to want to impose their model of therapy as treatment on everyone, as well as their particular definition of "empirically supported" on the basis of their choice of research criteria. I am not alone in questioning their tendency to use their research criteria to dismiss other forms of evidence (Orlinsky, Rønnestad, & Willutzki, 2004).

Beutler and Johannsen present the issue as a debate between competing worldviews: treatment versus relationship. They argue that a rapprochement can be achieved by developing empirically supported principles of change. Although I applaud this, I am less sure that a rapprochement is entirely desirable. I believe fundamental paradigm conflicts are at stake, and at least two viable but different paradigms of how psychotherapy works have been established. The first is the EST paradigm, patterned after the medical model and based on an unquestioned assumption that specific treatments are needed for specific disorders. The research method of choice is the RCT.

In contrast, various forms of relational paradigms exist. They put the personal relationship between the therapist and client at center stage. The relationship is egalitarian, collaborative, and nurturing. For many, the process is one of exploration and the discovery of personal meaning (e.g., Division 32 [Humanistic Psychology] Task Force, 2004), whereas others systematically use common factors (Duncan & Miller, 2000). Even though some therapists from this paradigm still refer to it as "treatment," it is not treatment in the same sense that an EST is treatment. ESTs may be used within this paradigm, but they are secondary to the relationship and collaboratively tailored to the individual. The expert therapist does not make decisions for the client on the basis of a recipe book of what is supposed to work with a given disorder. Furthermore, the idea of manualization is an oxymoron because the emphasis is on sensitive moment by moment responding rather than on applying a template for intervention. Conversation indicates what the therapist is doing better than "treatment."

Advocates of the relational paradigm tend to rely on evidence from a variety of research methods: meta-analysis, correlational studies, RCTs, qualitative methods, and case-based research (Miller, 2004). No one method has proven itself to be the gold standard. Elliott and Elliott (2004) argued that the gold standard metaphor is misguided and that a plurality of methods is needed. Conclusions are drawn by piecing together evidence from a variety of sources, each with its own limitations, which is how mature sciences like biology and physics proceed (Rozin, 2001). Clinical judgment may be trusted more than Chambless and Crits-Christoph (Miller, 2004) have indicated, and the tendency to denigrate human judgment and perception may be overdrawn (e.g., Coady, 1992). Kahneman (2002) thinks that highly skilled cognitive performances are often intuitive and rejects the idea that the availability and representative heuristics necessarily bias judgment.

Many clients find relational therapies useful, and increasing numbers of qualitative studies can back this up. Selby (2004), for instance, showed through intensive analyses of session tapes the kinds of creative accomplishments clients were able to make in a collaborative approach.

The paradigmatic nature of the controversy between the relational and EST worldviews needs to be taken seriously. Lakoff (2002) pointed out that proponents of a given worldview may try to incorporate elements stressed by another worldview. Chambless and Crits-Christoph illustrate this when they claim that the relationship is a form of treatment and should be included within their paradigm. The problem is, as Lakoff has noted, that when one assimilates an element into one worldview, its meaning changes. I do not believe that how I think of the relationship can meaningfully be viewed as "treatment."

Evidence supports both paradigms. It is premature to try to enshrine one model over another. Both can legitimately and scientifically form the basis of practice, and the most ethical position is to support therapists in being able to provide both models and for researchers to study both. In addition, I believe the pursuit of empirically supported principles of practice is valuable. Such principles could be productively used within a relational paradigm. It can only be to the good of our clients and field to embrace these coexisting, multiple paths.

Larry E. Beutler and Brynne E. Johannsen

The position papers in this chapter present many arguments that confirm our position that the role and definition of science should be extended beyond a particular research method. However, beyond this initial similarity, we note several disparities with our position among the contributors to this chapter.

It seems to us that, while acknowledging the complexity and multiplicity of factors that affect outcome, authors treat outcome analyses as if the contributions from different domains of variables are independent of one another and as if treatment or relationship variables are inherently more important than these complex interactions. We do not believe that any viable aspect of psychotherapy can be considered and studied independently of other influential variables. Acknowledgement of the complexity and interaction among different classes of variables should be present in how the research variables are selected, measured, analyzed, and discussed. Researchers should be encouraged to use methods that allow the interactions among the different variables and the moderating influences of these variables to emerge. Outcomes should also be seen as collective aspects of treatment technique, patient qualities, therapist factors, environments, and treatment relationships.

We also note that authors have a strong tendency to consider the contributors to therapeutic change in a very global manner. This leads to some premature conclusions, in our judgment. For example, Chambless and Crits-Christoph acknowledge that although extra treatment factors are important, treatment is "the only aspect that can be manipulated in a clinical experiment to test its worth, and, if proven valuable, the only aspect that can be disseminated to other psychotherapists" (pp. 199–200, this volume). This statement disparages efforts to train therapists to use personal styles that differentially strengthen the therapeutic relationship, to alter patient preferences, or to provide information that differentially impacts the therapist's attitude about treatment. We agree that one must use the best empirical knowledge available, but we believe that this includes the use of therapist selection and treatment-matching procedures whose relationship to outcome is also identifiable.

Ignoring research evidence on how complex variables affect outcome can be done in other ways as well. Norcross and Lambert illustrate this in their effort to assign percentages to various types of variables that contribute to outcome. Their subjective analysis advances a simplistic, additive model of psychotherapy in which patient, relationship, and technique factors add to the total of nonerror variance. This analysis tacitly assumes a linear addition of variables, a most unlikely model of the complexities of psychotherapeutic interactions. Not surprisingly, from such a model they conclude that interactions between what the therapist does and the patient's ability to receive it "may or may not account for 5%" (p. 209) of the total variance in outcomes. The demonstration (e.g., Beutler et al., 2000) that when one empirically adds a test of the effects of matching treatment and patient factors, explained variance is drawn not only from the error term but from the variability associated with patient, treatment, and therapist as well, highlights the erroneous assumptions that give rise to this latter conclusion.

Wampold approaches the same problem as Norcross and Lambert using a more sophisticated, statistical approach but falls error to some of the same tendency to assume that because matching effects don't automatically emerge, they must not be present. He, too, is pessimistic about the viability of therapy–patient or therapist–patient fit. In so doing, he ignores a large number of studies that have demonstrated the role of moderating (matching) effects (e.g., Beutler et al., 2003; Castonguay & Beutler, in press). Although these studies confirm that the interactive contributions of multiple domains of variables far surpass that associated with any one variable, they do not show up in Wampold's meta-analysis. One may conclude, as does Wampold, that they are unimportant, but more realistically it may simply be that to uncover them using this type of statistic requires that one look for them. To do this, each study must be coded for "fit" using a common set of dimensions. Any effort to do so would need a list of potential matching variables, an effort that would be complicated by the use of widely different measures and construct labels across studies. Because this is difficult, meta-analyses typically ignore all or most potential moderators of treatment effects. Beutler et al. (2000) inserted a step in which variables were defined and measured across studies and then were subjected to an independent test, the results of which confirmed the value of fitting the treatment to the patient.

Bohart's contribution illustrates still a different tendency among authors, that of allowing personal experiences and beliefs to supercede empirical demonstration in determining what works in psychotherapy. Bohart believes that the patient is the impetus of therapeutic change, raising a variety of largely unresearched and poorly measured patient variables to the highest position among contributors to change. Such a hypothesis is important and certainly deserves exploration, but in this context it is not advanced as a hypothesis, but as a fact. We cannot determine whether Bohart is right or wrong on the basis of available evidence because interactions among variable domains are infrequently addressed. However, we offer an alternative hypothesis. We suggest that Bohart's assertion is most likely to be accurate among patients who are informed, motivated, and self-aware. We propose that other variables, largely those drawn from the relationship, therapist–patient fit, and treatment fit, may be more important among patients who have low motivation, little insight, and no internal motivation for change (e.g., court-referred patients or seriously psychotic patients). In these cases, it might well be the treatment method, relationship, therapist, or contributions from all three that facilitate change. Although it is most certainly important to consider the patient because, after all, without him or her this would be a pointless discussion, other variables matter.

In sum, each of the position papers included in this chapter provides a piece to the puzzle. It is certainly important to research each of the factors of treatment, the relationship, the therapist, and the patient in isolation to attempt to understand how each contributes to therapeutic change. It is also necessary to understand that each of these factors does not exist in a bubble, protected from the influences of the others. Psychotherapy does not only involve a treatment method, relationship, participant, and environment factors. It involves all of the above, collectively and in complex patterns, and it is thus imperative that potentially viable and representative variables within each of these classes be taken into consideration when assigning responsibility for therapeutic change.

REFERENCES

American Psychological Association. (2002). Ethical principles of psychologists and code of conduct. *American Psychologist, 57*, 1060–1073.

Angus, L. E. (1992). Metaphor and the communication interaction in psychotherapy: A multimethodological approach. In S. G. Toukmanian & D. L. Rennie (Eds.), *Psychotherapy process research: Paradigmatic and narrative approaches* (pp. 187–210). Newbury Park, CA: Sage Press.

Arnkoff, D. B., Glass, C. R., & Shapiro, S. J. (2002). Expectations and preferences. In J. C. Norcross (Ed.), *Psychotherapy relationships that work* (pp. 335–356). New York: Oxford University Press.

Bachelor, A., & Horvath, A. (1999). The therapeutic relationship. In M. A. Hubble, B. L. Duncan, & S. M. Miller (Eds.), *The heart and soul of change: What works in therapy* (pp. 133–178). Washington, DC: American Psychological Association.

Barber, J. P., Connolly, M. B., Crits-Christoph, P., Gladis, L., & Siqueland, L. (2000). Alliance predicts patients' outcomes beyond in-treatment change in symptoms. *Journal of Consulting and Clinical Psychology, 68,* 1027–1032.

Barber, J. P., Crits-Christoph, P., & Luborsky, L. (1996). Therapist competence and treatment outcome in dynamic therapy. *Journal of Consulting and Clinical Psychology, 64,* 619–622.

Barber, J. P., & Muenz, L. R. (1996). The role of avoidance and obsessiveness in matching patients to cognitive and interpersonal psychotherapy: Empirical findings from the Treatment of Depression Collaborative Research Program. *Journal of Consulting and Clinical Psychology, 64,* 927–935.

Baron, J. (2000). *Thinking and deciding* (3rd ed.). Cambridge, England: Cambridge University Press.

Baskin, T. W., Tierney, S. C., Minami, T., & Wampold, B. E. (2003). Establishing specificity in psychotherapy: A meta-analysis of structural equivalence of placebo controls. *Journal of Consulting and Clinical Psychology, 71,* 973–979.

Beck, A. T., Rush, A. J., Shaw, B. F., & Emery, G. (1979). *Cognitive therapy of depression.* New York: Guilford Press.

Bergin, A. E. (1997). Neglect of the therapist and the human dimensions of change: A commentary. *Clinical Psychology: Science and Practice, 4,* 83–89.

Beutler, L. E., Clarkin, J. F., & Bongar, B. (2000). *Guidelines for the systematic treatment of the depressed patient.* New York: Oxford University Press.

Beutler, L. E., Engle, D., Mohr, D., Daldrup, R. J., Bergan, J., Meredith, K., et al. (1991). Predictors of differential response to cognitive, experiential, and self-directed psychotherapeutic techniques. *Journal of Consulting and Clinical Psychology, 59,* 333–340.

Beutler, L. E., & Harwood, T. M. (2000). *Prescriptive psychotherapy.* New York: Oxford University Press.

Beutler, L. E., Harwood, T. M., Alimohamed, S., & Malik, M. (2002). Functional impairment and coping style: Patient moderators of therapeutic relationships. In J. C. Norcross (Ed.), *Psychotherapy relationships that work* (pp. 145–170). New York: Oxford University Press.

Beutler, L. E., Malik, M., Alimohamed, S., Harwood, T. M., Talebi, H., Noble, S., et al. (2004). Therapist variables. In M. J. Lambert (Ed.), *Bergin and Garfield's handbook of psychotherapy and behavior change* (5th ed., pp. 227–306). New York: Wiley.

Beutler, L. E., Moleiro, C., Malik, M., Harwood, T. M., Romanelli, R., Gallagher-Thompson, D., et al. (2003). A comparison of the Dodo, EST, and ATI indicators among co-morbid stimulant dependent, depressed patients. *Clinical Psychology and Psychotherapy, 10,* 69–85.

Beutler, L. E., Moleiro, C. M., & Talebi, H. (2002a). How practitioners can systematically use empirical evidence in treatment selection. *Journal of Clinical Psychology, 58,* 1199–1212.

Beutler, L. E., Moleiro, C. M., & Talebi, H. (2002b). Resistance. In J. C. Norcross (Ed.), *Psychotherapy relationships that work.* New York: Oxford University Press.

Blatt, S. J., Sanislow, C. A., Zuroff, D. C., & Pilkonis, P. A. (1996). Characteristics of effective therapists: Further analyses of data from the National Institute of Mental Health Treatment of Depression Collaborative Research Program. *Journal of Consulting and Clinical Psychology, 64,* 1276–1284.

Bohart, A. (2005). Evidence-based psychotherapy means evidence-informed, not evidence-driven. *Journal of Contemporary Psychotherapy, 35,* 39–53.

Bohart, A., & Boyd, G. (1997, December). *Clients' construction of the therapy process: A qualitative analysis.* Paper presented at the Meeting of the North American Association of the Society for Psychotherapy Research, Tucson, AZ.

Bohart, A. C., Elliott, R., Greenberg, L. S., & Watson, J. C. (2002). Empathy. In J. C. Norcross (Ed.), *Psychotherapy relationships that work* (pp. 89–108). New York: Oxford University Press.

Bohart, A., & Tallman, K. (1999). *How clients make therapy work: The process of active self-healing.* Washington, DC: American Psychological Association.

Borkovec, T. D., & Costello, E. (1993). Efficacy of applied relaxation and cognitive–behavioral therapy in the treatment of generalized anxiety disorder. *Journal of Consulting and Clinical Psychology, 61,* 611–619.

Burlingame, G. M., Fuhriman, A., & Johnson, J. E. (2002). Cohesion in group psychotherapy. In J. C. Norcross (Ed.), *Psychotherapy relationships that work* (pp. 71–88). New York: Oxford University Press.

Busseri, M. A., & Tyler, J. D. (2004). Client–therapist agreement on target problems, working alliance, and counseling outcome. *Psychotherapy Research, 14,* 77–88.

Calvert, S. J., Beutler, L. E., & Crago, M. (1988). Psychotherapy outcomes as a function of therapist–patient matching on selected variables. *Journal of Social and Clinical Psychology, 6,* 104–117.

Cantor, N. (2003). Constructive cognition, personal goals, and the social embedding of personality. In L. G. Aspinwall & U. M. Staudinger (Eds.), *A psychology of human strengths* (pp. 49–60). Washington, DC: American Psychological Association.

Castonguay, L. G., & Beutler, L. E. (Eds.). *Principles of psychotherapy that work: Integrating relationship, treatment, client, and therapist factors.* Manuscript in preparation.

Castonguay, L. G., & Beutler, L. E. (Eds.). (in press). *Principles of therapeutic change that work.* New York: Oxford University Press.

Castonguay, L. G., Goldfried, M. R., Wiser, S., Raue, P. J., & Hayes, A. M. (1996). Predicting the effect of cognitive therapy for depression: A study of unique and common factors. *Journal of Consulting and Clinical Psychology, 65,* 497–504.

Chambless, D. L., & Hollon, S. D. (1998). Defining empirically supported therapies. *Journal of Consulting and Clinical Psychology, 66,* 7–18.

Chambless, D. L., & Ollendick, T. H. (2001). Empirically supported psychological interventions: Controversies and evidence. In S. T. Fiske, D. L. Schacter, & C. Zahn-Waxler (Eds.), *Annual Review of Psychology* (Vol. 52, pp. 685–716). Palo Alto, CA: Annual Reviews.

Chambless, D. L., & Peterman, M. (2004). Evidence on cognitive–behavioral therapy for generalized anxiety disorder and panic disorder: The second decade. In R. L. Leahy (Ed.), *Contemporary cognitive therapy* (pp. 86–115). New York: Guilford Press.

Coady, C. A. J. (1992). *Testimony: A philosophical study*. New York: Oxford University Press.

Cooney, N. L., Kadden, R. M., Litt, M. D., & Getter, H. (1991). Matching alcoholics to coping skills or interactional therapies: Two-year follow-up results. *Journal of Consulting and Clinical Psychology, 59*, 598–601.

Crits-Christoph, P. (1997). Limitations of the dodo bird verdict and the role of clinical trials in psychotherapy research: Comment on Wampold et al. (1997). *Psychological Bulletin, 122*, 216–220.

Crits-Christoph, P., Baranackie, K., Kurcias, J. S., Carroll, K., Luborsky, L., McLellan, T., et al. (1991). Meta-analysis of therapist effects in psychotherapy outcome studies. *Psychotherapy Research, 1*, 81–91.

Crits-Christoph, P., Connolly Gibbons, M. B., Narducci, J., Schamberger, M., & Gallop, R. (in press). Can therapists be trained to improve their alliances? A pilot study of Alliance-Fostering Therapy. *Psychotherapy Research*.

Crits-Christoph, P., & Mintz, J. (1991). Implications of therapist effects for the design and analysis of comparative studies of psychotherapies. *Journal of Consulting and Clinical Psychology, 59*, 20–26.

Cross, D. G., Sheehan, P. W., & Kahn, J. A. (1980). Alternative advice and counseling psychotherapy. *Journal of Consulting and Clinical Psychology, 48*, 615–625.

Deci, E. L., & Ryan, R. M. (1991). A motivational approach to self: Integration in personality. In R. A. Dienstbier (Ed.), *Perspectives on motivation: Nebraska Symposium on Motivation, 1990* (pp. 237–288). Lincoln: University of Nebraska Press.

DeRubeis, R. J., & Feeley, M. (1990). Determinants of change in cognitive behavioral therapy for depression. *Cognitive Therapy and Research, 14*, 469–482.

Division 32 Task Force. (2004). Recommended principles and practices for the provision of humanistic psychosocial services: Alternative to mandated practice and treatment guidelines. *Humanistic Psychologist, 32*, 3–75.

Dreier, O. (2000). Psychotherapy in clients' trajectories across contexts. In C. Mattingly & L. Garro (Eds.), *Narrative and the cultural construction of illness and healing* (pp. 237–258). Berkeley: University of California Press.

Duncan, B. L., & Miller, S. D. (2000). *The heroic client*. San Francisco: Jossey-Bass.

Edelman, R. E., & Chambless, D. L. (1993). Compliance during sessions and homework in exposure-based treatment of agoraphobia. *Behaviour Research and Therapy, 31*, 767–773.

Efran, J. S., & Blumberg, M. J. (1994). Emotion and family living: The perspective of structure determinism. In S. M. Johnson & L. S. Greenberg (Eds.), *The heart of the matter* (pp. 172–206). New York: Brunner/Mazel.

Elkin, I. (1999). A major dilemma in psychotherapy outcome research: Disentangling therapists from therapies. *Clinical Psychology: Science and Practice, 6*, 10–32.

Elkin, I., Shea, T., Watkins, J. T., Imber, S. D., Sotsky, S. M., Collins, I. F., et al. (1989). National Institute of Mental Health Treatment of Depression Collaborative Research Program: General effectiveness of treatments. *Archives General Psychiatry, 46*, 97–98.

Elliott, R. (1984). A discovery-oriented approach to significant change events in psychotherapy: Interpersonal process recall and comprehensive process analysis. In L. S. Greenberg & L. N. Rice (Eds.), *Patterns of change* (pp. 249–286). New York: Guilford Press.

Elliott, R., & Elliott, K. (2004, November). *The gold standard: Myth and metaphor in the EST/ESR debates.* Paper presented at the annual conference of the North American Society for Psychotherapy Research, Springdale, UT.

Elliott, R., & James, E. (1989). Varieties of client experience in psychotherapy: An analysis of the literature. *Clinical Psychology Review, 9*, 443–467.

Feeley, M., DeRubeis, R. J., & Gelfand, L. A. (1999). The temporal relation of adherence and alliance to symptom change in cognitive therapy for depression. *Journal of Consulting and Clinical Psychology, 67*, 578–582.

Finch, A. E., Lambert, M. J., & Brown, G. S. (2000). Attacking anxiety: A naturalistic study of a multimedia self-help program. *Journal of Clinical Psychology, 56*, 11–21.

Fisher, S., & Greenberg, R. P. (Eds.). (1997). *From placebo to panacea: Putting psychiatric drugs to the test.* New York: Wiley.

Garb, H. N. (1998). *Studying the clinician: Judgment research and psychological assessment.* Washington, DC: American Psychological Association.

Garfield, S. L. (1998). Some comments on empirically supported treatments. *Journal of Consulting and Clinical Psychology, 66*, 121–125.

Garfield, S. L. (1994). Research on client variables in psychotherapy. In A. E. Bergin & S. L. Garfield (Eds.), *Handbook of psychotherapy and behavior change* (4th ed., pp. 190–228). New York: Wiley.

Gaston, L., Marmar, L. R., Thompson, L., & Gallagher, D. (in press). The importance of the alliance in psychotherapy of elderly depressed patients. *Journal of Gerontology: Psychological Sciences.*

Gershefski, J. J., Arnkoff, D. B., Glass, C. R., & Elkin, I. (1996). Clients' perceptions of their treatment for depression: I. Helpful aspects. *Psychotherapy Research, 6*, 245–259.

Goin, M. K., Yamamoto, J., & Silverman, J. (1965). Therapy congruent with class-linked expectations. *Archives of General Psychiatry, 38*, 335–339.

Gold, J. R. (1994). When the patient does the integrating: Lessons for theory and practice. *Journal of Psychotherapy Integration, 4*, 133–158.

Gurin, J. (1990, March). Remaking our lives. *American Health*, 50–52.

Haas, E., Hill, R., Lambert, M. J., & Morrell, B. (2002). Do early responders to psychotherapy maintain treatment gains? *Journal of Clinical Psychology, 58,* 1157–1172.

Harding, C., Brooks, G. W., Ashikaga, T., Strauss, J. S., & Breier, A. (1987). The Vermont longitudinal study of persons with severe mental illness. I: Methodology, study sample, and overall status 32 years later. *American Journal of Psychiatry, 144,* 718–726.

Hirshoren, A., & Gregory, J. (1995). Further negative findings on facilitated communication. *Psychology in the School, 32,* 109–113.

Horvath, A. O., & Bedi, R. P. (2002). The alliance. In J. C. Norcross (Ed.), *Psychotherapy relationships that work* (pp. 37–69). New York: Oxford University Press.

Horvath, A. O., & Greenberg, L. S. (1986). The development of the Working Alliance Inventory. In L. S. Greenberg & W. M. Pinsof (Eds.), *The psychotherapeutic process: A research handbook* (pp. 529–556). New York: Guilford Press.

Horvath, A. O., & Luborsky, L. (1993). The role of the therapeutic alliance in psychotherapy. *Journal of Consulting and Clinical Psychology, 61,* 561–573.

Horvath, A. O., & Symonds, B. D. (1991). Relation between working alliance and outcome in psychotherapy: A meta-analysis. *Journal of Counseling Psychology, 38,* 139–149.

Huppert, J. D., Bufka, L. F., Barlow, D. H., Gorman, J. M., Shear, M. K., & Woods, S. W. (2001). Therapists, therapist variables, and cognitive–behavioral therapy outcomes in a multicenter trial for panic disorder. *Journal of Consulting and Clinical Psychology, 69,* 747–755.

Jacobson, N. S., & Truax, P. (1991). Clinical significance: A statistical approach to defining meaningful change in psychotherapy. *Journal of Consulting and Clinical Psychology, 59,* 12–19.

Kahneman, D. (2002). *Daniel Kahneman—Autobiography.* Retrieved March 1, 2005, from http://nobelprize.org/economics/laureates/2002/kahneman-autobio.html

Karno, M., Beutler, L. E., & Harwood, T. M. (2002). Interactions between psychotherapy process and patient attributes that predict alcohol treatment effectiveness: A preliminary report. *Addictive Behaviors, 27,* 779–797.

Karoly, P., & Anderson, C. W. (2000). The long and short of psychological change: Toward a goal-centered understanding of treatment and durability and adaptive success. In C. R. Snyder & R. E. Ingram (Eds.), *Handbook of psychological change* (pp. 154–176). New York: Wiley.

Kendall, P. C., Kipnis, D., & Otto-Salaj, L. (1992). When clients don't progress: Influences on and explanations for lack of therapeutic progress. *Cognitive Therapy and Research, 16,* 269–281.

Kim, D. M., Wampold, B. E., & Bolt, D. M. (in press). Therapist effects in psychotherapy: A random effects modeling of the NIMH TDCRP data. *Psychotherapy Research.*

Kirsch, I. (2002). Yes, there IS a placebo effect, but IS there a powerful antidepressant drug effect? *Prevention and Treatment, 5*(5), Article 0022. Retrieved July 15, 2002, from http://journals.apa.org/prevention/volume 5/pre 0050022i.html

Klein, D. N., Schwartz, J. E., Santiago, N. J., Vivian, D., Vocisano, C., Castonguay, L. G., et al. (2003). Therapeutic alliance in depression treatment: Controlling for prior change and patient characteristics. *Journal of Consulting and Clinical Psychology, 71*, 997–1006.

Kleinman, A. (1988). *Rethinking psychiatry: From cultural category to personal experience.* New York: Free Press.

Krupnick, J. L., Stotsky, S. M., Simmons, S., Moyer, J., Watkins, J., Elkin, I., et al. (1996). The role of the therapeutic alliance in psychotherapy and pharmacotherapy outcome: Findings in the National Institute of Mental Health Treatment of Depression Collaborative Research Program. *Journal of Consulting and Clinical Psychology, 64*, 532–539.

Kühnlein, I. (1999). Psychotherapy as a process of transformation: Analysis of post-therapeutic autobiographical narrations. *Psychotherapy Research, 9*, 274–288.

Lakoff, G. (2002). *Moral politics* (Rev. ed.). Chicago: University of Chicago Press.

Lambert, M. J. (1992). Psychotherapy outcome research: Implications for integrative and eclectic therapists. In J. C. Norcross and M. R. Goldfried (Eds.), *Handbook of psychotherapy integration* (pp. 94–129). New York: Basic Books.

Lambert, M. J. (2005). Enhancing psychotherapy outcome through feedback. *Journal of Clinical Psychology: In Session, 61.*

Lambert, M. J., Hansen, N. B., & Finch, A. E. (2001). Patient-focused research: Using patient outcome data to enhance treatment effects. *Journal of Consulting and Clinical Psychology, 69*, 159–172.

Lambert, M. J., & Ogles, B. M. (2004). The efficacy and effectiveness of psychotherapy. In M. J. Lambert (Ed.), *Bergin and Garfield's handbook of psychotherapy and behavior change* (5th ed., pp, 139–193). New York: Wiley.

Linehan, M. M. (1993). *Cognitive–behavioral treatment of borderline personality disorder.* New York: Guilford Press.

Luborsky, L. (1984). *Principles of psychoanalytic psychotherapy: A manual for supportive–expressive treatment.* New York: Basic Books.

Luborsky, L., Crits-Christoph, P., Mintz, J., & Auerbach, A. (1988). *Who will benefit from psychotherapy? Predicting therapeutic outcomes.* New York: Basic Books.

Luborsky, L., Rosenthal, R., Diguer, L., Andrusyna, T. P., Berman, J. S., Levitt, J. T., et al. (2001). The dodo bird verdict is alive and well—mostly. *Clinical Psychology: Science and Practice, 9*, 2–12.

Malik, M. L., Beutler, L. E., Gallagher-Thompson, D., Thompson, L., & Alimohamed, S. (2003). Are all cognitive therapies alike? A comparison of cognitive and non-cognitive therapy process and implications for the application of empirically supported treatments (ESTs). *Journal of Consulting and Clinical Psychology, 71*, 150–158.

Martin, D. J., Garske, J. P., & Davis, M. K. (2000). Relation of the therapeutic alliance with outcome and other variables: A meta-analytic review. *Journal of Consulting and Clinical Psychology, 68*, 438–450.

Masten, A. S., Best, K. M., Garmazy, N. (1990). Resilience and development: Contribution from the study of children who overcome adversity. *Development and Psychopathology, 2,* 425–444.

Matumoto, K., Jones, E., & Brown, J. (2003). Using clinical informatics to improve outcomes: A new approach to managing behavioral healthcare. *Journal of Information Technology in Health Care, 1,* 135–150.

McKeel, A. J. (1996). A clinician's guide to research on solution-focused brief therapy. In S. D. Miller, M. A. Hubble, & B. L. Duncan (Eds.), *Handbook of solution-focused brief therapy* (pp. 251–271). San Francisco: Jossey-Bass.

Michelson, L., Mavissakalian, M., & Marchione, K. (1985). Cognitive and behavioral treatments of agoraphobia: Clinical, behavioral, and psychophysiological outcomes. *Journal of Consulting and Clinical Psychology, 53,* 913–925.

Miller, R. B. (2004). *Facing human suffering: Psychology and psychotherapy as moral engagement.* Washington, DC: American Psychological Association.

Miller, S. D., Duncan, B. L., & Hubble, M. A. (in press). Outcome-informed clinical work. In J. C. Norcross & M. R. Goldfried (Eds.), *Handbook of psychotherapy integration* (2nd ed.). New York: Oxford University Press.

Miller, W. R. (Ed.). (2004). Quantum change. *Journal of Clinical Psychology: In Session, Special Issue, 60,* 453–541.

Miller, W. R., & Rollnick, S. (1991). *Motivational interviewing: Preparing people to change addictive behavior.* New York: Guilford Press.

Miller, W. R., Taylor, C. A., & West, J. C. (1980). Focused versus broad-spectrum behavior therapy for problem drinkers. *Journal of Consulting and Clinical Psychology, 48,* 590–601.

Moerbeek, M. (2004). The consequences of ignoring a level of nesting in multilevel analysis. *Multivariate Behavioral Research, 39,* 129–149.

Murphy, J. J. (1999). Common factors of school-based change. In M. A. Hubble, B. L. Duncan, & S. M. Miller (Eds.), *The heart and soul of change: What works in therapy* (pp. 361–388). Washington, DC: American Psychological Association.

Murphy, P. M., Cramer, D., & Lillie, F. J. (1984). The relationship between curative factors perceived by patients in their psychotherapy and treatment outcome: An exploratory study. *British Journal of Medical Psychology, 57,* 187–192.

Najavits, L. M., & Strupp, H. (1994). Differences in the effectiveness of psychodynamic therapists: A process–outcome study. *Psychotherapy, 31,* 114–123.

Nathan, P. E., & Gorman, J. M. (Eds.). (1998). *A guide to treatments that work.* New York: Oxford University Press.

Nathan, P. E., & Gorman, J. M. (Eds.). (2002). *A guide to treatments that work* (2nd ed.). New York: Oxford University Press.

Norcross, J. C. (Ed.). (2001). Empirically supported therapy relationships: Summary Report of the Division 29 Task Force. *Psychotherapy, 38,* 345–356.

Norcross, J. C. (Ed.). (2002). *Psychotherapy relationships that work: Therapist contributions and responsiveness to patient needs.* New York: Oxford University Press.

Norcross, J. C., Dryden, W., & DeMichele, J. T. (1992). British clinical psychologists and personal therapy: III. What's good for the goose? *Clinical Psychology Forum*, *44*, 29–33.

Norcross, J. C., Santrock, J. W., Campbell, L. F., Smith, T. P., Sommer, R., & Zuckerman, E. L. (2003). *Authoritative guide to self-help resources in mental health* (2nd ed.). New York: Guilford Press.

Norcross, J. C., Strausser-Kirtland, D., & Missar, C. D. (1988). The processes and outcomes of psychotherapists' personal treatment experiences. *Psychotherapy*, *25*, 36–43.

O'Donohue, W. T., Fisher, J. E., Plaud, J. J., & Link, W. (1989). What is a good treatment decision? The client's perspective. *Professional Psychology: Research and Practice*, *20*, 404–407.

Ogles, B. M., Anderson, T., & Lunnen, K. M. (1999). The contribution of models and techniques to therapeutic efficacy: Contradictions between professional trends and clinical research. In M. A. Hubble, B. L. Duncan, & S. M. Miller (Eds.), *The heart and soul of change: What works in therapy* (pp. 201–226). Washington, DC: American Psychological Association.

Orlinsky, D. E. (1989). Researchers' images of psychotherapy: Their origins and influences on research. *Clinical Psychology Review*, *9*, 413–442.

Orlinsky, D. E. (2000, August). *Therapist interpersonal behaviors that have consistently shown positive correlations with outcome.* Paper presented in a symposium on "Empirically Supported Therapy Relationships: Task Force of APA's Psychotherapy Division," at the annual convention of the American Psychological Association, Washington, DC.

Orlinsky, D. E., Grawe, K., & Parks, B. K. (1994). Process and outcome in psychotherapy—noch einmal. In A. E. Bergin & S. L. Garfield (Eds.), *Handbook of psychotherapy and behavior change* (4th ed., pp. 270–376). New York: Wiley.

Orlinsky, D. E., & Norcross, J. C. (2005). Outcomes and impacts of psychotherapists' personal therapy: A research review. In J. D. Geller, J. C. Norcross, & D. E. Orlinsky (Eds.), *The psychotherapist's personal therapy* (pp. 214–234). New York: Oxford University Press.

Orlinsky, D. E., Rønnestad, M. H., & Willutzki, U. (2004). Fifty years of psychotherapy process–outcome research: Continuity and change. In M. J. Lambert, (Ed.), *Bergin and Garfield's handbook of psychotherapy and behavior change* (5th ed., pp. 307–390). New York: Wiley.

Paivio, S. C., & Greenberg, L. S. (1995). Resolving "unfinished business": Efficacy of experiential therapy using empty-chair dialogue. *Journal of Consulting and Clinical Psychology*, *63*, 419–425.

Phillips, J. R. (1984). Influences on personal growth as viewed by former psychotherapy patients. *Dissertation Abstracts International*, *44*, 441A.

Prochaska, J. O., & Norcross, J. C. (2002). Stages of change. In J. C. Norcross (Ed.), *Psychotherapy relationships that work* (pp. 303–314). New York: Oxford University Press.

Prochaska, J. O., Norcross, J. C., & DiClemente, C. C. (1994). *Changing for good.* New York: Morrow.

Pulkkinen, L. (2001). Reveller or striver? How childhood self-control predicts adult behavior. In A. Bohart & D. Stipek (Eds.), *Constructive and destructive behavior* (pp. 167–186). Washington, DC: American Psychological Association.

Raine, R., Sanderson, C., Hutchings, A., Carter, S., Larkin, K., & Black, N. (2004). An experimental study of determinants of group judgments in clinical guideline development. *Lancet, 364,* 429–437.

Rennie, D. L. (1990). Toward a representation of the client's experience of the psychotherapy hour. In G. Lietaer, J. Rombauts, & R. Van Balen (Eds.), *Client-centered and experiential therapy in the nineties* (pp. 155–172). Leuven, Belgium; Leuven University Press.

Rennie, D. L. (1992). Qualitative analysis of the client's experience of psychotherapy: The unfolding of reflexivity. In S. G. Toukmanian & D. L. Rennie (Eds.), *Psychotherapy process research: Paradigmatic and narrative approaches* (pp. 211–233). Newbury Park, CA: Sage Press.

Rennie, D. L. (1994). Clients' deference in psychotherapy. *Journal of Counseling Psychology, 41,* 427–437.

Rennie, D. L. (2000). Aspects of the client's conscious control of the psychotherapeutic process. *Journal of Psychotherapy Integration, 10,* 151–168.

Roberts, A. H., Kewman, D. G., Mercier, L., & Hovell, M. F. (1993). The power of nonspecific effects in healing: Implications for psychosocial and biological treatments. *Clinical Psychology Review, 13,* 375–391.

Rogers, C. R. (1957). The necessary and sufficient conditions of therapeutic personality change. *Journal of Consulting Psychology, 22,* 95–103.

Rosen, C. S. (2000). Is the sequencing of change processes by stage consistent across health problems? A meta-analysis. *Health Psychology, 19,* 593–604.

Rozin, P. (2001). Social psychology and science: Some lessons from Solomon Asch. *Personality and Social Psychology Review, 5,* 2–14.

Sackett, D. L., Richardson, W. S., Rosenberg, W., & Haynes, R. B. (1997). *Evidence-based medicine.* New York: Churchill Livingstone.

Safran, J. D., & Wallner, L. K. (1991). The relative predictive validity of two therapeutic alliance measures in cognitive therapy. *Psychological Assessment: A Journal of Consulting and Clinical Psychology, 3,* 188–195.

Schön, D. A. (1983). *The reflective practitioner: How professionals think in action.* New York: Basic Books.

Serlin, R. C., Wampold, B. E., & Levin, J. R. (2003). Should providers of treatment be regarded as a random factor? If it ain't broke, don't "fix" it: A comment on Siemer and Joorman (2003). *Psychological Methods, 8,* 524–534.

Shaffer, D. R. (2000). *Social and personality development* (4th ed.). Belmont, CA: Wadsworth Press.

Shaw, B. F., Elkin, I., Yamaguchi, J., Olmsted, M., Vallis, T. M., Dobson, K. S., et al. (1999). Therapist competence ratings in relation to clinical outcome in cognitive therapy of depression. *Journal of Consulting and Clinical Psychology, 67,* 837–846.

Shirk, S. R., & Karver, M. (2003). Prediction of treatment outcome from relationship variables in child and adolescent therapy: A meta-analytic review. *Journal of Consulting and Clinical Psychology, 71,* 452–464.

Siemer, M., & Joormann, J. (2003). Power and measures of effect size in analysis variance with fixed versus random nested factors. *Psychological Methods, 8,* 497–517.

Silverman, W. K., Kurtines, W. M., Ginsburg, G. S., Weems, C. F., Rabian, B., & Serafini, L. T. (1999). Contingency management, self-control, and education support in the treatment of childhood phobic disorders: A randomized clinical trial. *Journal of Consulting and Clinical Psychology, 67,* 675–687.

Sloane, R. B., Staples, F. R., Cristol, A. H., Yorkston, N. J. I., & Whipple, K. (1975). *Short-term analytically oriented psychotherapy vs. behavior therapy.* Cambridge, MA: Harvard University Press.

Smith, M. L., Glass, G. V., & Miller, T. (1980). *The benefits of psychotherapy.* Baltimore: Johns Hopkins University Press.

Snyder, C. R., Michael, S. T., & Cheavens, J. S. (1999). Hope as a psychotherapeutic foundation of common factors, placebos, and expectancies. In M. A. Hubble, B. L. Duncan, & S. M. Miller (Eds.), *The heart and soul of change: What works in therapy* (pp. 179–200). Washington, DC: American Psychological Association.

Snyder, M., & Thomsen, C. J. (1988). Interactions between therapists and clients: Hypothesis testing and behavioral confirmation. In D. C. Turk & P. Salovey (Eds.), *Reason, inference, and judgment in clinical psychology* (pp. 125–152). New York: Free Press.

Stevens, S. E., Hynan, M. T., & Allen, M. (2000). A meta-analysis of common factor and specific treatment effects across outcome domains of the phase model of psychotherapy. *Clinical Psychology: Science and Practice, 7,* 273–290.

Suinn, R. M. (1999, September). President's column. *American Psychological Association Monitor, 30,* 2.

Talmon, M. (1990). *Single session therapy.* San Francisco: Jossey-Bass.

Task Force on Promotion and Dissemination of Psychological Procedures, Division of Clinical Psychology of the American Psychological Association. (1995). Training and dissemination of empirically-validated psychological treatments: Report and recommendations. *The Clinical Psychologist, 48,* 3–23.

Tedeschi, R. G., Park, C. L., & Calhoun, L. G. (Eds.). (1998). *Posttraumatic growth.* Mahwah, NJ: Erlbaum.

Trierweiler, S. J., & Stricker, G. (1998). *The scientific practice of professional psychology.* New York: Plenum Press.

Tryon, G. S., & Winograd, G. (2002). Goal consensus and collaboration. In J. C. Norcross (Ed.), *Psychotherapy relationships that work* (pp. 109–128). New York: Oxford University Press.

Turk, D. C., & Salovey, P. (Eds.). (1988). *Reason, inference, and judgment in clinical psychology.* New York: Free Press.

Vessey, J. T., Howard, K. I., Lueger, R. J., Kachele, H., & Mergenthaler, E. (1994). The clinician's illusion and the psychotherapy practice: An application of stochastic modeling. *Journal of Consulting and Clinical Psychology, 62,* 679–685.

Vocisano, C., Klein, D. F., Arnow, B., Rivera, C., Blalock, J., Rothbaum, B., et al. (2004). Therapist variables that predict symptom change in psychotherapy with chronically depressed outpatients. *Psychotherapy: Theory, Research, Practice, Training, 41,* 255–265.

Wampold, B. E. (2001a). Contextualizing psychotherapy as a healing practice: Culture, history, and methods. *Applied and Preventive Psychology, 10,* 69–86.

Wampold, B. E. (2001b). *The great psychotherapy debate: Models, methods, and findings.* Mahwah, NJ: Erlbaum.

Wampold, B. E., & Bhati, K. S. (2004). Attending to the omissions: A historical examination of the evidence-based practice movement. *Professional Psychology: Research and Practice, 35,* 563–570.

Wampold, B. E., & Brown, G. S. (in press). Estimating therapist variability: A naturalistic study of outcomes in managed care. *Journal of Consulting and Clinical Psychology.*

Wampold, B. E., Mondin, G. W., Moody, M., Stich, F., Benson, K., & Ahn, H. (1997). A meta-analysis of outcome studies comparing bona fide psychotherapies: Empirically, "all must have prizes." *Psychological Bulletin, 122,* 203–215.

Wampold, B. E., & Serlin, R. C. (2000). The consequences of ignoring a nested factor on measures of effect size in analysis of variance. *Psychological Methods, 5,* 425–433.

Watson, J. C., & Rennie, D. L. (1994). Qualitative analysis of clients' subjective experience of significant moments during the exploration of problematic reactions. *Journal of Counseling Psychology, 41,* 500–509.

Westen, D., Novotny, C. M., & Thompson-Brenner, H. (2004). The empirical status of empirically supported psychotherapies: Assumptions, findings, and reporting in controlled clinical trials. *Psychological Bulletin, 130,* 631–663.

6

WHAT ELSE MATERIALLY INFLUENCES WHAT IS REPRESENTED AND PUBLISHED AS EVIDENCE?

Theoretical Allegiance

Lester B. Luborsky and Marna S. Barrett

In this position paper we argue that a researcher's theoretical allegiance contributes to treatment outcome and thereby influences what is presented as evidence for treatment benefits. It is designed to facilitate dialogue among researchers with different perspectives.

A well-known conclusion in psychotherapy research is that nearly two thirds of all patients experience a positive outcome from treatment. Moreover, evidence-based reviews show similar degrees of benefits from differing theoretical models (Lambert & Bergin, 1994). However, treatment benefits, as evidenced in comparative trials, are so influenced by the researcher's theoretical allegiance that in many comparisons differences between treatments lessen or become negligible when the influence of allegiance is considered.

Allegiance refers to the degree of loyalty or commitment a person has for a particular ideal or philosophy. In the context of therapy research, theoretical allegiance is the degree of loyalty a researcher expresses for a specific theory of behavior change. A researcher may hold allegiance to any one of the myriad theoretical models proposed. However, in comparative treatment trials the most frequent theoretical comparisons are for the broad categories of dynamic, cognitive, behavioral, or pharmacological (Luborsky et al., 2002). In conducting clinical trials of competing therapies, most researchers attempt to control for the degree to which a person's bias or allegiance for one therapy over another might influence the resulting findings. For example, experts within a particular therapy are often used to train therapists, and all participants are kept blind to treatment assignment. Despite such efforts, the researcher's allegiance can, and often does, influence the resulting findings.

INTERCOMPARISON AMONG 24 COMPARATIVE PSYCHOTHERAPY STUDIES

We begin with a systematic comparison of researcher allegiance for outcomes from different psychotherapy groups for 24 studies involving 29 treatment comparisons: cognitive versus behavioral, dynamic versus behavioral, dynamic versus cognitive, and pharmacotherapy versus psychotherapy (Luborsky et al., 1999). The studies of each pair of treatments were identified through a computerized search of the literature for the years 1965–1995. The analysis of researcher allegiance was assessed in three related ways: the reprint measure, the self-measure, and the colleague measure, as shown in Table 6.1 and elaborated later in this section.

Reprint Measure

Early measures of allegiance relied on ratings of treatment preference on the basis of the extent to which a particular theory was emphasized in the introduction of the paper. However, concern was raised that a particular treatment may be emphasized not because of researcher allegiance but due to the researcher's knowledge of the results. In response to these concerns, several investigators (Berman, Miller, & Massman, 1985; Luborsky et al., 1999; Robinson, Berman, & Neimeyer, 1990) began assessing allegiance by reviewing previous articles published by the authors of the study. Using this method, independent judges were asked to rate the degree to which earlier reprints emphasized one theoretical idea more than another. All ratings of allegiance were standardized to allow for comparison on our 4-point allegiance scale. The rating system follows the guide by Gaffan, Tsaousis, and Kemp-Wheeler,

(1995), which is a slightly more systematic version of the usual reprint ratings system.

1. Relying on this revised reprint measure, the largest allegiance differences emerge from comparisons between dynamic and behavioral treatments. As can be seen in Table 6.1, a difference between treatments of 2.5 was found in the Gallagher and Thompson (1982) study, in which a stronger allegiance to behavioral therapy yielded an advantage to outcome for behavioral treatments.

2. Four comparisons of dynamic and cognitive therapies were found. Although the study by Gallagher and Thompson (1982) found a difference in ratings of allegiance in favor of cognitive therapy, a mean difference of only 0.7 was identified across the four studies.

3. For the comparison of cognitive and behavioral treatments, the study by Biran and Wilson (1981) demonstrated the largest difference in reprint ratings of allegiance. Although allegiance ratings favored behavioral therapy more than cognitive (behavioral therapy was rated a 3 and cognitive a 1) the effect size was 0. In other words, despite a bias for behavioral treatments, this allegiance did not seem to influence the outcome.

4. Among the studies comparing pharmacotherapy and psychotherapy, the study by Dunn (1979) demonstrated the greatest difference in allegiance. In this study the researchers more strongly favored psychotherapy than pharmacotherapy (2.5 vs. 0.5). Not surprisingly, the effect on outcome also favored psychotherapy.

Self-Measure

Because reprints are a somewhat indirect measure of allegiance and may not accurately reflect the true bias of a researcher, ratings of allegiance were also obtained from the researchers themselves. For the self-measure, researchers were asked to rate their allegiance to a particular theory on a 5-point scale, with 5 indicating a very strong allegiance. These ratings were obtained from first and second authors of 16 comparative studies.

1. Utilizing the self-ratings of allegiance, the middle column of Table 6.1 shows that the largest differences were evidenced in the comparisons between behavioral and cognitive treatments. For example, Butler and colleagues (1991) had the greatest allegiance difference with behavioral treatment rated a 3 and cognitive rated a 5. Overall, the self-rated allegiance to

TABLE 6.1
Studies Included in the Treatment Comparisons for Researcher Therapeutic Allegiance

Study	Effect size (r)	Allegiance difference (reprint)	Allegiance difference (self)[1]	Allegiance difference (colleague)[2]
Cognitive (+) versus behavioral (−)				
Barlow, Rapee, & Brown (1992)	−.021	0	0	−0.9
Biran & Wilson (1981)	0	−2.0	0.5	−0.4
Butler, Fennell, Robson, & Gelder (1991)	.437	0	2.0	1.1
Gallagher & Thompson (1982)	.107	0	0	−0.6
McNamara & Horan (1986)	−.135	0		
Moleski & Tosi (1976)	.503	0.5		
Taylor & Marshall (1977)	.054	−0.5		
Wilson, Goldin, & Charbonneau–Powis (1983)	−.108	1.0	0	−1.4
Zeiss, Lewinsohn, & Munoz (1979)	0	0.5	−1.0	−1.5
Dynamic (+) versus behavioral (−)				
Brom, Kleber, & Defares (1989)	.002	0		
Cross, Sheehan, & Khan (1982)	.219	0	1.0	0
Gallagher & Thompson (1982)	−.183	−2.5	−1.0	−1.9
Pierloot & Vinck (1978)	−.128	−0.5		
Sloane et al. (1975)	.070	−0.5	1.0	−2.0
Thompson, Gallagher, & Breckenridge (1987)	−.103	−1.0	−1.0	−1.9
Zitrin, Klein, & Woerner (1978)	.025	−1.0	−1.0	−1.0
Dynamic (+) versus cognitive (−)				
Elkin et al. (1989)	.102	0	0	0.8
Gallagher & Thompson (1982)	−.376	−2.5	−1.0	−1.3
Thompson et al. (1987)	.001	0	−1.0	−1.3
Woody et al. (1983)	.317	−0.5	1.25	3.0

Pharmacotherapy (+) versus psychotherapy (−)				
Blackburn, Bishop, Glen, Whalley, & Christie (1981)	−.426	−1.0	−1.0	−2.5
DiMascio et al. (1979)	.110	0.5		−0.8
Dunn (1979)	−.611	−2.0		
Elkin et al. (1989) (vs. IPT)	.031	1.0	0	−0.9
Elkin et al. (1989) (vs. cognitive)	.134	1.0	0	−0.1
Hollon et al. (1992)	−.054	0	−1.5	−1.8
Murphy, Simons, Wetzel, & Lustman (1984)	−.009	0	−1.0	−1.7
Power, Jerrom, Simpson, Mitchell, & Swanson (1989)	−.465	−1.5		
Rush, Beck, Kovacs, & Hollon (1977)	−.360	−1.0	0	−1.3

[1]Self-ratings of allegiance by the first or second authors were unable to be obtained for 8 of the studies.
[2]Colleague ratings for seven studies could not be done because none of the 24 judges were familiar with the researcher's work.

cognitive treatments was relatively higher than the allegiance to behavioral treatments, although the resulting effect size was close to zero (0.069).

2. For the dynamic versus behavioral comparisons, all studies evidenced allegiance differences of 1, although two studies favored dynamic treatments and three favored behavioral treatments. The effect sizes for these comparisons were relatively small, ranging from 0.02 to 0.2, with the favored treatment for allegiance also demonstrating the advantage in outcome. That is, the three comparisons with allegiance ratings in support of behavioral therapy had effect sizes that slightly favored behavioral treatments.

3. Among the studies comparing dynamic and cognitive treatments, Woody and colleagues (1983) demonstrated the greatest disparity in allegiance ratings, with an allegiance difference of 1.25 favoring dynamic therapy. The outcome of treatment also favored the treatment with the advantage in allegiance, although the effect size was only 0.3.

4. There were six comparisons for pharmacotherapy and psychotherapy. The mean difference in allegiance was 0.58 in favor of psychotherapy with the study by Hollon et al. (1992) showing a difference of 1.5 between treatments. As with the previous comparisons, the treatment with the greatest allegiance was also the treatment favored in outcome. A greater effect on outcome was seen for psychotherapy with a relatively small effect size of 0.2.

Colleague Measure

In addition to the reprint and self-rated measures of allegiance, it is also helpful to have a rating from professional colleagues who know the work of a researcher apart from any one particular study. Therefore, a special sample of judges composed of 24 experienced psychotherapy researchers rated the allegiance of each researcher with whom they were familiar. Ratings were made on a 5-point scale in which higher scores indicated a greater allegiance to that theory. The colleague measure is the mean ratings of allegiance for all judges with both the first and second authors combined.

Within the 47 first and second authors of the research studies reviewed, each colleague was able to rate only 5 to 10 people whose type of therapy allegiance was well known to them (either behavioral, cognitive, dynamic, or pharmacological). The agreement of judges was very good (an intraclass correlation of .79, $p < .001$) with agreement for the first author of .83 and agreement for the second author of .77.

1. Colleague ratings of allegiance produced somewhat similar results to those found for self-ratings of allegiance. For example, the comparison between cognitive and behavioral treatments in the study by Butler and colleagues (1991) resulted in allegiance ratings of 4.9 for cognitive therapy and 3.8 for behavioral. Although both represent fairly high levels of allegiance (ratings based on a 5-point scale), allegiance ratings were stronger for cognitive therapy, and the effect size favored cognitive therapy.

2. For the seven studies comparing dynamic and behavioral therapies, Sloane and associates (1975) demonstrated the largest difference in allegiance ratings with a 2-point range in favor of behavioral therapy. Despite this difference, the effect on outcome was minimal (effect size = .070). Furthermore, across all studies differences in treatment outcome were negligible (ES = 0.014).

3. Among the four studies comparing dynamic and cognitive treatments, the study of opiate abuse by Woody et al. (1983) showed a strong allegiance for dynamic treatments with allegiance ratings of 5, as compared to ratings of 2 for the cognitive therapies. This corresponds with the trend found for all such allegiant samples in that the effect size more strongly favors dynamic therapy (0.3).

4. Comparing the seven studies of pharmacotherapy with psychotherapy, Blackburn et al. (1981) evidenced the greatest allegiance difference with ratings of 4.6 for psychotherapy and 2.1 for pharmacotherapy. As seen in previous comparisons, the treatment to which researchers were most allegiant also showed the greatest effect on outcome (effect size = .43). Across the seven studies psychotherapy was more effective than pharmacotherapy with an effect size of 0.2.

Summary of Measures

When assessing a theoretical construct such as allegiance, it is appropriate to use multiple measures of the construct to demonstrate its validity and reliability. To this end, we used three measures of allegiance: reprint ratings, self-ratings, and ratings by knowledgeable colleagues. Although a sizeable correlation was found between self-ratings of allegiance and colleagues' allegiance ratings of the first and second authors across different therapies ($r = .48, p < .01$), reprint ratings of allegiance were not significantly correlated with self-ratings ($r = .10, p < .05$) and were minimally correlated with colleague ratings ($r = .37, p < .05$). Moreover, colleagues' ratings of allegiance and researchers' self-ratings of allegiance were highly correlated with the effect size of treatment outcomes ($r = .73$ and $.68$, respectively, $ps < .001$).

Furthermore, combining the three measures of allegiance offers a more dramatic demonstration of the influence of researcher allegiance on outcome. Mean ratings of allegiance correlated $.85$ with the outcome of the 29 treatment comparisons. What this means is that nearly two thirds of the variability in treatment outcome was due to theoretical allegiance. This finding suggests that the usual comparison of psychotherapies without regard to researcher allegiance has limited validity.

Effect Sizes

Allegiance ratings based on the reprint, self-, and colleague measures were all conducted on comparative treatment studies that yielded small effect sizes. The largest effect, that between pharmacotherapy and psychotherapy, had an effect size of about 0.2, which, though small, was the most sizeable of all comparisons (the largest effect size for these psychotherapy comparisons was that between cognitive and behavioral treatments, ES = 0.1). Thus, it is not surprising that the correction for allegiance resulted in only slight changes in the effect size. For example, the effect size for cognitive versus behavioral treatments was 0.102. When corrected for allegiance using the reprint measure, the effect size was still only 0.107. Using the self-ratings of allegiance, the corrected effect size was 0.076, and for the colleague ratings the effect size was 0.15.

OTHER STUDIES OF THEORETICAL ALLEGIANCE

For this position paper, we not only wanted to determine if more recent studies of allegiance had been done but also to determine whether any comparative treatment trials conducted since Luborsky et al.'s (1999) review had taken researcher allegiance into account either in their design or by an assessment of allegiance. We identified seven meta-analyses (Babcock, Green, & Robie, 2004; Casacalenda, Perry, & Looper, 2002; DiGuiseppe & Tafrate, 2003; Elliott, Greenberg, & Lietaer, 2003; Ghahramanlou, 2003; Prendergast, Podus, Chang, & Urada, 2002; Wampold, Minami, Baskin, & Tierney, 2002) and 14 comparative trials of psychotherapy or psychotherapy and pharmacotherapy (Agras, Walsh, Fairburn, Wilson, & Kraemer, 2000; Browne et al., 2002; Hirschfeld et al., 2002; Ironson, Freund, Strauss, & Williams, 2002; Keller et al., 2000; Largo-Marsh & Spates, 2002; Maxfield & Hyer, 2002; Otto et al. 2000; Szapocznik et al., 2004; Thase et al., 2000; Thompson, Coon, Gallagher-Thompson, Sommer, & Koin, 2001; Warner et al., 2001; Watson, Gordon, Stermac, Kalogerakos, & Steckley, 2003; Wilfley et al., 2002) that met the criteria used in the previous review (see Luborsky et al.,

1999). Despite the degree to which researcher allegiance was acknowledged to be an important factor in determining the "true" effectiveness of a treatment (see Hollon, 1999; Jacobson, 1999; Lambert, 1999; Shaw, 1999; Shoham & Rohrbaugh, 1999; Thase, 1999b), only 4 of the 21 studies reviewed addressed the influence of researcher allegiance (Elliott, Greenberg, & Lietaer, 2003; Ghahramanlou, 2003; Prendergast et al., 2002; Watson et al., 2003).

Elliott and colleagues (2003) conducted what has been by far the most comprehensive assessment of allegiance effects since that of Luborsky, et al (1999). They conducted a meta-analytic review of 79 controlled studies in which at least one of the treatments was an experiential therapy (humanistic, person-centered, Gestalt, emotion-focused). Although a difference between treatments was initially found (favoring nonexperiential therapies), once researcher allegiance was taken into account, experiential therapies were found to be equally effective as the treatments to which they were compared.

Although not correcting for allegiance effects, two studies alluded to the influence of researcher allegiance in the data analysis. Whether examining the outcome of various treatments for drug abuse (Prendergast et al., 2002) or cognitive–behavioral therapy for anxiety disorders (Ghahramanlou, 2003), larger outcome effect sizes were associated with greater researcher allegiance. It should be noted, however, that in the Prendergast study allegiance ratings were based only on the articles included in the review (no reprint, self-, or colleague ratings).

Despite the number of ways allegiance can be accounted for in the design of a study (Luborsky et al., 1999), only one such study was found (Watson et al., 2003). Comparing a cognitive–behavioral psychotherapy with a process–experiential approach, Watson and colleagues sought to control for allegiance effects by balancing the number of researchers adhering to a process–experiential approach with those holding a more cognitive–behavioral position. Moreover, experts in each therapy conducted the training of therapists, and all therapists were adherents of the treatment they provided. Consistent with findings from meta-analyses that controlled for allegiance (e.g., Elliott et al., 2003; Luborsky et al., 1999; Luborsky et al., 2002; Robinson et al., 1990), Watson and colleagues found the two treatments generally equivalent in outcome.

Although few studies have addressed the influence of allegiance on treatment outcome, researchers have continued to comment on the problem. For instance, in a clinical trial of pharmacotherapy versus cognitive–behavioral therapy for depression in men (Thase et al., 2000), the potential influence of researcher allegiance on outcome was discussed, and the authors acknowledged their bias toward cognitive–behavioral therapy, despite the greater effect for pharmacotherapy. Shapiro and Paley (2002) offered a lengthy discussion about the "equivalent outcomes paradox" and researcher allegiance, particularly as it relates to psychotherapeutic treatments for schizophrenia. They argue that in this age of evidence-based practice (EBP), clinical trials must consider numerous methodological challenges, of which researcher allegiance is a part. In an earlier commentary, Jacobson and Hollon (1996) discussed ways to control for allegiance in multisite comparative trials, namely that researchers with allegiance to both treatments be included at each site.

Summarizing these more recent findings, we find that the conclusions of Luborsky et al. (1999, 2002) remain: (a) researcher allegiance is associated with treatment outcomes, although the effect is variable; (b) controls for allegiance can be included in study designs; (c) the most accurate assessment of allegiance resides in a threefold approach that incorporates ratings of reprints, self-ratings, and colleague ratings; and most importantly (d) nearly two thirds of the variance in reported outcome differences among therapies is due to researchers' own theoretical allegiances. Thus, evidence from comparative trials can be most informative when the allegiance of all participating researchers is taken into account.

CONCLUSIONS

In sum, these results provide strong evidence for the importance of researcher theoretical allegiance as a factor influencing treatment outcome and thus what is promulgated as evidence. Not only has allegiance shown a strong association with outcome but in many studies it equalizes treatment differences when taken into account. Despite this evidence, few clinical trials assessed theoretical allegiance in their analysis prior to the 1999 Luborsky et al. study. We therefore looked at all the comparative psychotherapy and psychotherapy versus pharmacotherapy studies conducted in the last few years. Surprisingly, there continues to be little evidence that researchers account for the moderating effect of their theoretical allegiance when analyzing comparative treatment trials.

A multifaceted approach to rating researcher allegiance yields a more precise assessment than that of the reprint method previously advocated. In other words, combining ratings of reprints with ratings by colleagues and self is a more accurate method for assessing the influence of allegiance on outcome than relying solely on reprints. One caveat to consider is that in most comparative studies the differences in outcome among treatments is quite small. In fact, the smaller the effect size, the less of an effect allegiance is likely to have on the resulting outcomes. However, allegiance remains a powerful influence on outcome accounting for nearly two thirds of the variance.

For the practitioner, theoretical allegiance represents a special consideration in evaluating evidenced-based research. Although not directly affecting the practice of psychotherapy, clinicians need to recognize the potential moderating effect of allegiance on treatment outcomes. The issues to consider when evaluating the degree of allegiance in a study include the following: (a) Is there a balance of researchers with allegiance to each treatment comparison? (b) Have the results been corrected for researcher allegiance? (c) Are therapists experienced in the treatment provided and supervised by experts apart from the researchers? (d) How similar are the allegiances of each researcher?

Whether or not a study directly acknowledges the role of allegiance, and most studies do not, our findings suggest that allegiance is an important factor in comparative trials and can influence treatment outcome.

Impact of Funding Source on Published Research

David O. Antonuccio and Deacon Shoenberger

Science is not just a matter of collecting data and seeing where the chips fall. The interests of the funding source often shape the questions that are asked and the data that are highlighted. This position paper addresses the question "What materially influences what is represented and published as evidence?" by reviewing the evidence for the powerful effect of funding sources.

One of the most powerful funding sources in the science of mental health is the pharmaceutical industry. The extensive financial reach of the drug industry has created conflicts of interest that have undermined the evidence base on which we rely to guide clinical practice (Antonuccio, Danton, & McClanahan, 2003). Although we also acknowledge the importance of nonfinancial (e.g., interest in career advancement) conflicts of interest (Levinsky, 2002), we have narrowed the scope of this paper to address the financial conflicts of interest related to the drug industry, because they are more easily measurable, voluntary, and often unrecognized unless disclosed (Bekelman, Li, & Gross, 2003).

The pharmaceutical industry has contributed to many innovations in medicine that have been healing (e.g., antibiotics for infections and chemotherapy for certain cancers), life enhancing (e.g., anesthesia and other medication for pain), and life extending (e.g., insulin for diabetes and thrombolytic therapies for vascular disease). Partly as a result of this success, the industry generated more than $400 billion in annual revenue worldwide in 2002 according to pharmaceutical consulting firm IMS Health, with the United States accounting for about one third of all pharmaceutical sales (Louie, 2001). It is America's most profitable industry in terms of return on revenues, return on assets, and return on equity (*Fortune*, 2000). From a business perspective, it is arguably the most successful industry in the world.

Although many lives are saved by pharmaceutical innovations, many lives are also put at risk. For example, it has been estimated that as many as 100,000 hospitalized patients die each year in the United States from adverse prescription drug reactions (Lazarou, Pemeranz, & Corey, 1998). In an ambulatory clinical setting, adverse drug events are common and often preventable (Gandhi et al., 2003), especially among elderly patients (Gurwitz et al., 2003; Juurlink et al., 2003). Some harmful reactions cannot be foreseen because the medications are only tested on an average of 3,000 people prior to approval, causing a reliance on postmarketing data to identify less common reactions (Friedman, 2002). Up to 20% of approved drugs subsequently require a new black box warning about life-threatening drug reactions or are withdrawn from the market (Lasser et al., 2002). Such medications can generate substantial revenue before being withdrawn. For example, seven potentially lethal drugs (among them the diet pill Redux and the diabetes medication Rezulin) generated more than $5 billion in sales revenue before they were ultimately withdrawn from the market between 1997 and 2000 (Willman, 2000).

TARGETING SCIENTISTS

It is difficult to think of any arena involving information about medications that does not have significant industry financial or marketing influences. Industry financial ties extend to federal regulatory agencies, professional organizations, continuing medical education, researchers, media experts, and consumer advocacy organizations (Antonuccio et al., 2003). Such widespread corporate interests may contribute to self-selecting academic oligarchies and to narrowing the range of acceptable clinical and scientific inquiry (Fava, 1998; Marks et al., 1993b). This can lead to legal, professional, or even personal attacks, directly or indirectly financed by the industry for those who deliver information or produce data that conflict with corporate interests (e.g., Boseley, 2002; Deyo, Psaty, Simon, Wagner, & Omenn, 1997; Healy, 2002; Marks et al., 1993b; Monbiot, 2002; Nathan & Weatherall, 2002; Rennie, 1997).

As one example, Marks and colleagues (1993a) conducted one of the most carefully designed and executed studies ever done on the treatment of panic disorder with agoraphobia. Initially, Upjohn, the maker of Xanax (alprazolam) supported the design, execution, analysis, and quality assurance of this multisite study comparing (a) alprazolam plus exposure, (b) alprazolam plus relaxation (psychological placebo), (c) placebo plus exposure, and (d) placebo plus relaxation (double placebo). At some point it was discovered that the results were going to favor exposure plus relaxation and that the alprazolam actually seemed to interfere with the treatment outcome. Marks et al. (1993b, p. 792) wrote that "monitoring and support stopped abruptly when the results became known. Thereafter, Upjohn's response was to invite professionals to critique the study they had nurtured so carefully before. The study is a classic demonstration of the hazards of research funded by industry."

Another troubling example of constraints on academic freedom in psychiatry involved psychiatrist David Healy, who publicly presented data linking Selective Serotonin Reuptake Inhibitors (SSRIs) to an increased risk for suicidal behavior in a subset of susceptible patients (Healy, 2002, 2003). This resulted in the rescission by the university of an already accepted job offer for him to head a depression research unit at the University of Toronto. This led to an outpouring of support for Healy from other scientists around the world (Axelrod et al., 2001) and a lawsuit filed by Healy for breach of contract, libel, and a first-ever suit for breach of academic freedom. The suit was resolved by representatives of the university clarifying what had happened and responding to the issues of libel and breach of academic freedom by making Healy a visiting professor. At the heart of what had happened were representations to the university by academics with close contacts with the industry. In such an environment, large doses of integrity, courage, and stamina may be required if one decides to present data that conflict with corporate interests.

CONFLICTS OF INTEREST IN RESEARCH

Widely acknowledged publication biases (e.g., Blumenthal, Campbell, Anderson, Causino, & Louis, 1997; Callaham, Wears, Weber, Barton, & Young, 1998; Chalmers, 2000; Gilbody & Song, 2000; Krzyzanowska, Pintilie, & Tannock, 2003; Lexchin, Bero, Djulbegovic, & Clark, 2003; Misakian & Bero, 1998; Rennie, 1999; *The Lancet*, 2001; Wise & Drury, 1996) are often related to conflicts of interest (Campbell, Louis, & Blumenthal, 1998; Cech & Leonard, 2001; Chopra, 2003; DeAngelis, Fontanarosa, & Flanagin, 2001; Fava, 2001; Lo, Wolf, & Berkeley, 2000) that favor pharmaceutical industry products (Als-Nielsen, Chen, Gluud, & Kjaergard, 2003; Bekelman et al., 2003). In fact, these biases have so eroded the credibility of the medical literature (Quick, 2001), including the psychiatry literature (e.g., Torrey, 2002), that recent proposals call for stringent accountability guidelines (e.g., Davidoff et al., 2001; Moses & Martin, 2001) to ensure researcher independence in study design, access to data, and right to publish. So far, American medical schools have demonstrated minimal adherence to the standards embodied by these guidelines (Schulman et al., 2002).

Data may be withheld or delayed if they reflect unfavorably on the sponsor's products (Blumenthal et al., 1997). For example, the publication of data (from a study sponsored by a nicotine patch manufacturer) showing a nicotine patch to be ineffective without behavioral counseling (Joseph & Antonuccio, 1999) was delayed for several years after favorable safety data from the same study were published (Joseph et al., 1996), which is not an isolated delay in the nicotine replacement literature (Vergano, 2001).

In the antidepressant literature, an indirect estimate of publication bias is possible by examining the Food and Drug Administration (FDA) antidepressant database for medications in the initial approval process when all data from every study must be submitted, whether the study is ultimately published or not. Several independent analyses of the FDA antidepressant database have shown that study medications had a significant advantage over inert placebos in less than half (as few as 43%) of randomized controlled trials (RCTs; Khan, Khan, & Brown, 2002; Kirsch, Moore, Scoboria, & Nicholls, 2002; Laughren, 2001). In the published literature, antidepressants are significantly more effective than inert placebos in about two thirds of the studies (Thase, 1999a). Such a pattern would be consistent with a failure to publish results from as many as 35% of the antidepressant trials (mostly those showing no advantage to the antidepressant), which is somewhat higher than previous estimates of up to 20% (Gram, 1994). The discrepancy between the FDA database and the published literature may also reflect duplicate publication, selective publication, or selective reporting as has recently been found in SSRI studies submitted to the Swedish drug regulatory authority (Melander, Ahlqvist-Rastad, Meijer, & Beermann, 2003).

Roughly one quarter of biomedical investigators have industry affiliations, and roughly two thirds of academic institutions hold equity in startup companies that sponsor research at the same institutions (Bekelman et al., 2003). Although most clinical researchers recognize the risks associated with conflicts of interest, they tend to feel that they are not personally at risk (Boyd, Cho, & Bero, 2003). One study (Krimsky, Rothenberg, Stott, & Kyle, 1998) examined research conducted by 1,000 Massachusetts scientists who were lead authors on articles published in major scientific and medical journals during 1992. The report concluded that more than a third of the articles had lead authors with a financial interest in the research (defined as investment in a related patent, on a scientific advisory board of a related biotechnology company, or serving as an officer or major shareholder in a commercially related firm), even without considering honoraria and consultancies. Another study (Choudhry, Stelfox, & Detsky, 2002) found that the vast majority of authors of clinical practice guidelines had financial relationships (mostly undisclosed in the guidelines) with companies whose drugs were considered in the guidelines. Even leading bioethicists, whose objectivity is crucial to their role as ethical watchdogs, have developed financial conflicts in the form of consulting fees, contracts, honoraria, and salaries from the drug industry (Elliot, 2001). Conflicts of interest can occur at the level of the individual scientist or at the level of the academic institution itself, resulting in calls for divestiture and oversight by an independent review panel (e.g., Johns, Barnes, & Florencio, 2003).

Some top journals require the disclosure of financial conflicts of interest. For example, the *New England Journal of Medicine* revealed that 11 of the 12 authors of an article about the efficacy of nefazadone and behavior analytic therapy (Keller et al., 2000) had financial ties to Bristol Myers Squibb, the drug's manufacturer. In fact, the authors' ties with companies that make antidepressant medications were so extensive that it was decided to summarize them on the journal's Web site rather than take up journal space to detail them fully (Angell, 2000). The journal even had trouble finding psychiatric researchers who met their standard of independence from manufacturers of antidepressants to write an accompanying editorial (Angell). In fact, because the editors of the *New England Journal of Medicine* concluded that they could not find enough experts without financial ties to the drug industry, the journal soon thereafter relaxed its strict policy against financial conflicts of interest by editorial and review authors (Drazen & Curfman, 2002), bringing it in line with most other medical journals. This example gives a clear indication of just how pervasive the industry ties are. This is a challenging and important issue, because it has long been established that public relations firms for major drug companies are willing to pay professionals to write articles, such as editorials designed to favor their clients' products (Brennan, 1994).

Industry support has shifted from academic medical centers to private research companies called contract research organizations (CROs) and site–management organizations (SMOs), both of which have grown tremendously in recent years (Bodenheimer, 2000). In 1991, 80% of industry money for clinical trials went to academic medical centers; in 1998, only 40% went there (Bodenheimer).

Subtle biases in industry-funded research may influence the results that are produced (Bodenheimer, 2000; Safer, 2002). Drug company marketing departments may rule out funding studies that might reduce sales of their products. The companies may design studies likely to favor their products. A new medication may be tested on a population who is healthier than those who will actually receive the drug, or a new medication may be compared with an insufficient or excessive dose of an older one. Clinical trials may use surrogate end points or "markers" instead of clinical end points (e.g., measuring blood pressure as a surrogate for heart attacks or measuring suicidal ideation as a surrogate for suicidal behavior) or certain data analysis strategies (e.g., the last observation carried forward instead of observed cases; see Kirsch et al., 2002) to get the most favorable outcome. A recent meta-analysis found that 61% of the trials funded solely by the industry had major discrepancies between the primary outcomes specified in the protocols and those defined in the published articles, suggesting an effort to "cherry pick" the most favorable results, a scientifically unsound practice (Chan,

Hrobjartsson, Haahr, Gotzsche, & Altman, 2004). In drug company studies, investigators may receive only portions of the data. In fact, industry sponsorship has been associated with restrictions on publication and data sharing (Bekelman et al., 2003). Drug companies have even been hiring advertising companies that are buying or investing in other companies that perform clinical trials of experimental drugs in an attempt to get "closer to the test tube" (Petersen, 2002).

Several other questionable practices can bias the scientific literature toward products favored by the marketing departments of such companies (Bodenheimer, 2000). Professional medical writers (ghostwriters) are often paid by a drug company to write an article but not be named as an author. Sometimes a clinical investigator (guest author) will appear as an author of a paper on which they did not contribute or analyze the original data (Bates, Anic, Marusic, & Marusic, 2004). This practice can be akin to a celebrity endorsement of a product or idea and might be more appropriately considered advertising than science. In one study, 19% of the articles had guest authors who did not sufficiently contribute (did not help conceive the study, analyze the data, or contribute to the writing), and 11% had ghostwriters who were not named as authors (Flanagin et al., 1998). Healy (2001) estimated that up to 50% of the review articles about new drugs in respectable Medline journals appear as supplements (i.e., are not adequately peer reviewed), are ghostwritten, or are written by company personnel. Such supplements and reprints of actual articles can be a rich source of revenue for scientific journals. Sometimes an apparently independent journal can have strong undisclosed editorial ties to the industry that can influence the content and emphasis of articles that appear in the journal (Letter to Academic Press, 2002). One study found that in journals with policies calling for disclosure of conflicts of interest, only 0.5% of the authors made such disclosure (Krimsky & Rothenberg, 2001), most likely reflecting a poor compliance with such policies. As yet, not enough data exist to evaluate the impact of ghost writing on the literature. However, because the ghostwriters generally work for the marketing departments of the drug companies themselves, it is probable that the articles may selectively report data that favor the manufacturer's product (Healy & Catell, 2003).

POTENTIAL METHODOLOGICAL BIASES

Recent methodological analyses of RCTs suggest that design flaws and reporting omissions are associated with biased estimates of the treatment outcome (Moher, Schulz, & Altman, 2001). This has led to the publication of the Consolidated Standards of Reporting Trials (CONSORT) statement, developed by an international group of clinical trial specialists, statisticians, epidemiologists, and biomedical editors (Moher et al., 2001). The CON-

SORT statement, adopted by many leading medical journals, specifies the design and reporting standards for selection criteria, intervention details, randomization, blinding procedures, and intent-to-treat analyses in randomized trials.

Some of the methodological biases are subtle and woven into the fabric of study design. For example, in antidepressant research it is common to use a "placebo washout" procedure prior to randomization (Antonuccio, Danton, DeNelsky, Greenberg, & Gordon, 1999). This procedure typically involves a 1- to 2-week single blind trial during which all prospective subjects are placed on a placebo. Any patients who improve during this washout period are excluded from the study before randomization. Such a procedure may subtly favor the drug condition by, among other things, eliminating placebo responders before the study even starts (Antonuccio, Burns, & Danton, 2002).

The double blind in antidepressant studies is likely to be unintentionally penetrated due to the pattern of side effects in the active and inactive drug conditions (Greenberg & Fisher, 1997; White, Kando, Park, Waternaux, & Brown, 1992). Research clinicians routinely educate themselves and patients about potential side effects as part of the standard informed consent process. Further, these studies tend to rely on measures by clinicians who often have a major allegiance or stake in the outcome, resulting in larger differences than with patient-rated measures (Greenberg, Bornstein, Greenberg, & Fisher, 1992; Moncrieff, 2001). Efforts to ensure the integrity of the blind tend to diminish estimates of drug efficacy. For example, a review of the Cochrane database of antidepressant studies using "active" placebos (i.e., placebos with side effects, making side effect differences more difficult to detect) found very small or nonsignificant outcome differences, suggesting that trials using inert placebos may overestimate drug effects (Moncrieff, Wessely, & Hardy, 2001).

Also, antidepressant studies do not adequately evaluate the efficacy of medication alone because most of these studies allow the prescription of a sedative (Kirsch et al., 2002; Walsh, Seidman, Sysko, & Gould, 2002). If patients in the drug condition are most likely to take sedatives or antidepressants with sedative properties, this could distort the results because at least 6 points on the Hamilton Depression Rating Scale favor medications with sedative properties (Moncrieff, 2001). Many of these studies provide concurrent supportive psychotherapy, giving a distorted picture of the effectiveness of these medications in a typical managed primary care environment where mental health support may be offered on a more limited basis or even not at all (Antonuccio et al., 2002).

Klein (2000) and Quitkin (1999) argued that, because antidepressants have been established as effective in the treatment of depression, trials that do not find a statistical advantage of antidepressants over placebos lack "assay sensitivity" (the ability to detect specific treatment effects). In other words, they argue that something is wrong with the sampling or methodology of such trials, and the results should be discounted or discarded. If that logic had been applied to the recent meta-analysis of the FDA antidepressant database (Kirsch et al., 2002), more than half the studies would have been discarded, a strategy that would have seriously distorted the overall results (Antonuccio et al., 2002; Otto & Nierenberg, 2002).

RESEARCH SAFEGUARDS

At a minimum, reports of all drug treatment trials should conform to the CONSORT guidelines (Moher et al., 2001). The following requirements are designed to complement those standards.

1. All initiated clinical trials should be listed in a public registry such as the Current Controlled Trials Meta-Register as a condition for Institutional Review Board approval or publication (DeAngelis et al., 2004; Dickersin & Rennie, 2003). This will ensure that all initiated trials are a matter of public record and reduce the probability of data suppression.

2. All studies claiming double blind status should test and report whether the blind was penetrated to pass peer review for a mental health journal (Piasecki, Antonuccio, Steinagel, & Kohlenberg, 2002). This could be done by asking research subjects and clinicians to attempt to identify the actual treatment condition while analyzing the impact of accurate identification on outcome. A simple blindness assessment and protection checklist has been established to help facilitate this process (Even, Siobud-Dorocant, & Dardennes, 2000).

3. No patients should be excluded from any study on the basis of improvement during placebo washout (see Antonuccio et al., 2002)

4. All studies should include patient-rated self-report measures in addition to clinician-rated measures.

5. The use of any concurrent medication or concurrent treatment of any kind should be specified in the analysis and abstract of all RCTs.

6. All raw data for any study published in a mental health journal should be made available on a publicly accessible Web site, allowing for independent review of the data and data analysis (Bekelman et al., 2003; Klein et al., 2002). The data would be stripped of any patient-identifying information.

7. Research protocols should be made available to journal reviewers and be published online concurrently with the publication

of all outcome studies to ensure congruence between planned analyses and published analyses.

8. Research contracts should explicitly exclude industry control of publication or data ownership (Schulman et al., 2002) in order for a study to qualify for publication in a mental health journal. All authors should offer signed assurance that they had independent access to all data and contributed to the writing of any manuscript for any published study.

CONCLUSIONS

Conflicts of interest in research due to funding sources lead to probable biases in the production and publication of scientific data. These biases can distort the evidence base that clinicians use to determine best practices. The "evidence" is not pure science; rather it is part science and part marketing. This situation is quite often analogous to buying a car but relying only on information provided by the dealer to make the decision. Smart buyers also look for independent sources of data. Although the focus of this position paper was on drug treatment, similar influences are also probably operating in the production and publication of scientific data on psychological assessments and psychotherapy as well. We need to keep these lessons in mind when we interpret what is dispassionately purported to be the best evidence in a field.

A Poor Fit Between Empirically Supported Treatments and Psychotherapy Integration

George Stricker

Definitions of what constitutes evidence, and therefore which treatments are likely to receive the endorsement of science, vary as a function of the group constructing the list (Chambless & Ollendick, 2001). The gold standard for most of the groups is the presence of at least two RCTs with either a credible placebo or an alternative treatment as a control factor. The crucial question is whether this standard is the uniformly highest form of evidence that can be presented for every approach to treatment or if it is differentially suitable for some psychotherapy approaches. The position that I will put forward in this paper is that the extant evidence-based compilations have unnecessarily privileged manualized, outcome-oriented, pure-form therapies to the detriment of more flexible and more widely practiced integrative–eclectic therapies.

Even among pure-form treatments, it is important to distinguish between the outcome-oriented and process-oriented approaches to psychotherapy (Gold, 1995). The outcome-oriented approaches include the behavioral and cognitive orientations for the most part, and they focus on precise interventions as they relate to specific and defined outcome variables. Clearly, they are well suited to the RCT format and indeed emerge as dominant on most evidence-based lists. The process-oriented approaches include the psychodynamic and humanistic orientations as well as integrative–eclectic efforts for the most part, and they focus on inner states and interpersonal relationships. Outcome variables for these approaches are most likely to refer to quality of life, self-experience, and awareness. These are much more difficult to quantify, both as to the intervention and the outcome, and so they tend to be underrepresented on conventional lists.

Outcome-oriented treatments almost always have symptom reduction as the primary dependent variable (this is not necessary, but it is usually the case). However, many of the process-oriented approaches, including most of the integrative approaches, do not focus exclusively on symptom reduction, and many patients do not enter psychotherapy with an eye toward such change. Relationship conflicts, patterns of relating, and quality of life also bring patients to treatment, and the value of that treatment is not captured by a research study that does not evaluate change on these dimensions. Once again, this is a methodological dimension that favors one approach to treatment at the expense of another. However, a choice does not have to be made, and a full appreciation of the multiplicity of the therapeutic endeavor is best approached by a range of dependent variables, perhaps tailored to the individual goals of the specific treatment.

INTEGRATIVE PSYCHOTHERAPIES

Although the pure-form orientations are easily classified, the plurality of psychotherapists ascribes to an integrative or eclectic orientation, and their practice is not as simple to characterize. According to a recent survey of members of the APA Society of Clinical Psychology (Santoro, Lister, Karpiak, & Norcross, 2004), 29% of the respondents consider their theoretical orientation to be eclectic–integrative, and this is consistent with the results of a series of studies with a similar sample over the years, almost all of which found the percentage of integrative–eclectic respondents to range between one quarter and one third. An earlier study (Milan, Montgomery, & Rogers, 1994) based on psychologists listed in the National Register of Health Service Providers found that the largest single grouping, 39%, listed eclectic as their primary theoretical orientation. This percentage hovered about 40% for the decade preceding this listing. Furthermore, approximately 90% of the registrants listed more than one orientation, an indication that practice according to strict adherence to a single orientation is rare. In a summary of 11 surveys completed in the past decade (Norcross, in press), practitioners who identify as integrative or eclectic ranged from 7% (in Australia) to 42% (in Britain), with a median of about a third.

The question then must be raised as to the transportability of the empirically supported treatment (EST) findings to the world of practice. Although clearly delineated and narrowly defined interventions may be presented on EST lists, most practitioners are unlikely to base their practice on this narrow list, even though they are well advised to include these in their armamentarium when relevant. Instead, practitioners are more likely to pick and choose, using some techniques because of compelling evidentiary data, some because of favorable past clinical experience, some because of theoretical allegiance, and some because of personal preference. The evaluation of treatment constructed in such a manner is a heady task.

The term *eclectic* varies in meaning and can range from having a clear rationale for the choice of a variety of interventions to a generally uninformed choice on the basis of personal predilection with little in the way of research support. In contrast, psychotherapy integration has a more specific, if varied, meaning and is usually rooted in a theoretical understanding of the person and the treatment. Four different approaches to psychotherapy integration have been identified (Stricker & Gold, 2003): technical eclecticism, common factors, theoretical integration, and assimilative integration. In reviewing these, it also would behoove us to examine the implications of ESTs for each of these.

Technical eclecticism is the approach to psychotherapy integration that is closest to what traditionally has been called eclecticism. It is relatively free of theory, but not of systematic coherence in its best versions (Beutler & Harwood, 2000; Lazarus, 1981). This approach chooses freely among techniques, using whatever, in the judgment and experience of the practitioner, would best serve the interests of the patient. Generally, such an individualistic approach to interventions cannot be reduced to a manual and therefore would not be assessed properly by an RCT. Although some systematic attempts have been made to document the effectiveness of technically eclectic approaches (e.g., Beutler, Moliero, & Talebi, 2002), these, as with many RCTs, require such a specification of eligible patients that generalizability may be compromised. For example, if RCTs were required to show efficacy, the multimodal therapy of Lazarus would fall by the wayside (Schottenbauer, Glass, & Arnkoff, in press).

The common factors approach (Frank, 1973) begins by identifying those aspects of therapy that are shared by almost every orientation (e.g., developing a relationship and instilling hope). The treatment is based on some combination of these generally effective factors, and the importance of specific techniques is minimized. Specific techniques, of course, are the focus of ESTs, so that it is unlikely that proponents of common factors will be well served by the movement toward developing these lists.

Theoretical integration is a complex and sophisticated approach to psychotherapy integration. It involves the integration of several theories, producing a hybrid that takes more factors into account than any single approach does. Practitioners have made a great many attempts at theoretical integration, beginning with a landmark work (Wachtel, 1977) that provided the impetus for much of the contemporary integrative movement, and an effort that shows little RCT support (Schottenbauer et al., in press). Most of the attempts at theoretical integration can be classified as process-oriented and, as such, focus on internal processes and outcome variables, making them unlikely to emerge from an RCT with an appropriate degree of endorsement. However, it should be noted that cognitive–behavior therapy (CBT; Beck, Rush, Shaw, & Emery, 1979) is a theoretically integrated treatment, combining cognitive factors with more traditional behavioral approaches. CBT, of course, dominates most lists of ESTs (Chambless & Ollendick, 2001) and is the exception to the rule that psychotherapy integration suffers as a result of the movement toward ESTs.

Finally, assimilative integration (Messer, 1992) is the most recent addition to the collection of integrative approaches. Here a single, central theoretical orientation is maintained, but techniques generated by other orientations are assimilated as needed to facilitate progress in the patient (Stricker & Gold, 1996, 2002). Many of the examples of assimilative integration are process oriented, and each retains an individualistic character, with techniques being assimilated as needed, so manualization is unlikely.

This brief summary of the approaches to psychotherapy integration makes it clear that integration, although endorsed by a significant number of practitioners and probably practiced by a majority, is unlikely to receive strong representation on EST lists, with the significant exception of CBT. This is because ESTs focus on specific techniques that can be reduced to a manual and be assessed in an RCT, with a specific behavioral outcome goal delineated. Despite my preference for an integrative approach, it would be folly for any responsible psychotherapist to ignore the findings of sound research. It is often necessary to practice without specific knowledge, but it is unethical to ignore contradictory data (Stricker, 1992).

The critical issue, then, is not whether research should inform practice to the greatest extent possible, which is a proposition that hardly seems debatable. Rather, the concern is the types of psychotherapy (practice and research) that are privileged by the current preferred research methodology. The answer, in my view, is that multiple approaches to psychotherapy are desirable. Moreover, any answer that emphasizes a single theoretical approach is bound to be overly simplistic and limited.

ASSUMPTIONS OF THE RCT

The RCT is an elegant design in which patients are randomly assigned to different treatments, and then differences in outcome are measured. The design allows for conclusions as to differential efficacy among the treatments and, because of the randomization, it avoids many of the problems that occur in a more naturalistic research approach. The various stages of this design are (a) the random assignment of selected patients; (b) different treatments, usually manual based; and (c) outcome measurement. I would like to look at the implications of each of these for the assessment of the impact of psychotherapy integration.

Random assignment is a process that trades veridicality for precision. In the typical clinical situation, patients are not assigned randomly to therapists. They choose their therapist and, by doing so, assume some measure of expectation and hope for their chosen healer. Furthermore, in the clinical situation, they are not selected carefully. Rather, with exceptions dictated by the boundaries of competence of the practitioner, all patients are seen. The problem this creates, however, does not differentially affect the integrative–eclectic therapies. The problems of generalizability are common to any treatment, regardless of the orientation of the practitioner, and so this is not a dimension that prejudices the integrative–eclectic style.

The assignment to different treatments is a critical matter. The assumptions of this step are that treatments are more different than similar, and that there is value in accentuating the differences rather than the similarities. This is precisely the opposite of the foundation of psychotherapy integration, which recognizes and values the extent to which treatments are similar, either because of common factors or by the means of combining treatments. Furthermore, treatments fare best in RCTs if they can be reduced to a manual. This is an interesting step, and the manual may be a solution to a problem that does not exist. Initially, psychotherapy research compared treatments by having people of declared orientations serve as therapists. It was quite correctly noted that what people say they do may differ from what they actually do, and to compare Treatment X with Treatment Y, it would be necessary to do a validity check and ensure that Treatments X and Y were being implemented. This led to the construction of manuals that would prove true to the orientation being described and allow for neatly demarcated distinctions between the therapies. However, it would have equally been possible, and more profitable, if the correct recognition of the problem had led to the conclusion that Treatments X and Y do not exist as pure forms when actually implemented by practitioners, and the focus should shift to treatment as practiced, with an emphasis on the integrative and eclectic.

An assumption underlying the comparison of different interventions, as embodied by a pure-form orientation, is that the interventional technique per se is the mutative factor. However, it is not unusual for investigators to find that specific techniques account for only 10% to 15% of the relevant variance in psychotherapeutic change (Norcross, in press) and that common factors, patient variables, and relationship variables, none of which ordinarily are captured in manuals, are more powerful. Even more interestingly, a well-regarded and specific set of techniques that have been found to be effective, such as CBT, may not have the effect on the basis of the techniques after all. For example, the reduction in depression attributed to CBT occurred prior to the introduction of specific cognitive techniques and is likely to be due in large part to common factors (Ilardi & Craighead, 1994). The less important specific techniques are, the less valuable manuals and RCTs will be, and consequently the more we need to recognize that EBP can be compatible with a greater breadth of approaches to psychotherapy, both integrative–eclectic and pure-form but process-oriented.

Although RCTs focus on techniques, a major source of change is due to the therapeutic relationship. A task force established by APA Division 29 (Psychotherapy; Norcross, 2002) developed an effort parallel to that of the Division of Clinical Psychology (which produced the original list of ESTs), but it emphasized the therapeutic relationship rather than the specific intervention. This group especially emphasized the therapeutic alliance, cohesion in group therapy, empathy, and goal consensus and collaboration. These are factors that are much more likely to appear in psychotherapy integration efforts than specific and isolated interventions, and research methods are needed that will do more justice to efforts emphasizing these factors. It thus appears that the investigator might do better by focusing on the similarities between treatments (the relationship and other common factors) than on the differences (specific techniques). This strategy would favor more integrative–eclectic efforts and not the pure-form approaches favored by the RCT. It also would lead to conclusions that give far more weight to the value of a greater breadth of treatment approaches.

Finally, there is the measurement of the outcome of the treatments being compared. As long as the outcome being measured is specific, the approach that develops specific focused interventions will be most likely to prevail. However, if the goals of treatment are based more on the process, with changes desired in the internal and interactional dimensions, a broader set of dependent variables will be necessary. Because the integrative–eclectic approaches tend to adopt such broader goals, they are not served well by the standard design of the RCT.

It is necessary to acknowledge that the RCT is a source of information and is not to be dismissed even by those who do not prize it as highly as the people who have constructed lists of ESTs. The RCT does provide information about the effect of a specific technique, usually administered in a brief period of time, on a specific outcome goal with a specific population of patients. For those therapists wishing to accomplish that goal with such a patient, it may be a valuable source of information. Within psychotherapy integration, the theoretically integrative CBT approach fares well when so evaluated, but many of the other approaches, particularly the process-oriented ones, are not judged appropriately by this methodology.

In a comprehensive review of the empirical status of ESTs (Westen, Morrison, & Thompson-Brenner, in press), the authors conclude that

> Any treatment that (a) requires principle-based rather than intervention-based manualization, (b) prescribes a large set of interventions from which clinicians must choose based on the material the patient presents, or (c) allows the patient to structure the session will introduce too much within-condition variability to permit the optimal use of EST designs.

Of course, much of psychotherapy integration is principle based, allows the clinician to choose from a large variety of possible interventions, and follows the lead of the patient.

Finally, the emphasis I have placed on the value of added sources of data to properly evaluate and support psychotherapy integration should not be taken to reflect a paucity of more traditional supportive data. In a recent review (Schottenbauer et al., in press), and one that does not include CBT as a type of psychotherapy integration, nine separate psychotherapy integration approaches were classified as receiving substantial empirical support, meeting a criterion of four or more RCTs, which exceeds the requirements of the initial list of ESTs (Task Force on Promotion and Dissemination of Psychological Procedures, 1995). These integrative approaches included dialectical behavior therapy, EMDR, cognitive analytic therapy, prescriptive psychotherapy, and transtheoretical therapy. In addition, 13 integrative approaches were classified as receiving some empirical support, meeting a criterion of one to three RCTs. Despite this large number of empirically supported integrative approaches, this still represents a minority of the systematic approaches to psychotherapy integration extant and does not include the myriad eclectic approaches that are not systematic and cannot be classified. Some of these studies did use specific symptom remission, such as depression and anxiety, as dependent variables, but they included a much wider variety of dependent variables, such as global functioning, life satisfaction, and metacognitive awareness, thus beginning to capture the richness of the integrative approach.

The conclusion we must reach on the basis of the narrow scope of the RCT and the resultant lists of ESTs is that these lists favor pure-form, outcome-oriented approaches at the expense of integrative–eclectic and pure-form, process-oriented approaches. Given the nature of psychotherapy as practiced, the goals that patients bring to the treatment setting, and the success achieved by therapists in the natural setting, it would behoove us to endorse approaches that are more in line with the needs of the patient and the practices of the therapist, and to develop research methodology that captures these practices.

SUMMARY

To sum up, research is universally accepted as an important building block toward an EBP. However, an overemphasis on manualized, pure-form therapies neglects integrative approaches, which constitute the modal clinical practice. An emphasis on relationships as well as techniques, on process-oriented as well as outcome-oriented approaches, and on the establishment of therapeutic principles as well as clinical techniques will likely be much more supportive of psychotherapy integration, including eclecticism. Research then will point toward the value of treatment as it actually occurs, without the pejorative implications of the current emphasis on ESTs. By doing so, the development of more integrative–eclectic approaches will be encouraged, and the evaluation of these approaches can be accomplished in a more veridical manner.

A psychotherapist who functions in an empirically informed manner will take into account the research data as they exist, but he or she will also attend to carefully documented experience, clinical theory, and any other source of knowledge that will contribute to the well-being of the patient. This therapist is functioning as a local clinical scientist (Stricker & Trierweiler, 1995; Trierweiler & Stricker, 1998), a stance that can serve as a bridge between science and practice. It is just such a bridge that psychotherapy integration promotes, and that seems far superior to erecting a dam between science and practice, something that may be the inadvertent effect of restricting prized practice to ESTs.

Dialogue: Convergence and Contention

Lester B. Luborsky and Marna S. Barrett

From the evidence presented in these position papers, it is clear that researcher allegiance to a theory, the source of study funding, and EST guidelines do represent biases that must be considered when interpreting the results from a particular study. Antonuccio and Shoenberger have offered a cogent and detailed argument concerning the degree to which conflicts of interest between a research funding source and an investigator can bias the publication or other presentation of results. Moreover, they highlight the breadth of the problem by suggesting areas of potential bias in the design, analysis, and interpretation of the research. Despite these well-reasoned arguments, it is clear that few empirical studies have directly assessed the impact of these biases on outcomes. Certainly, requiring adherence to the CONSORT guidelines as well as to the additional protections suggested by the authors will help minimize a potential funding source bias. However, if we are to effect change in this area, the evidence at hand documenting a funding source bias must be used to demonstrate empirically the degree to which such bias influences the resulting findings.

In his discussion of ESTs and their usefulness in guiding treatment, Stricker makes several points substantiating the potential bias of RCTs for manualized treatments with behavioral outcomes. We agree that the relational and intrapsychic focus of many psychodynamic, humanistic, and eclectic–integrative models make manualization difficult. However, greater difficulty in operationalization does not preclude the development of manuals for conducting RCTs of these approaches. In fact, Stricker fails to recognize that several of these approaches have already been manualized (e.g., supportive–expressive psychotherapy or a short-term dynamic therapy; Luborsky, 1984; Luborsky & Crits-Christoph, 1990; Luborsky et al., 1995) and tested in RCTs (e.g., Brom, Kleber, & Defares, 1989; Elkin et al., 1989; Gallagher & Thompson, 1982; Pierloot & Vinck, 1978; Thompson, Gallagher, & Breckenridge, 1987; Woody et al., 1983; Zitrin, Klein, & Woerner, 1978). Furthermore, most of these studies demonstrated the initial superiority of psychodynamic models over either behavioral or cognitive approaches.

Also, it should be recognized that the limited focus of RCTs on interpersonal or quality-of-life outcomes does not rule out the use of at least some behavioral measures in assessing outcome. Indeed, many of the RCTs of dynamic therapies include a behavioral outcome measure. Furthermore, as discussed in our position paper on theoretical allegiance, despite any possible biases of the RCTs towards a particular model of treatment, once researcher allegiance is considered in the analyses, initial treatment differences cease to exist. Thus, the initial superiority of one treatment over another has frequently not held up.

Despite these concerns, we agree that psychotherapy research would be advanced if research focused more on the similarities among treatments than on potential differences. Moreover, all treatment packages tested in comparative trials need to be more consistent with "real world" practices and the decision-making of therapists. They should also incorporate outcome measures assessing the key components of change within each treatment tested and should use designs that seek to control for the potential influence of theoretical allegiance.

David O. Antonuccio and Deacon Shoenberger

If you are reading this commentary, you must read a lot of books! The position paper by Luborsky and Barrett on theoretical allegiance highlighted the important relationship between theoretical allegiance and treatment outcome. It left us wondering whether the relationship might be reciprocal; that is, allegiance may drive the outcomes we see, not necessarily for nefarious reasons, but perhaps because we are likely to be better at implementing treatments we believe in. Conversely, outcome may drive allegiance, perhaps because we are prone to develop more allegiance to treatments that work particularly well for us.

Stricker has made a persuasive argument that randomized controlled designs may favor manualized treatments and encourage horse-race studies where the differences in treatment efficacy are likely to be much smaller than the nonspecific treatment effects. Small and specific treatment effects have also been found in the controlled antidepressant trials where the placebo effects (psychological effects) duplicate 82% of the drug effects (Kirsch, Moore, Scoboria, & Nicholls, 2002). It is quite likely that the specific advantages for most psychological treatments are similarly small. One possible drawback of an overemphasis on specific techniques of limited, added value is that clinical training programs may not spend enough time on general psychotherapy skills that apparently account for the vast majority of treatment effects.

One nuance not addressed by Stricker has to do with the usefulness of a placebo concept in psychological research. Kirsch (in press) has argued that to establish efficacy in psychological research, a no-treatment, waiting list, or natural history control makes more sense than a placebo control as a comparison because with a placebo control one is simply comparing more psychological treatment (the "active" psychological treatment) with less psychological treatment (the placebo). Clearly, placebos do make a great deal of sense in drug studies because the goal is to separate out the "true" drug effect from the nonspecific psychological effects. Placebos in medical research have all of the psychological characteristics of the drug condition without the chemical. Because psychotherapy has no chemical, it may be considered a placebo by definition, making a comparison with another "psychological placebo" illogical unless one is simply interested in the relative efficacy of psychological interventions.

It seems to us that allegiance, the funding source, and the small specific treatment advantages are all linked by the therapeutic alliance. Allegiance may matter in treatment studies because of the superior therapeutic alliance generated in the context of a treatment that one believes in. Through the possibility of future funding, the funding source may reinforce provider behaviors that generate a better alliance, resulting in a better treatment outcome. Finally, the powerful effects of the therapeutic alliance appear to dwarf the small, specific treatment effects found for most treatments (Martin, Garske, & Davis, 2000).

Another hidden wild card affecting our evidence base and cutting across all these topics is the apparent active suppression of unfavorable data. This has apparently occurred in the antidepressant literature (e.g., Melander, Ahlqvist-Rastad, Meijer, & Beermann, 2003) and with other pharmaceuticals (Fontanarosa, Rennie, & DeAngelis, 2004). Data suppression is not likely to be limited to the drug industry. The best hope for preserving the integrity of our science may involve total transparency by requiring that all initiated clinical trials be publicly registered and that all raw data involving human subjects be made publicly accessible.

George Stricker

There seems to be a convergence among these three seemingly different position papers. In each case, a different factor is considered that serves to compromise the body of evidence contributing to any list of ESTs. For Antonuccio and Schoenberger, the problem lies with what they see as the distortions introduced by the funding source, particularly the pharmaceutical industry. For Luborsky and Barrett, the difficulty is related to the theoretical allegiance of the investigator. I discuss the theoretical orientation of the therapist, with particular reference to the problems of integrative and eclectic psychotherapists. Despite this convergence on a higher level of abstraction, some differences exist among the presentations.

Antonuccio and Schoenberger point to the conscious and venal motives of the pharmaceutical companies that provide the funding for the research they sponsor. The research is designed and published in a manner that highlights the efficacy of the drugs they are producing to the detriment of alternative treatments, including placebos and competing drugs. The research is designed to demonstrate such efficacy, suppressed if it does not do so, and selectively presented so as to appear most favorable to the target product. To the extent that this occurs, this unquestionably is a pernicious practice, as it undercuts any semblance of science while being clothed in scientific objectivity. It strikes me as a crass and extreme example of the allegiance effect, in which the prior commitments of the investigator are related to the outcome of the study. I hope that these practices do not occur in more traditional research on psychosocial interventions, but even in those interventions, often economic and reputational factors are at issue, and these may lead to some distortions in presentation and publication.

Luborsky and Barrett directly address the more subtle manifestations of the allegiance effect. Their major finding is that the allegiance of the investigator is correlated with the outcome of the study, although it is not clear whether and how this allegiance is causal. The accumulating evidence they have gathered and inspired requires that allegiance be taken into account in interpreting the findings of psychotherapy research, and many apparent differences may wash out when the variance contributed by allegiance is controlled. Thus, and optimistically, a sound research design can remove the most obvious confounds of allegiance. The finding of an allegiance effect is consistent with my view that technique is not a major source of variance for outcome, and it pales when compared to relationship factors.

What I find most interesting about the allegiance effect is speculation about the mechanism by which it occurs. It clearly is not due to magic, and I hope we can dismiss the conscious manipulation of the data in psychosocial studies, although Antonuccio and Schoenberger assert that it is precisely such conscious motives that govern the findings concerning pharmaceuticals. I would suggest two possible sources of influence, although it is not clear the extent to which either is operative. The first concerns the possibility of experimenter bias, by means of which the experimenter or therapist transmits his or her expectations to the research participant or patient who then performs in a way that conforms to those expectations. To the extent that the investigator is the therapist, chooses the therapist, or trains the therapist, experimenter bias may well operate. A second possibility rests with the research design chosen for the study. If the study is designed in a way to ignore the therapeutic relationship or process in favor of the intervention technique, or if the dependent variable focuses on changes in symptom rather than including more internal or self-reflective processes, the study is only likely to find results that support possible differences in technique and overlook any contributions from the relationship or other common factors. It may be this flaw that has led to findings that support differences in intervention and minimize findings due to the therapeutic process.

Finally, there is the important matter of the relation of this controversy to clinical practice. We can assume that every practitioner has a strong allegiance to his or her own treatment approach, whether that approach is based on orientation or is more eclectic in nature. This conviction undoubtedly is conveyed to the patient and has a salutary effect in that it instills hope in the patient and through this may lead to promoting a positive outcome (Frank, 1973). Interestingly, this positive outcome then serves to reinforce the initial allegiance of the therapist. Thus, the allegiance effect not only is a significant confound in therapeutic research but it also may be a significant contributor to therapeutic success. To the extent that this is the case, it would argue for a more eclectic or integrative approach to practice, for it is in the attitude and stance of the therapist, rather than in specific techniques, that the heart of therapeutic success lies.

REFERENCES

Ackerman, S. J., Benjamin, L. S., Beutler, L. E., Gelso, C. J., Goldfried, M. R., Hill, C., et al. (2001). Empirically supported therapy relationships: Conclusions and recommendations of the Division 29 Task Force. *Psychotherapy: Theory, Research, Practice, Training, 38*, 495–497.

Agras, W. S., Walsh, T., Fairburn, C. G., Wilson, G. T., & Kraemer, H. C. (2000). A multicenter comparison of cognitive–behavioral therapy and interpersonal psychotherapy for bulimia nervosa. *Archives of General Psychiatry, 57*, 459–466.

Als-Nielsen, B., Chen, W., Gluud, C., & Kjaergard, L. L. (2003). Association of funding and conclusions in randomized drug trials: A reflection of treatment effect or adverse events? *Journal of the American Medical Association, 290*, 921–928.

Angell, M. (2000). Is academic medicine for sale? *New England Journal of Medicine, 342*, 1516–1518.

Antonuccio, D. O., Burns, D. D., & Danton, W. G. (2002). Antidepressants: A triumph of marketing over science? *Prevention and Treatment, 5*, Article 25. Retrieved from http://www.journals.apa.org/prevention/volume5/pre0050025c.html

Antonuccio, D. O., Danton, W. G., DeNelsky, G. Y., Greenberg, R. P., & Gordon, J. S. (1999). Raising questions about antidepressants. *Psychotherapy and Psychosomatics, 68*, 3–14.

Antonuccio, D. O., Danton, W. G., & McClanahan, T. M. (2003). Psychology in the prescription era: Building a firewall between marketing and science. *American Psychologist, 58*, 1028–1043.

Axelrod, J., Ban, T.A., Battegay, R., Bech, P., Berrios, G.E., Bolwig, T., et al. (2001). *Academic freedom: Eminent physicians protest treatment of Dr. David Healy.* Retrieved July 1, 2003, from http://www.caut.ca/english/issues/acadfreedom/healyletter.asp

Babcock, J. C., Green, C. E., & Robie, C. (2004). Does batterer's treatment work? A meta-analytic review of domestic violence treatment. *Clinical Psychology Review, 23*, 1023–1053.

Barlow, D. H., Rapee, R. M., & Brown, T. A. (1992). Behavioral treatment of generalized anxiety disorder. *Behavior Therapy, 23*, 551–570.

Bates, T., Anic, A., Marusic, M., & Marusic, A. (2004). Authorship criteria and disclosure of contributions. *Journal of the American Medical Association, 292*, 86–88.

Beck, A. T., Rush, A. J., Shaw, B. F., & Emery, G. (1979). *Cognitive therapy of depression.* New York: Guilford Press.

Bekelman, J. E., Li, Y., & Gross, C.P. (2003). Scope and impact of financial conflicts of interest in biomedical research. *Journal of the American Medical Association, 289*, 454–465.

Berman, J. S., Miller, R. C., & Massman, P. J. (1985). Cognitive therapy versus systematic desensitization: Is one treatment superior? *Psychological Bulletin, 97*, 451–461.

Beutler, L. E., & Harwood, T. M. (2000). *Prescriptive psychotherapy: A practical guide to systematic treatment selection.* New York: Oxford University Press.

Beutler, L. E., Moliero, C., & Talebi, H. (2002). How practitioners can systematically use empirical evidence in treatment selection. *Journal of Clinical Psychology, 58,* 1199–1212.

Biran, M., & Wilson, G. T. (1981). Treatment of phobic disorders using cognitive and exposure methods: A self-efficacy analysis. *Journal of Consulting and Clinical Psychology, 49,* 886–889.

Blackburn, I. M., Bishop, S., Glen, A. I. M., Whalley, L. J., & Christie, J. E. (1981). The efficacy of cognitive therapy in depression: A treatment trial using cognitive therapy and pharmacotherapy, each alone and in combination. *British Journal of Psychiatry, 139,* 181–189.

Blumenthal, D., Campbell, E. G., Anderson, M. S., Causino, N., & Louis, K. S. (1997). Withholding research results in academic life science: Evidence from a national survey of faculty. *Journal of the American Medical Association, 277,* 1224–1228.

Bodenheimer, T. (2000). Uneasy alliance—clinical investigators and the pharmaceutical industry. *New England Journal of Medicine, 342,* 1539–1544.

Boseley, S. (2002, May 21). Bitter pill. *The Guardian.* Retrieved May 21, 2002, from http://www.guardian.co.uk/Archive/Article/0,4273,4417163,00.html

Boyd, E. A., Cho, M. K., & Bero, L. A. (2003). Financial conflict-of-interest policies in clinical research: Issues for clinical investigators. *Academic Medicine, 78,* 769–774.

Brennan, T. A. (1994). Buying editorials. *The New England Journal of Medicine, 331,* 673–675.

Brom, D., Kleber, R. J., & Defares, P. B. (1989). Brief psychotherapy for posttraumatic stress disorders. *Journal of Consulting and Clinical Psychology, 57,* 607–612.

Browne, G., Steiner, M., Roberts, J., Gafni, A., Byrne, C., Dunn, E., et al. (2002). Sertraline and/or interpersonal psychotherapy for patients with dysthymic disorder in primary care: 6-month comparison with longitudinal 2-year follow-up of effectiveness and costs. *Journal of Affective Disorders, 68,* 317–330.

Butler, G., Fennell, M., Robson, P., & Gelder, M. (1991). Comparison of behavior therapy and cognitive behavior therapy in the treatment of generalized anxiety disorder. *Journal of Consulting and Clinical Psychology, 59,* 167–175.

Callaham, M. L., Wears, R. L., Weber, E. J., Barton, C., & Young, G. (1998). Positive-outcome bias and other limitations in the outcome of research abstracts submitted to a scientific meeting. *Journal of the American Medical Association, 280,* 254–257.

Campbell, E. G., Louis, K. S., & Blumenthal, D. (1998). Looking a gift horse in the mouth: Corporate gifts supporting life sciences research. *Journal of the American Medical Association, 279,* 995–999.

Casacalenda, N., Perry, C. J., & Looper, K. (2002). Remission in major depressive disorder: A comparison of pharmacotherapy, psychotherapy, and control conditions. *American Journal of Psychiatry, 159,* 1354–1360.

Cech, T. R., & Leonard, J. S. (2001). Conflict of interest—Moving beyond disclosure. *Science, 291,* 989–990.

Chalmers, I., (2000). Current controlled trials: An opportunity to help improve the quality of clinical research. *Current Controlled Trials in Cardiovascular Medicine, 1*, 3–8.

Chambless, D. C., & Ollendick, T. H. (2001). Empirically supported psychological interventions: Controversies and evidence. *Annual Review of Psychology, 52*, 685–716.

Chan, A., Hrobjartsson, A., Haahr, M., Gotzsche, P. C., & Altman, D. G. (2004). Empirical evidence for selective reporting of outcomes in randomized trials: Comparison of protocols to published articles. *Journal of the American Medical Association, 291*, 2457–2465.

Chopra, S. S. (2003). Industry funding of clinical trials. *Journal of the American Medical Association, 290*, 113–114.

Choudhry, N. K., Stelfox, H. T., & Detsky, A. S. (2002). Relationships between authors of clinical practice guidelines and the pharmaceutical industry. *Journal of the American Medical Association, 287*, 612–617.

Cross, D. G., Sheehan, P. W., & Kahn, J. A. (1982). Short- and long-term follow-up of clients receiving insight-oriented therapy and behavior therapy. *Journal of Consulting and Clinical Psychology, 50*, 103–112.

Davidoff, F., DeAngelis, C. D., Drazen, J. M., Nicholls, M. G., Hoey, J., Hojgaard, L., et al. (2001). Sponsorship, authorship, and accountability. *New England Journal of Medicine, 345*, 825–827.

DeAngelis, C. D., Drazen, J. M., Frizelle, F. A., Haug, C., Hoey, J., Horton, R., et al. (2004). Clinical trial registration: A statement from the International Committee of Medical Journal Editors. *Journal of the American Medical Association, 292*, 1363.

DeAngelis, C. D., Fontanarosa, P. B., & Flanagin, A. (2001). Reporting financial conflicts of interest and relationships between investigators and research sponsors. *Journal of the American Medical Association, 286*, 89–91.

Deyo, R. A., Psaty, B. M., Simon, G., Wagner, E. H., & Omenn, G. S. (1997). The messenger under attack—Intimidation of researchers by special-interest groups. *New England Journal of Medicine, 336*, 1176–1179.

Dickersin, K., & Rennie, D. (2003). Registering clinical trials. *Journal of the American Medical Association, 290*, 516–523.

DiGuiseppe, R., & Tafrate, R. C. (2003). Anger treatment for adults: A meta-analytic review. *Clinical Psychology: Science and Practice, 10*, 70–84.

DiMascio, A., Weissman, M. M., Prusoff, B. A., Neu, C., Zwilling, M., & Klerman, G. (1979). Differential symptom reduction by drugs and psychotherapy in acute depression. *Archives of General Psychology, 36*, 1450–1456.

Drazen, J. M., & Curfman, G. D. (2002). Financial associations of authors. *New England Journal of Medicine, 346*, 1901–1902.

Dunn, R. J. (1979). Cognitive modification with depression-prone psychiatric patients. *Cognitive Therapy and Research, 3*, 307–317.

Editorial: The tightening grip of big pharma. (2001). *The Lancet, 357,* 1141.

Elkin, I., Shea, T., Watkins, J., Imber, S., Sotsky, S., Colins, J., et al. (1989). National Institute of Mental Health Treatment of Depression Collaborative Research Program—general effectiveness of treatments. *Archives of General Psychiatry, 46,* 966–980.

Elliot, C. (2001). Pharma buys a conscience. *The American Prospect, 12,* 1–9.

Elliott, R., Greenberg, L. S., & Lietaer, G. (2003). Research on experiential psychotherapies. In M. J. Lambert (Ed.), *Bergin and Garfield's handbook of psychotherapy and behavior change* (5th ed., pp. 493–539). New York: Wiley.

Even, C., Siobud-Dorocant, E., & Dardennes, R. M. (2000). Critical approach to antidepressant trials: Blindness protection is necessary, feasible, and measurable. *British Journal of Psychiatry, 177,* 47–51.

Fava, G. A. (1998). All our dreams are sold. *Psychotherapy and Psychosomatics, 67,* 191–193.

Fava, G. A. (2001). Conflict of interest in special interest groups: The making of a counter culture. *Psychotherapy and Psychosomatics, 70,* 1–5.

Flanagin, A., Carey, L. A., Fontanarosa, P. B., Phillips, S. G., Pace, B. P., Lundberg, G. D., et al. (1998). Prevalence of articles with honorary authors and ghost authors in peer-reviewed medical journals. *Journal of the American Medical Association, 280,* 222–224.

Fontanarosa, P. B., Rennie, D., & DeAngelis, C. D. (2004). Postmarketing surveillance—Lack of vigilance, lack of trust. *Journal of the American Medical Association, 292,* 2647–2650.

Fortune. (2000, April 17). How the industries stack up. Retrieved July 1, 2001, from www.fortune.com/indexw.jhtml?channel=artcol.jhtml& doc_id=00001423

Frank, J. D. (1973). *Persuasion and healing* (2nd ed.). Baltimore: Johns Hopkins University Press.

Friedman, R. A. (2002, December 17). Curing and killing: The perils of a growing medicine cabinet. *The New York Times.* Retrieved June 20, 2005, from www.3sistersapothcary.com/html/resources/library/curing.cfm

Gaffan, E. A., Tsaousis, I., & Kemp-Wheeler, S. N. (1995). Researcher allegiance and meta-analysis: The case of cognitive therapy for depression. *Journal of Consulting and Clinical Psychology, 63,* 966–980.

Gallagher, D. E., & Thompson, L. W. (1982). Treatment of major depressive disorder in adult outpatients with brief psychotherapies. *Psychotherapy: Theory, Research, and Practice, 19,* 482–490.

Gandhi, T. K., Weingart, S. N., Borus, J., Seger, A. C., Peterson, J., Burdick, E., et al. (2003). Adverse drug events in ambulatory care. *New England Journal of Medicine, 348,* 1556–1564.

Ghahramanlou, M. (2003). Cognitive behavioral treatment efficacy for anxiety disorders: A meta-analytic review. *Dissertation Abstracts International: Section B: The Sciences and Engineering, 64,* 1901.

Gilbody, S. M., & Song, F. (2000). Publication bias and the integrity of psychiatry research. *Psychological Medicine, 30,* 253–258.

Gold, J. R. (1995). The place of process-oriented psychotherapies in an outcome-oriented psychology and society. *Applied and Preventive Psychology, 4*, 61–74.

Gram, L. F. (1994). Fluoxetine. *New England Journal of Medicine, 331*, 1354–1361.

Greenberg, R. P., Bornstein, R. F., Greenberg, M. D., & Fisher, S. (1992). A meta-analysis of antidepressant outcome under "blinder" conditions. *Journal of Consulting and Clinical Psychology, 60*, 664–669.

Greenberg, R. P., & Fisher, S. (1997). Mood-mending medicines: Probing drug, psychotherapy, and placebo solutions. In S. Fisher & R. P. Greenberg (Eds.), *From placebo to panacea: Putting psychiatric drugs to the test* (pp. 115–172). New York: Wiley.

Gurwitz, J. H., Field, T. S., Harrold, L. R., Rothschild, J., Debellis, K., Seger, A. C., et al. (2003). Incidence and preventability of adverse drug events among older persons in the ambulatory setting. *Journal of the American Medical Association, 289*, 1107–1116.

Healy, D. (2001). The dilemmas posed by new and fashionable treatments. *Advances in Psychiatric Treatment, 7*, 322–327.

Healy, D. (2002). Conflicting interests in Toronto: Anatomy of a controversy at the interface of academia and industry. *Perspectives in Biology and Medicine, 45*, 250–263.

Healy, D. (2003). Lines of evidence on the risks of suicide with selective serotonin reuptake inhibitors. *Psychotherapy and Psychosomatics, 72*, 71–79.

Healy, D., & Catell, D. (2003). Interface between authorship, industry and science in the domain of therapeutics. *British Journal of Psychiatry, 183*, 22–27.

Hirschfeld, R., Dunner, D. L., Keitner, G., Klein, D. N., Koran, L. M., Kornstein, S. G., et al. (2002). Does psychosocial functioning improve independent of depressive symptoms? A comparison of nefazodone, psychotherapy, and their combination. *Biological Psychiatry, 51*, 123–133.

Hollon, S. D. (1999). Allegiance effects in treatment research: A commentary. *Clinical Psychology: Science and Practice, 6*, 107–112.

Hollon, S. D., DeRubeis, R. J., Evans, M. D., Wiemer, M. J., Garvey, M. J., & Tuason, V. B. (1992). Cognitive therapy and pharmacotherapy for depression: Singly and in combination. *Archives of General Psychiatry, 49*, 774–781

Ilardi, S. S., & Craighead, W. E. (1994). The role of nonspecific factors in cognitive behavioral therapy for depression. *Clinical Psychology: Science and Practice, 1*, 138–156.

Ironson, G., Freund, B., Strauss, J. L., & Williams, J. (2002). Comparison of two treatments for traumatic stress: A community-based study of EMDR and prolonged exposure. *Journal of Clinical Psychology, 58*, 113–128.

Jacobson, N. S. (1999). The role of the allegiance effect in psychotherapy research: Controlling and accounting for it. *Clinical Psychology: Science and Practice, 6*, 116–119.

Jacobson, N. S., & Hollon, S. D. (1996). Prospects for future comparisons between drugs and psychotherapy: Lessons from the CBT-versus-pharmacotherapy exchange. *Journal of Consulting and Clinical Psychology, 64*, 104–108.

Johns, M. M. E., Barnes, M., & Florencio, P. S. (2003). Restoring balance to industry–academia relationships in an era of institutional financial conflicts of interest: Promoting research while maintaining trust. *Journal of the American Medical Association, 289*, 741–746.

Joseph, A. M., & Antonuccio, D. O. (1999). Lack of efficacy of transdermal nicotine in smoking cessation. *New England Journal of Medicine, 341*, 1157–1158.

Joseph, A. M., Norman, S. M., Ferry, L. H., Prochazka, A. V., Westman, E. C., Steele, B. G., et al. (1996). The safety of transdermal nicotine as an aid to smoking cessation in patients with cardiac disease. *New England Journal of Medicine, 335*, 1792–1798.

Juurlink, D. N., Mamdani, M., Kopp, A., Laupacis, A., & Redelmeier, D. A. (2003). Drug–drug interactions among elderly patients hospitalized for drug toxicity. *Journal of the American Medical Association, 289*, 1652–1658.

Keller, M. B., McCullough, J. P., Klein, D. N., Arnow, B., Dunner, D. L., Gelenberg, A. J., et al. (2000). A comparison of nefazodone, the cognitive–behavioral analysis system of psychotherapy, and their combination for the treatment of chronic depression. *New England Journal of Medicine, 342*, 1462–1470.

Khan, A., Khan, S., & Brown, W. A. (2002). Are placebo controls necessary to test new antidepressants and anxiolytics? *International Journal of Neuropsychopharmacology, 5*, 193–197.

Kirsch, I. (in press). Placebo psychotherapy: Synonym or oxymoron? *Journal of Clinical Psychology.*

Kirsch, I., Moore, T. J., Scoboria, A., & Nicholls, S. S. (2002). The emperor's new drugs: An analysis of antidepressant medication data submitted to the U.S. Food and Drug Administration. *Prevention and Treatment, 5*, Article 23. Retrieved July 1, 2004, from http://www.journals.apa.org/prevention/volume5/pre0050023a.html

Klein, D. F. (2000). Flawed meta-analyses comparing psychotherapy with pharmacotherapy. *American Journal of Psychiatry, 157*, 1204–1211.

Klein, D. F., Thase, M. E., Endicott, J., Adler, L., Glick, I., Kalali, A., et al. (2002). Improving clinical trials: American Society of Clinical Psychopharmacology recommendations. *Archives of General Psychiatry, 59*, 272–278.

Krimsky, S., & Rothenberg, L. S. (2001). Conflict of interest policies in science and medical journals: Editorial practices and author disclosures. *Science and Engineering Ethics, 7*, 205–218.

Krimsky, S., Rothenberg, L. S., Stott, P., & Kyle, G. (1998). Scientific journals and their authors' financial interests: A pilot study. *Psychotherapy and Psychosomatics, 67*, 194–201.

Krzyzanowska, M. E., Pintilie, M., & Tannock, I. F. (2003). Factors associated with failure to publish large randomized trials presented at an oncology meeting. *Journal of the American Medical Association, 290*, 495–501.

Lambert, M. J. (1999). Are differential treatment effects inflated by researcher therapy allegiance? Could clever Hans count? *Clinical Psychology: Science and Practice, 6,* 127–130.

Lambert, M. J., & Bergin, A. E. (1994). The effectiveness of psychotherapy. In A. E. Bergin and S. L. Garfield (Eds.), *Handbook of psychotherapy and behavior change* (pp. 143–149). New York: Wiley.

Largo-Marsh, L., & Spates, C. R. (2002). The effects of writing therapy in comparison to EMDR on traumatic stress: The relationship between hypnotizability and client expectancy to outcome. *Professional Psychology: Research and Practice, 6,* 581–586.

Lasser, K. E., Allen, P. D., Woolhandler, S. J., Himmelstein, D. U., Wolfe, S. M., & Bor, D. H. (2002). Timing of new black box warnings and withdrawals for prescription medications. *Journal of the American Medical Association, 287,* 2215–2220.

Laughren, T. P. (2001). The scientific and ethical basis for placebo-controlled trials in depression and schizophrenia: An FDA perspective. *European Psychiatry, 16,* 418–423.

Lazarou, J., Pemeranz, B., & Corey, P. N. (1998). Incidence of adverse drug reactions in hospitalized patients: A meta-analysis of prospective studies. *Journal of the American Medical Association, 279,* 1200–1205.

Lazarus, A. A. (1981). *The practice of multimodal therapy.* New York: McGraw–Hill.

Letter to Academic Press. (2002, November 19). Re: Regulatory Toxicology and Pharmacology. Retrieved from www.cspinet.org/new/pdf/final_letter_academic _press_rtp.pdf

Levinsky, N. G. (2002). Nonfinancial conflicts of interest in research. *New England Journal of Medicine, 347,* 759–761.

Lexchin, J., Bero, L. A., Djulbegovic, B., & Clark, O. (2003). Pharmaceutical industry sponsorship and research outcome and quality: Systematic review. *British Medical Journal, 326,* 1167–1170.

Lo, B., Wolf, L. E., & Berkeley, A. (2000). Conflict-of-interest policies for investigators in clinical trials. *New England Journal of Medicine, 343,* 1643–1645.

Louie, L. (2001, May). A prescription for profits. *Upside,* 102–107.

Luborsky, L. (1984). *Principles of psychoanalytic psychotherapy: A manual for supportive–expressive (SE) treatment.* New York: Basic Books.

Luborsky, L., & Crits-Christoph, P. (1990). *Understanding transference: The CCRT Method (The Core Conflictual Relationship Theme).* New York: Basic Books.

Luborsky, L., Diguer, L., Seligman, D. A., Rosenthal, R., Krause, E. D., Johnson, S., et al. (1999). The researcher's own therapy allegiances: A "wild card" in comparisons of treatment efficacy. *Clinical Psychology: Science and Practice, 6,* 95–132.

Luborsky, L., & Luborsky, E. (in preparation). *SE dynamic psychotherapy: Clinical principles and research discoveries.*

Luborsky, L., Mark, D., Hole, A. V., Popp, C., Goldsmith, B., & Cacciola, J. (1995). Supportive–expressive dynamic psychotherapy of depression: A time-limited version. In J. P. Barber & P. Crits-Christoph (Eds.), *Psychodynamic psychotherapies for psychiatric disorders (Axis I)* (pp. 13–42). New York: Basic Books.

Luborsky, L., Rosenthal, R., Diguer, L., Andrusyna, T. P., Levitt, J. T., Seligman, D. A., et al. (2002). The Dodo Bird Verdict is alive and well—mostly. *Clinical Psychology: Science and Practice, 9,* 2–12.

Marks, I. M., Swinson, R. P., Basoglu, M., Kuch, K., Noshirvani, H., O'Sullivan, G., et al. (1993a). Alprazolam and exposure alone and combined in panic disorder with agoraphobia: A controlled study in London and Toronto. *British Journal of Psychiatry, 162,* 776–787.

Marks, I. M., Swinson, R. P., Basoglu, M., Noshirvani, H., Kuch, K., O'Sullivan, G., et al. (1993b). Reply to comment on the London/Toronto Study. *British Journal of Psychiatry, 162,* 790–794.

Martin, D. J., Garske, J. P., & Davis, M. K. (2000). Relation of the therapeutic alliance with outcome and other variables: A meta-analytic review. *Journal of Consulting and Clinical Psychology, 68,* 438–449.

Maxfield, L., & Hyer, L. (2002). The relationship between efficacy and methodology in studies investigating EMDR treatment of PTSD. *Journal of Clinical Psychology, 58,* 23–41.

McNamara, K., & Horan, J. J. (1986). Experimental construct validity in the evaluation of cognitive and behavioral treatments for depression. *Journal of Consulting and Clinical Psychology, 33,* 23–30.

Melander, H., Ahlqvist–Rastad, J., Meijer, G., & Beermann, B. (2003). Evidence b(i)ased medicine-selective reporting from studies sponsored by pharmaceutical industry: Review of studies in new drug applications. *British Medical Journal, 326,* 1171–1173.

Messer, S. B. (1992). A critical examination of belief structures in interpretive and eclectic psychotherapy. In J. C. Norcross & M. R. Goldfried (Eds.), *Handbook of psychotherapy integration* (pp. 130–165). New York: Basic Books.

Milan, M. A., Montgomery, R. W., & Rogers, E. C. (1994). Theoretical orientation revolution in clinical psychology: Fact or fiction? *Professional Psychology: Research and Practice, 25,* 398–402.

Misakian, A. L., & Bero, L. A. (1998). Publication bias and research on passive smoking: Comparison of published and unpublished studies. *Journal of the American Medical Association, 280,* 250–253.

Moher, D., Schulz, K. F., & Altman, D. G. (2001). The CONSORT statement: Revised recommendations for improving the quality of reports of parallel-group randomized trials. *Annals of Internal Medicine, 134,* 657–662.

Moleski, R., & Tosi, D. J. (1976). Comparative psychotherapy: Rational–emotive therapy versus systematic desensitization in the treatment of stuttering. *Journal of Consulting and Clinical Psychology, 44,* 309–311.

Monbiot, G. (2002, May 14). The fake persuaders: Corporations are inventing people to rubbish their opponents on the internet. *The Guardian.* Retrieved May 14, 2002, from http://politics.guardian.co.uk/green/comment/0,9236,715160,00.html

Moncrieff, J. (2001). Are antidepressants overrated? A review of methodological problems in antidepressant trials. *Journal of Nervous and Mental Disorders, 189,* 288–295.

Moncrieff, J., Wessely, S., & Hardy, R. (2001). Antidepressants using active placebos (Cochrane review). *Cochrane Database Systematic Review, 2,* CD003012.

Moses, H., & Martin, J. B. (2001). Academic relationships with industry: A new model for biomedical research. *Journal of the American Medical Association, 285,* 933–935.

Murphy, G. E., Simons, A. D., Wetzel, R. D., & Lustman, P. J. (1984). Cognitive therapy and pharmacotherapy: Singly and together in the treatment of depression. *Archives of General Psychiatry, 41,* 33–41.

Nathan, D. G., & Weatherall, D. J. (2002). Academic freedom in clinical research. *New England Journal of Medicine, 347,* 1368–1371.

Norcross, J. C. (Ed.). (2002). *Psychotherapy relationships that work: Therapist contributions and responsiveness to patients.* New York: Oxford University Press.

Norcross, J. C. (in press). A primer on psychotherapy integration. In J. C. Norcross & M. R. Goldfried (Eds.), *Handbook of psychotherapy integration* (2nd ed.). New York: Oxford University Press.

Otto, M. W., & Nierenberg, A. A. (2002). Assay sensitivity, failed clinical trials, and the conduct of science. *Psychotherapy and Psychosomatics, 71,* 241–243.

Otto, M. W., Pollack, M. H., Gould, R. A., Worthington, J. J., III, McArdle, E. T., Rosenbaum, J. F., et al. (2000). A comparison of the efficacy of clonazepam and cognitive–behavioral group therapy for the treatment of social phobia. *Journal of Anxiety Disorders, 14,* 345–358.

Petersen, M. (2002, November 22). Madison Ave. plays growing role in drug research. *The New York Times,* p. A1.

Piasecki, M., Antonuccio, D. O., Steinagel, G., & Kohlenberg, B. (2002). Penetration of the blind in a controlled study of paxil used to treat cocaine addiction. *Journal of Behavior Therapy and Experimental Psychiatry, 33,* 67–71.

Pierloot, R., & Vinck, J. (1978). Differential outcome of short-term dynamic psychotherapy and systematic desensitization in the treatment of anxious outpatients: A preliminary report. *Psychology Belgium, 18,* 87–98.

Power, K. G., Jerrom, D. W. A., Simpson, R. J., Mitchell, M. J., & Swanson, V. (1989). A controlled comparison of cognitive–behaviour therapy, diazepam and placebo in the management of generalized anxiety. *Behavioural Psychotherapy, 17,* 1–14.

Prendergast, M. L., Podus, D., Chang, E., & Urada, D. (2002). The effectiveness of drug abuse treatment: A meta-analysis of comparison group studies. *Drug and Alcohol Dependence, 67,* 53–72.

Quick, J. (2001, December). Maintaining the integrity of the clinical evidence base. *Bulletin of the World Health Organization,* Reference No. 01–1602.

Quitkin, F. M. (1999). Placebos, drug effects, and study design: A clinician's guide. *American Journal of Psychiatry, 156,* 829–836.

Rennie, D. (1997). Thyroid storm. *Journal of the American Medical Association, 277,* 1238–1243.

Rennie, D. (1999). Fair conduct and fair reporting of clinical trials. *Journal of the American Medical Association, 282,* 1766–1768.

Robinson, L. A., Berman, J. S., & Neimeyer, R. A. (1990). Psychotherapy for the treatment of depression: A comprehensive review of controlled outcome research. *Psychological Bulletin, 108,* 30–49.

Rush, A. J., Beck, A. T., Kovacs, M., & Hollon, S. (1977). Comparative efficacy of cognitive therapy and pharmaco–therapy in the treatment of depressed patients. *Cognitive Therapy and Research, 1,* 17–37.

Safer, D. (2002). Design and reporting modifications in industry-sponsored comparative psychopharmacology trials. *Journal of Nervous and Mental Disease, 190,* 583–592.

Santoro, S. O., Lister, K. M., Karpiak, C. P., & Norcross, J. C. (2004, April). *Clinical psychologists in the 2000s: A national study.* Paper presented at the annual meeting of the Eastern Psychological Association, Washington, DC.

Schottenbauer, M. A., Glass, C. R., & Arnkoff, D. B. (in press). Outcome research on psychotherapy integration. In J. C. Norcross & M. R. Goldfried (Eds.), *Handbook of psychotherapy integration* (2nd ed.). New York: Oxford University Press.

Schulman, K. A., Seils, D. M., Timbie, J. W., Sugarman, J., Dame, L. A., Weinfurt, K. P., et al. (2002). A national survey of provisions in clinical–trial agreements between medical schools and industry sponsors. *New England Journal of Medicine, 347,* 1335–1341.

Shapiro, D., & Paley, G. (2002). The continuing potential relevance of equivalence and allegiance to research on psychological treatment of psychosis: Reply. *Psychology and Psychotherapy: Theory, Research and Practice, 75,* 375–379.

Shaw, B. F. (1999). How to use the allegiance effect to maximize competence and therapeutic outcomes. *Clinical Psychology: Science and Practice, 6,* 131–132.

Shoham, V., & Rohrbaugh, M. J. (1999). Beyond allegiance to comparative outcome studies. *Clinical Psychology: Science and Practice, 6,* 120–123.

Sloane, R., Staples, F., Cristol, A., Yorkston, N., & Whipple, K. (1975). *Psychotherapy vs. behavior therapy.* Cambridge, MA: Harvard University Press.

Stricker, G. (1992). The relationship of research to clinical practice. *American Psychologist, 47,* 543–549.

Stricker, G., & Gold, J. R. (1996). Psychotherapy integration: An assimilative, psychodynamic approach. *Clinical Psychology: Science and Practice, 3,* 47–58.

Stricker, G., & Gold, J. R. (2002). An assimilative approach to integrative psychodynamic psychotherapy. In J. Lebow (Ed.), *Integrative/eclectic* (Vol. 4, pp. 295–315). New York: Wiley.

Stricker, G., & Gold, J. R. (2003). Integrative approaches to psychotherapy. In A. S. Gurman & S. B. Messer (Eds.), *Essential psychotherapies: Theory and practice* (2nd ed., pp. 317–349). New York: Guilford Press.

Stricker, G., & Trierweiler, S. J. (1995). The local clinical scientist: A bridge between science and practice. *American Psychologist, 50,* 995–1002.

Szapocznik, J., Feaster, D. J., Mitrani, V. B., Prado, G., Smith, L., Robinson-Batista, C., et al. (2004). Structural ecosystems therapy for HIV–Seropositive African

American women: Effects on psychological distress, family hassles, and family support. *Journal of Consulting and Clinical Psychology, 72,* 288–303.

Task Force on Promotion and Dissemination of Psychological Procedures. (1995). Training in and dissemination of empirically-validated psychological treatments. *The Clinical Psychologist, 48,* 3–23.

Taylor, F. G., & Marshall, W. L. (1977). Experimental analysis of cognitive–behavioral therapy for depression. *Cognitive Therapy and Research, 1,* 59–72.

Thase, M. E. (1999a). How should efficacy be evaluated in randomized clinical trials of treatments for depression? *Journal of Clinical Psychiatry, 60,* 23–31.

Thase, M. E. (1999b). What is the investigator allegiance effect and what should we do about it? *Clinical Psychology: Science and Practice, 6,* 113–115.

Thase, M. E., Friedman, E. S., Fasiczka, A. L., Berman, S. R., Frank, E., Nofzinger, E. A., et al. (2000). Treatment of men with major depression: A comparison of sequential cohorts treated with either cognitive–behavioral therapy or newer generation antidepressants. *Journal of Clinical Psychiatry, 61,* 466–472.

Thompson, L. W., Coon, D. W., Gallagher-Thompson, D., Sommer, B. R., & Koin, D. (2001). Comparison of desipramine and cognitive/behavioral therapy in the treatment of elderly outpatients with mild-to-moderate depression. *American Journal of Geriatric Psychiatry, 9,* 225–240.

Thompson, L. W., Gallagher, D., & Breckenridge, J. S. (1987). Comparative effectiveness of psychotherapies for depressed elders. *Journal of Consulting and Clinical Psychology, 55,* 385–390.

Torrey, E. F. (2002). The going rate on shrinks: Big Pharma and the buying of psychiatry. *The American Prospect, 13.* Retrieved July 1, 2002, from www.prospect.org/print/V13/13/torrey-e.html

Trierweiler, S. J., & Stricker, G. (1998). *The scientific practice of professional psychology.* New York: Plenum Press.

Vergano, D. (2001, May 16). Filed under F (for forgotten). *USA Today.* Retrieved May 16, 2001, from http://www.usatoday.com/news/health/2001-05-17-drug-companies.htm

Wachtel, P. L. (1977). *Psychoanalysis and behavior therapy: Toward an integration.* New York: Basic Books.

Walsh, B. T., Seidman, S. N., Sysko, R., & Gould, M. (2002). Placebo response in studies of major depression. *Journal of the American Medical Association, 287,* 1840–1847.

Wampold, B. E., Minami, T., Baskin, T. W., & Tierney, S. C. (2002). A meta-(re)analysis of the effects of cognitive therapy versus "other therapies" for depression. *Journal of Affective Disorder, 68,* 159–165.

Warner, L. K., Herron, W. G., Javier, R. A., Patalano, F., Sisenwein, F., & Primavera, L. H. (2001). A comparison of dose–response curves in cognitive–behavioral and psychodynamic psychotherapies. *Journal of Clinical Psychology, 57,* 63–73.

Watson, J. C., Gordon, L. B., Stermac, L., Kalogerakos, F., & Steckley, P. (2003). Comparing the effectiveness of process–experiential with cognitive–behavioral psychotherapy in the treatment of depression. *Journal of Consulting and Clinical Psychology, 71*, 773–781.

Westen, D., Morrison, K., & Thompson-Brenner, H. (in press). The empirical status of empirically supported psychotherapies: Assumptions, findings, and reporting in clinical trials. *Psychological Bulletin.*

White, K., Kando, J., Park, T., Waternaux, C., & Brown, W. A. (1992). Side effects and the "blindability" of clinical drug trials. *American Journal of Pyschiatry, 149,* 1730–1731.

Wilfley, D. E., Welch, R. R., Stein, R. I., Spurrell, E. B., Cohen, L. R., Saelens, B. E., et al. (2002). A randomized comparison of group interpersonal psychotherapy for the treatment of overweight individuals with binge-eating disorder. *Archives of General Psychiatry, 59,* 713–721.

Willman, D. (2000, December 20). How a new policy led to seven deadly drugs. *Los Angeles Times.* Retrieved from www.msbp.com/fda.htm

Wilson, P. H., Goldin, J. C., & Charbonneau-Powis, M. (1983). Comparative efficacy of behavioral and cognitive treatments of depression. *Cognitive Therapy and Research, 7,* 111–124.

Wise, P., & Drury, M. (1996). Pharmaceutical trials in general practice: The first 100 protocols. An audit by the clinical research ethics committee of the Royal College of General Practitioners. *British Medical Journal, 313,* 1245–1248.

Woody, G., Luborsky, L., McLellan, A. T., O'Brien, C., Beck, A. T., Blaine, J., et al. (1983). Psychotherapy for opiate addicts: Does it help? *Archives of General Psychiatry, 40,* 639–645.

Zeiss, A. M., Lewinsohn, P. M., & Munoz, R. F. (1979). Non-specific improvement effects in depression using interpersonal skills training, pleasant activity schedules, or cognitive training. *Journal of Consulting and Clinical Psychology, 47,* 427–439.

Zitrin, C. M., Klein, D. F., & Woerner, M. G. (1978). Behavior therapy, supportive psychotherapy, imipramine, and phobias. *Archives of General Psychiatry, 35,* 307–316.

7

DO THERAPIES DESIGNATED AS EMPIRICALLY SUPPORTED TREATMENTS FOR SPECIFIC DISORDERS PRODUCE OUTCOMES SUPERIOR TO NON-EMPIRICALLY SUPPORTED TREATMENT THERAPIES?

Not a Scintilla of Evidence to Support Empirically Supported Treatments as More Effective Than Other Treatments

Bruce E. Wampold

A psychological treatment for a particular disorder that has not been designated as an empirically supported treatment (EST) does not imply that this treatment is not efficacious or as efficacious as an EST. Simply, it may be that this treatment has not been subjected to the test required for designation as an EST. There is no requirement that a particular treatment be superior to another treatment to be designated as an EST. According to the criteria for a well-established treatment published in 1998 (see Chambless et al., 1998), (a) the treatment must be superior to a pill or psychological placebo or (b) the treatment must be superior to another treatment or be

equivalent to an already established treatment. Thus, no structural requirement ensures that an EST is superior to any other treatment. Nevertheless,
designation as an EST confers a privileged status (Wampold & Bhati, 2004),
as if such a treatment were superior.

The EST movement and the criteria used to designate treatments as
ESTs have been criticized on many bases (e.g., Henry, 1998; Wampold, 1997;
Westen, Novotny, & Thompson-Brenner, 2004). However, in this position
paper, only one issue will be addressed: What is the evidence that proves ESTs
are superior to treatments not so designated? For the purpose of this comment, the evidence used to answer this question will be derived from clinical
trials of individual psychotherapy for adults.

EVIDENCE ACROSS DISORDERS

The general equivalence of all psychological treatments across disorders
in terms of outcomes has been called the Dodo Bird Effect, a term coined by
Saul Rosenzweig (1936) to denote that "All have won and all must have
prizes." The Dodo Bird Effect has been meta-analytically examined since the
initial application of meta-analysis as a means to assess psychotherapy efficacy (in 1977 by Smith & Glass), and generally it has been found that all
treatments are generally equivalent. The various meta-analyses will be summarized chronologically (see Wampold, 2001).

Smith, Glass, and colleagues (Smith & Glass, 1977; Smith, Glass, &
Miller, 1980) collected and analyzed every counseling and psychotherapy
outcome study available at the time and found some differences among types
of therapy. Overall, cognitive, cognitive–behavioral, and behavioral treatments produced larger effects than other types of therapy. However, after
adjusting the effect sizes for differences in the reactivity of the measures used
in the studies, the differences disappeared because the studies of cognitive
and behavioral treatments used more reactive measures.

Shapiro and Shapiro (1982) improved on the Smith and Glass meta-
analyses by including several behavioral studies that were previously omitted
and by examining direct comparisons of two or more treatments, which eliminated much of the confounding that Smith and Glass handled by statistical
means. Shapiro and Shapiro classified each treatment into the following
types: (a) rehearsal, self-control, and monitoring; (b) biofeedback; (c) covert
behavioral; (d) relaxation; (e) systematic desensitization; (f) social skills
training; (g) cognitive; (h) dynamic–humanistic; (i) mixed; (j) unclassified;
and (k) minimal. Then the effect sizes for direct comparisons of treatments
that fell into different classes were examined. Eliminating the minimal therapies, which were not intended to be therapeutic, and the mixed therapies,
which were not "pure" treatment types, the only comparison that showed a
statistically significant difference was an advantage of cognitive therapy over

systematic desensitization. However, Berman, Miller, and Massman (1985) showed that this difference was due to the fact that researchers conducted the studies comparing cognitive and systematic desensitization in the Shapiro and Shapiro meta-analysis with an allegiance to cognitive therapies. When later studies conducted by advocates of systematic desensitization were included, the effect for the differences across all studies was near zero.

The meta-analysis conducted by Wampold, Mondin, Moody, Stich, et al. (1997) also examined only direct comparisons between treatments, but it eliminated the problem of classifying treatments into types by including every comparison (even within a class) and only including treatments that were bona fide (i.e., treatments intended to be therapeutic). When all such comparisons were aggregated, the best estimate of the effect size for the differences among treatments was zero. Under the most liberal assumptions, the effect size was of the order designated as a small effect, accounting for less than 1% of the variability in outcomes. Moreover, the dissimilarity of the treatments was not related to the effect size (i.e., the results were not due to comparisons within classes of treatments).

Although the reviewed meta-analyses, as well as others (e.g., Grissom, 1996), have consistently demonstrated uniform efficacy, for several reasons these results do not completely address the question of whether ESTs are superior to non-ESTs for particular disorders. First, many of the comparisons in these meta-analyses were either among ESTs (e.g., many of the treatments in Wampold et al., 1997, were behavioral or cognitive–behavioral; see Crits-Christoph, 1997) or were between non-ESTs. Second, the meta-analyses aggregated studies without regard to disorder. These issues are addressed in the next two sections.

ESTS VERSUS PLACEBOS

One of the ways a treatment can qualify as an EST is to demonstrate that it is more effective than a psychological placebo (Chambless et al., 1998). Many conceptual and methodological problems occur with placebos as controls for common factors in psychotherapy (Basham, 1986; Baskin, Tierney, Minami, & Wampold, 2003; Borkovec & Nau, 1972; Brody, 1980; Horvath, 1988; O'Leary & Borkovec, 1978; Shepherd, 1993; Wampold, 1997, 2001). Most problematic in terms of the outcomes produced by the psychological placebo is that the basic design requirement of blinding is absent; the therapists in the placebo condition are aware they are providing a sham treatment. Exacerbating that and other problems is the fact that some of these psychological placebos are poorly designed in that (a) the placebos did not provide an equal dose of treatment (the placebo had fewer or shorter sessions), (b) the format in the placebo was different than the format used in the treatment (e.g., the group rather than individual therapy), (c) the placebo therapists had less skill or training, and (d) the design enjoined placebo therapists from using therapeutic actions that therapists would typically use in any type of therapy (see Baskin et al., 2003).

Recently, Baskin et al. (2003) investigated the efficacy of commonly accepted treatments, most of which were ESTs, vis-à-vis psychological placebos that were structurally equivalent to the established treatment. Structurally equivalent placebos had the same number and length of sessions as the active treatment, used the same format (e.g., group, family, or individual), and used therapists with training comparable to therapists of the active treatment. These placebos also involved treatments that were individualized to the patient, allowed patients to discuss topics logical to the treatment, and did not constrain the interaction to neutral topics. It was found that the active treatments (all behavioral and cognitive–behavioral) were only negligibly better than the structurally equivalent placebos. This finding suggests that ESTs for particular disorders are only marginally superior to well-designed psychological placebos.

ESTS FOR DEPRESSION AND ANXIETY

To answer the question of whether ESTs for particular disorders are superior to other treatments, I will examine evidence for two particular disorders, depression and anxiety. These two disorders were chosen because depression and anxiety are the most commonly occurring disorders, because most ESTs exist for treatments of these disorders, and because it has been claimed that, although the common factors are sufficient to treat mild disorders, they are not effective in treating more debilitating disorders (e.g., obsessive–compulsive disorder [OCD] or major depressive disorder [MDD]).

Studies Used to Designate Treatments as "Well-Established Treatments"

As indicated earlier, a treatment can qualify as a well-established EST by either being superior to a placebo (pill or psychological) or to another treatment. Table 7.1 presents the well-established ESTs for depression and anxiety, the citations that provide the evidence (see Chambless et al., 1998), and the comparison group used to establish the EST. Four of the ESTs (exposure for agoraphobia, exposure–response prevention for OCD, stress inoculation for coping with stressors, and cognitive–behavior therapy [CBT] for depression) were established by reference to meta-analyses of primary studies, rather than by reference to primary studies. Only the meta-analysis for CBT for depression indicated that the EST being investigated was superior to another treatment. Dobson (1989) found that CBT was superior to behavioral treatments for depression, a result that has not stood the test of time (see the following). Three of the studies in Table 7.1 used comparisons with

TABLE 7.1
Analysis of Research Cited for EST

Disorder	EST	Citation	Comparison	Type of psychological comparison	EST superior to bona fide treatment
Panic disorder with or without agoraphobia	CBT	Barlow et al. (1989)	Relaxation	Bona fide	NO
Panic disorder with or without agoraphobia	CBT	Clark et al. (1994)	Applied relaxation (AR)	Bona fide	YES
GAD	CBT	Butler, Fennell, Robson, & Gelder (1991)	BT	Bona fide	YES
Agoraphobia	CBT	Borkovec et al. (1987)	Non directive	Psych Placebo	
Agoraphobia	Exposure	Trull, Nietzel, & Main (1988)	Meta-analysis		
Specific phobia	Exp./guided mastery	Bandura, Blanchard, & Ritter (1969)	Symbolic modeling, symbolic desensitization	Bona fide	YES
Specific phobia	Exp./guided mastery	Öst et al. (1991)	Self-directed exp.	Not bona fide	
OCD	Exp./response prevention	Van Balkom et al. (1994)	Meta-analysis		
Coping with stressors	Stress inoculation	Saunders, Driskell, Hall, & Salas (1996)	Meta-analysis		
Depression	BT	Jacobson et al. (1996)	CBT	Bona fide	NO
Depression	BT	McLean & Hakstian (1979)	Relaxation	Not bona fide	NO
Depression	CBT	Dobson (1989)	Meta-analysis		
Depression	IPT	DiMascio et al. (1979)	None		
Depression	IPT	Elkin et al. (1989)	CBT	Bona fide	NO

Note. The studies listed here were designated by Chambless et al., 1998. Some treatments were established by meta-analysis and thus the control group designation is not relevant; these meta-analyses are discussed in the text.

treatments that would not be classified as bona fide psychotherapy using Wampold, Mondin, Moody, and Ahn's (1997) definition of treatments intended to be therapeutic: nondirective therapy for agoraphobia (Borkovec et al., 1987), self-directed exposure for specific phobia (no therapist; Öst, Salkovskis, & Hellstrom, 1991), and relaxation for depression (no rationale for its mechanism; McLean & Hakstian, 1979). In three cases within the study used to establish the EST, the comparison treatment was not found to be inferior to the EST, and these cases were CBT and relaxation for panic disorder (Barlow, Craske, Cerny, & Klosko, 1989), BT and CBT for depression (Jacobson et al., 1996), and interpersonal therapy (IPT) and CBT for depression (Elkin et al., 1989). It should be noted that in all three cases the comparison treatment either was already a "well-established" EST or became at least a "probably efficacious treatment" (Chambless et al., 1998).

In three cases within the studies used to establish an EST, the EST was found to be superior to another treatment intended to be therapeutic: CBT was more effective than applied relaxation (AR) for panic disorder (Clark et al., 1994), exposure and guided mastery were more effective than symbolic treatments for a specific phobia (Bandura et al., 1969), and CBT was more effective than behavioral therapy for generalized anxiety disorder (GAD; Butler et al., 1991). In the first instance, AR has now been designated as a probably efficacious treatment (Chambless et al., 1998), nullifying this comparison as an example of a non-EST as being inferior (an issue to be discussed later). Moreover, at least two other studies have found no differences between CBT and AR (Öst & Westling, 1995; Öst, Westling, & Hellstrom, 1993). Bandura's findings suggested that exposure in vivo is superior to covert exposure for a simple phobia, which is an examination of the intricacies of a particular treatment, rather than a comparison between an EST and a non-EST. The final study that showed the superiority of an EST (viz., CBT for GAD over BT) has also been shown to be inconsistent with several other studies that have shown an equivalence between CBT and BT for GAD (see Emmelkamp, 2004).

The point here is that the studies used to designate treatments as well-established ESTs for depression and anxiety have not shown that the EST was superior to a non-EST. In the few cases where the well-established EST was superior to another treatment, later studies either contradicted the original result or demonstrated an equivalence of the EST and non-EST, often resulting in the comparison treatment then appearing on an EST list (see next section).

Depression and the Proliferation of ESTs

The treatment of depression illustrates a dilemma inherent in making the case that non-ESTs are as effective as ESTs. If all bona fide treatments of depression are equally effective, then one would expect to see a proliferation of ESTs as each treatment is standardized and the appropriate clinical trials conducted. By 1998, behavior therapy, cognitive therapy, interpersonal therapy, brief dynamic therapy, reminiscence therapy (for geriatric patients), self-control therapy, and social problem-solving therapy had all been designated as well-established or probably efficacious treatments for depression (Chambless et al., 1998).

Meta-analyses of depression treatments have shown that all treatments are equivalent when various confounds are taken into account (Wampold, 2001). For example, Robinson, Berman, and Neimeyer (1990) found the superiority of behavioral and cognitive–behavioral treatments was due to the allegiance of the researchers. Dobson (1989), as indicated previously, found that cognitive therapy was superior to behavior therapy, but Gaffan, Tsaousis, and Kemp-Wheeler (1995) found the opposite. Gloaguen, Cottraux, Cucherat, and Blackburn (1998) found that behavioral and cognitive–behavioral treatments were equivalent, but that cognitive therapies were superior to a class of "other" therapies, which were noncognitive, nonbehavioral, and primarily "verbal." However, many of the treatments in the latter group were not intended to be therapeutic and were used to control common factors; when these treatments were eliminated, cognitive therapy was not superior to noncognitive, nonbehavioral therapies (Wampold, Minami, Baskin, & Tierney, 2002). Elliott, Greenberg, and Lietaer (2004) found meta-analytically that bona fide experiential psychotherapies were as effective as other therapies for the treatment of depression.

Anxiety and the Hegemony of Behavioral and Cognitive–Behavioral Treatments

A threat to the Dodo Bird Effect is that some relatively benign disorders are treatable via the common factors of psychotherapy, but that more severe pathology requires specific treatment (e.g., Crits-Christoph, 1997). The anxiety disorders are often presented as those that require specific treatments. However, precious little data suggest that any treatment of any anxiety disorder is more effective than any other. Wampold (2001) reviewed eight meta-analyses of the treatment of anxiety disorders that compared various psychological treatments and found few differences between any treatments.

The treatment of OCD is often raised as the perspicuous example of the superiority of an EST: exposure and response prevention (ERP). However, early on ERP became generally accepted as the treatment of choice, and researchers were not interested in (or could not obtain funding) to develop and test other therapies, with the exception of CBT. Initially, it appeared that ERP was superior to CBT, but recent trials have suggested an equivalence (some trials favoring CBT, some favoring ERP; Emmelkamp, 2004). No reasonably conducted clinical trial comparing CBT or ERP to any nonbehavioral, noncognitive treatment intended to be therapeutic for OCD has been conducted due to the hegemony of CBT and ERP. It may well be that directive, focused treatments are superior to more insight and experiential therapies for the treatment of OCD, as suggested by Elliott, Greenberg, and Lietaer (2004), but the existing evidence does not show that this is true.

Despite the hegemony of cognitive and behavioral treatments in clinical trials, exceptions exist. Meta-analyses tend to support the efficacy of social skill training for social phobia (Taylor, 1996), eye movement desensitization and reprocessing (EMDR) for posttraumatic stress disorder (PSTD; Sherman, 1998), and experiential therapies for GAD (Elliott et al., 2004). Whether these treatments are as efficacious as cognitive and behavioral ESTs for the respective disorders has not been addressed extensively; nevertheless, these treatments have not been shown to be inferior to the ESTs. It is worth noting that it has been claimed that EMDR is effective because it involves exposure, a primary behavioral component; however, it also could be claimed that experiencing the painful event in an experiential therapy involves exposure. The conclusion at the end of that slippery slope is that exposure of some form is a powerful common factor in the treatment of anxiety.

METHODOLOGICAL ISSUES

Two methodological issues are critical to any comparison of EST and non-EST treatments. The first is that researcher allegiance has been found reliably to exert a strong influence on the outcomes of clinical trials (Luborsky & Barrett, chap. 6, this volume; Luborksy et al., 1999; Wampold, 2001). The literature is replete with examples of studies that favor a particular treatment conducted by advocates of that treatment, whereas studies conducted by advocates of an alternative treatment favor the alternative. Evidence shows that the size of the allegiance effect is several times as great as the effect for differences among treatments (Wampold, 2001). Given that researchers conduct most investigations of ESTs with an allegiance to the EST being investigated, allegiance has to be taken into account in any apparent superiority of an EST over a non-EST. The National Institute of Mental Health (NIMH) Treatment of Depression Collaborative Research Program (TDCRP) was commendable in that the therapists for CBT and IPT had allegiance to the treatments, respectively (Elkin et al., 1989), providing a fair comparison between the treatments (and yielding no significant differences). Another study that deliberately balanced allegiance compared process–experiential (a non-EST) and cognitive–behavioral treatments for depression and found no differences as well (Watson, Gordon, Stermac, Kalogerakos, & Steckley, 2003).

The second issue is that ignoring therapist effects results in an overestimation of treatment effects and an inflation of error rates (Crits-Christoph & Mintz, 1991; Moerbeek, 2004; Wampold, chap. 7, this volume; Wampold

& Serlin, 2000). In clinical trials, observed differences between treatments are due to random variations among therapists as well as true differences between treatments. The variability in outcomes due to therapists within treatments in clinical trials is in the neighborhood of 8% (Kim, Wampold, & Bolt, in press), which is sufficient to result in significantly biased estimates of treatment superiority. For example, in a study by Durham and colleagues (1994) used to establish cognitive therapy as an EST for GAD, the observed superiority of cognitive therapy to analytic therapy could be explained by therapist variability. When such variability was modeled, the two treatments were not significantly different (Wampold & Serlin, 2000).

CONCLUSIONS

The scientific method stipulates that the null hypothesis be retained until such time that sufficient evidence justifies rejection and acceptance of the alternative hypothesis. That is, the scientific community should not disseminate a claim as being established if the evidence is not strong. In the present case, the null hypothesis is that ESTs and other psychotherapies intended to be therapeutic (i.e., bona fide treatments) are equally effective. Evidence has been presented that psychotherapies compared in clinical trials are equally efficacious, in general and specifically for depression and anxiety disorders. Most clinical trials investigate behavioral or cognitive behavioral treatments and most of these treatments meet the criteria for being an EST, but the lack of trials involving non-ESTs intended to be therapeutic is not a reason to reject the null hypothesis. Moreover, when advocates of these treatments conduct trials of non-ESTs, the treatments produce effects comparable to those produced by ESTs.

The EST movement clearly stated criteria by which a treatment could be designated as empirically supported. Comparable criteria should be used to designate that a non-EST is inferior to an EST:

A non-EST is empirically established as inferior to an EST provided

A. the non-EST is a bona fide treatment proffered as a treatment for the disorder.
B. two trials are conducted that compare the treatments and
   1. allegiance is controlled in both trials, or
   2. an advocate of the EST conducts one trial and an advocate of the non-EST conducts the other trials.
C. therapist effects are considered in the design and analysis.
D. both trials favor the EST using a multivariate test (i.e., a linear combination of the outcome variables) modeling therapist effects and the size of the difference is clinically significant.

Evidence for the inferiority of non-ESTs has never approached meeting these criteria. The null hypothesis that ESTs are equivalent to non-ESTs must not be rejected in general or in any particular instance. Consequently, no claim for the superiority of ESTs should be made in the scientific community or to the public.

Empirically Supported Treatments Typically Produce Outcomes Superior to Non-Empirically Supported Treatment Therapies

Thomas H. Ollendick and Neville J. King

In this position paper, we address the question of whether those treatments that have been identified as empirically supported (ESTs) produce outcomes superior to those treatments that have not been identified as empirically supported (non-ESTs). At some level, the answer to this question is patently obvious and resoundingly in the affirmative. After all, the 1995 Task Force Report on Promotion and Dissemination of Psychological Procedures (Task Force, 1995) indicated that the designation of a well-established treatment could be confirmed only by showing that the treatment was "superior to pill or psychological placebo or to another treatment" (see Table 1, p. 21, Task Force). Thus, by definition, a treatment receiving EST status had to be shown to be more effective than a placebo control treatment or some "other" treatment. It was further specified that such superiority should be shown in "two good between-group design experiments" using treatment manuals and that the efficacy should be demonstrated by "at least two different investigators or investigatory teams" (Table 1, Task Force). On the other hand, if the treatment was shown to be more effective than a wait-list control or no treatment, this level of evidence would suggest that the treatment was only "probably efficacious" but not well established (see Table 2, Task Force). In the Task Force report, an attempt was made to identify psychotherapies of proven worth that emanated from different theoretical perspectives. To this end, the original task force was composed of members who represented a number of theoretical perspectives, including psychodynamic, interpersonal, behavioral, and cognitive–behavioral orientations.

Although at first blush the answer to the question at hand may seem obvious, the answer is much more complex largely because not all psychotherapies of different theoretical persuasions have been subjected to "good between-group design experiments," let alone by two or more different investigators or investigatory teams. Thus, it may never be the case that ESTs will be shown to be superior to some commonly practiced and nonempirically supported psychosocial treatments, simply because they have not been, and perhaps never will be, subjected to randomized clinical trials (RCTs) using treatment manuals. This state of affairs is unfortunate for the practice of psychotherapy, and we can only encourage research to occur with these commonly practiced psychotherapies to determine the evidentiary support for their ongoing use.

In this position paper, we review available evidence for the superiority of ESTs. Specifically, we examine (a) whether any evidence proves that they work better than treatment as usual (TAU) in clinical settings, and (b) whether they work better than treatments of some "other" theoretical orientation. We illustrate these developments primarily with two commonly occurring disorders, panic disorder and major depression, but we also comment on other disorders as appropriate.

DO ESTS WORK?

A little over 50 years ago, Eysenck (1952) wrote his now (in)famous review of the effects of adult psychotherapy. He asserted that psychotherapy, as practiced at that time, was no more effective than the simple passage of time. A few years later, Levitt (1957) reviewed the child psychotherapy literature and arrived at a similar verdict. These conclusions were unsettling, but at the same time they served as a stimulus for increased research activity. Although the reviews led many to question the continued viability of the practice of child and adult psychotherapy, they energized others to address the challenges inherent in establishing the efficacy of psychotherapy. Thus, these seminal reviews served as a wake-up call and, in no small way, led to a revolution in psychotherapy research. As a result, we have moved beyond the simple question, "Does psychotherapy work?" to identify the efficacy of specific treatments for individuals who present with specific behavioral and emotional disorders.

The movement to develop, identify, disseminate, and use ESTs (initially referred to as "empirically validated treatments;" Task Force, 1995) has not been without controversy. On the surface, it hardly seems possible that anyone could or would object to the initial report issued by the Society of Clinical Psychology of the American Psychological Association (APA) 10 years ago. Surely, identifying, developing, and disseminating treatments that possess empirical support should be encouraged, not discouraged, especially by a profession committed to the welfare of those whom it serves. However, as we have witnessed in recent years, the Task Force report has served to deeply divide the profession of clinical psychology and related mental health disciplines.

In a series of papers over the years, Chambless and her colleagues have reviewed the literature and provided updated lists of ESTs. In the original

Task Force Report (1995), 25 treatments that met the criteria of an EST were identified. In 1998, the list had grown to 71 treatments (Chambless & Hollon, 1998), and by 2001 the list mushroomed to 108 treatments for adults and 37 for children (Chambless & Ollendick, 2001). As is evident, the designation of treatments as ESTs has been an active, dynamic process. Although the majority of treatments identified as empirically supported over the past 10 years have been behavioral and cognitive–behavioral ones, treatments emanating from other theoretical persuasions have been identified and included on the EST lists as well. For example, although Chambless and Ollendick reported that empirical support for the treatment of panic disorder was available only for behavioral and cognitive–behavioral psychotherapies, they identified evidentiary support for (in alphabetical order) behavior therapy, brief psychodynamic therapy, CBT, interpersonal psychotherapy, and problem-solving therapy in the treatment of adult depression. These developments are good testimony to the dynamic and inclusive nature of the designation process, as well as the healthy state of psychotherapy research. Quite obviously, a number of specific treatments for specific disorders have been identified and have been implemented in community mental health and primary care settings, both for adults (e.g., Craske et al., 2002; Merrill, Tolbert, & Wade, 2003; Persons, Bostrom, & Bertagnolli, 1999; Peterson & Halstead, 1998; Stuart, Treat, & Wade, 2000; Wade, Treat, & Stuart, 1998) and children (e.g., Taylor, Schmidt, Pepler, & Hodgins, 1998; Tynan, Schuman, & Lampert, 1999; Weersing & Weisz, 2002).

DO ESTS WORK BETTER THAN TAU IN COMMUNITY PRACTICE SETTINGS?

The studies used to establish the evidentiary base of treatments have not typically evaluated the effectiveness of the designated ESTs when compared to routine clinical practice in mental health and primary care settings. Such a direct comparison is desirable, though infrequently pursued. In recent years, regulatory boards and funding agencies have eschewed such comparisons, yet such studies are clearly needed to establish whether the ESTs truly perform better than practice as usual in those settings.

Two questions must be raised here: How effective are TAUs? And do ESTs perform better than TAUs? Evidence on the effectiveness of TAUs is surprisingly scant in the adult literature. A notable early exception, of course, is the seminal review completed by Eysenck in 1952 that suggested that clinic-based therapy was no better than the passage of time. In the child and adolescent literature, however, Weisz, Donenberg, Han, and Kauneckis (1995) searched for studies that might fairly be called "clinic therapy." Specifically, they searched for studies that involved (a) the treatment of clinic-referred youngsters, not recruited ones, (b) treatments that were conducted in service-oriented clinics, not research settings, (c) therapy that was provided by practicing clinicians, not graduate students or residents, and (d) therapy that was delivered as part of the ongoing services of the clinic, not special research programs. For inclusion, they retained studies that involved direct comparisons between youngsters who received TAU and a control group who received no treatment or a placebo control condition. Nine studies were identified, including one of their own (Weisz & Weiss, 1989) that met these exacting criteria. The studies all compared treatment and control groups, but with different methodologies. The effect sizes ranged from $-.40$ to $+.29$, with a mean effect size for the nine studies of .01, suggesting that if the treated child were placed in the control group after treatment, he or she would be no better off than the average child in the control group (essentially no effect due to treatment). This effect size fell well below the mean effect size of four broad-based meta-analyses of child and adolescent treatment outcome (.77) reviewed by Weisz, Huey, and Weersing (1998). These results indicate that "clinic-based" TAU therapy was much less effective than therapy as delivered in randomized clinical control efficacy studies. Similar reviews of the literature for adults receiving TAU in community clinics are greatly needed at this time.

How do ESTs compare to TAUs in clinical settings? Studies that directly compare the outcomes of ESTs with existing clinical services provide one of the true litmus tests for the effectiveness of ESTs (Addis, 1997; Chambless & Ollendick, 2001; Ollendick & King, 2004). Although not many such studies have been reported, a limited number of studies suggest that ESTs compare quite well. In one of the first such studies, Teasdale and associates (Teasdale, Fennel, Hibbert, & Amies, 1984) compared the CBT of depression to TAU in a clinical setting and found the subsequently established EST to be more effective. Similarly, Linehan and colleagues (Linehan, Armstrong, Suarez, Allmon, & Heard, 1991) examined the efficacy of dialectical behavior therapy (DBT) to TAU in the treatment of parasuicidal behavior (any intentional, acute self-injurious behavior with or without suicidal intent) in women with borderline personality disorder. The treatment lasted 1 year, with assessments conducted every 4 months. At most assessment points and during the entire year, the women who received DBT had fewer incidences of parasuicide and less medically severe parasuicides, they were more likely to stay in psychotherapy, and they had fewer psychiatric inpatient days. For example, the women who received DBT had a median of 1.5 parasuicide acts per year compared with 9.0 acts per year for the women who received TAU. Although decreases on self-report measures of depression, hopelessness, and suicidal ideation did not favor DBT, in none of the measures did TAU outperform DBT.

In a recent study, Addis and colleagues (Addis et al., 2004) determined the effectiveness of CBT for panic disorder versus TAU in a managed care setting. Panic control therapy (PCT) was the CBT intervention selected for evaluation. In brief, PCT is a 12 to 15 session manual-based treatment that integrates psychoeducational, cognitive, and exposure-based (agoraphobic and interoceptive) treatment components (see Barlow et al., 1989; Barlow, Gorman, Shear, & Woods, 2000). Therapists in this condition were informed that the treatment typically required approximately 15 weekly sessions; however, they were not required to schedule a specific number of sessions. Rather, they were instructed to adapt the standard treatment protocol and to use it as they saw fit. As such, they were requested to use the treatment protocol in a flexible and clinically sensitive manner. The TAU therapists, on the other hand, were instructed to provide whatever treatment they deemed appropriate. They were given no special instructions about the length or type of treatment to be used. For both groups, decisions about medication use were left up to the clients and their caregivers; that is, clients were free to obtain medications in both conditions. Although clients in both conditions showed significant changes from pre- to posttreatment on a number of outcome measures, those receiving PCT showed greater levels of change than those receiving TAU. Overall, 42.9% of those in the PCT condition and 18.8% of those in the TAU condition achieved clinically significant changes across outcome measures. Importantly, these differences were obtained, even though strategies for agoraphobic exposure, one of the key components in PCT, were used infrequently by the CBT therapists.

Therapists in this EST–TAU trial were 10 master's-level practitioners who were employed by a managed care company. Reportedly, none of them identified their primary theoretical orientation as cognitive–behavioral and as a group they described themselves as being equally distributed among eclectic, family systems, psychodynamic, and humanistic orientations. The therapists, matched on the number of years of experience, were randomly assigned to one of the two conditions. The PCT treatment was manualized, but the TAU was not. Credibility measures were obtained, and therapist adherence to PCT was determined (competence in the implementation of treatment was not measured, however).

Addis and colleagues (2004) commented on a number of methodological limitations in their study, including the absence of a no-treatment or wait-list control group, the nonspecific aspects of therapist training that might have favored the therapists in the CBT condition, the lack of a competence measure for the CBT condition, and expectancy effects associated with feedback and the monitoring of the therapists in the CBT but not TAU condition. Still, they argued these limitations are likely to characterize all attempts to implement ESTs in clinical practice settings and that these "realities" are the very ones that must be considered in evaluating the ESTs in those settings. In effect, internal and external validity must be jointly considered.

Taken together, these few studies provide a rich glimpse into the potential efficacy of ESTs in comparison to "other" treatments, defined as TAU in those settings. However, it should be noted that comparing a structured EST to a TAU does not allow definitive conclusions because the TAU is typically unspecified and its ingredients are not well known. More reliable conclusions are likely to be drawn from comparisons of one specified treatment (a potential EST) with another specified treatment that has already been established as an EST.

DO ESTS FOR SPECIFIC DISORDERS WORK BETTER THAN "OTHER" TREATMENTS?

As noted earlier, by definition, ESTs work better than a pill, psychological placebo, or "other" treatments to which they have been compared in RCTs. In many of these studies, a potent form of intervention was compared to a less potent form, such as when systematic desensitization or graduated exposure was compared to relaxation training alone. In other studies, treatment on the basis of one theoretical orientation was compared to treatment emanating from another orientation, such as when CBT was compared to nondirective therapy, and in still other studies a candidate treatment was compared to an education support or psychological placebo treatment. Many authors have commented on the methodological problems inherent in several of these studies and question whether they truly provide support for the efficacious nature of the "empirically supported" treatments (e.g., Wampold et al., 1997; Westen et al., 2004). In doing so, these reviewers also question whether any meaningful differences exist among the various types of treatment and whether the infamous Dodo Bird Effect ought to apply (i.e., the equivalence of outcomes in psychotherapy research: All have won and all ought to receive prizes). Others have supplied commentaries on these reviews and have challenged the substance of the reviews themselves (e.g., Crits-Christoph, 1997; Haaga, 2004).

Crits-Christoph (1997), for example, suggested that Wampold, Mondin, Moody, Stitch, et al.'s (1997) reliance on follow-up assessments versus posttreatment assessments may have affected their conclusion about the equivalence of different psychotherapies. For example, some patients who were well at the end of treatment relapsed, and others may have received effective intermediate treatments. He also suggested that Wampold et al.'s decision to average effect sizes across outcome measures within a study may have been flawed because, for example, some measures are more important than others (some measure core symptoms, whereas others measure associated phenomena). Crits-Christoph also commented on the actual studies reviewed by Wampold and colleagues. Of the 114 articles used in the meta-analysis, Crits-Christoph noted that only 51 articles (about 45%) examined treatments for more severe problems that could be viewed as "disorders," and 79 (about 69%) of the studies involved comparisons of one form of behavioral or cognitive–behavioral treatment to another form of behavioral or cognitive–behavioral treatment. Finally, Crits-Christoph argued that the Dodo bird conclusion of equivalence did not apply when he examined studies that compared a cognitive–behavioral treatment to a bona fide noncognitive–behavioral treatment, such as nondirective psychotherapy. Fourteen such studies were identified. For these studies, the effect size was large in magnitude and demonstrated the superiority of behavioral and cognitive–behavioral interventions over noncognitive–behavioral ones. Hence, although Wampold and colleagues concluded that equivalence existed among the psychotherapies and that all should receive prizes, Crits-Christoph challenged that conclusion. We do as well.

A couple of studies will be presented that illustrate the superiority of ESTs over bona fide treatments. It is important to note here that the comparison treatments in these studies are not sham placebos; rather, they are thought to be structurally equivalent therapies. In one of the first such studies, Borkovec and colleagues (Borkovec et al., 1987) assigned 30 clients who met criteria for GAD to progressive muscle relaxation with cognitive therapy (PMR + CT) or to PMR with nondirective therapy (PMR + ND). Although both groups improved at posttreatment and follow-up, the PMR + CT group was superior to the PMR + ND group on almost all the treatment outcome measures. Borkovec and colleagues concluded that the addition of CT to PMR was not only more effective than the addition of ND but also that CT contained specific effective components of change that ND did not. In a second study, Borkovec and Costello (1993) found that CBT, without AR, was significantly superior to ND at both posttreatment and 1-year follow-up. Clients in CBT and ND were comparable in their ratings of expectancy of change and in both conditions treatment manuals guided therapists. In addition, the authors verified that treatment effects were consistent across therapists. Consistent with the theory underlying ND, observers rated clients in that condition as having a greater depth of experiencing than clients in the CBT condition. Nonetheless, these clients failed to improve as much on outcome measures as those in CBT. Over 61% of those receiving ND requested and received additional treatment, compared to 16% of those receiving CBT. Similarly, Craske, Maidenberg, and Bystritsky (1995) showed that brief CBT treatment was more effective than brief nondirective supportive therapy in the treatment of panic disorder.

Similarly, in the child and adolescent arena, Kazdin, Esveldt-Dawson, French, and Unis (1987) showed that a cognitive–behavioral intervention (problem-solving therapy) was more effective than relationship therapy in the treatment of conduct-disorder children. Stark, Rouse, and Livingston (1991) also indicated that CBT was more effective than nondirective, supportive therapy in the treatment of children who reported high levels of depressive symptoms. At posttreatment and at 7-month follow-up, children in the CBT group reported fewer depressive symptoms on a semistructured interview and indicated fewer depressive symptoms on a depression questionnaire than children in the nondirective, supportive condition. In both of these studies, CBT or some variant of it was compared to a bona fide treatment and significant differences were obtained.

Of course, differences between ESTs and "other" treatments have not always been found. In such instances, these direct comparisons have led to the "comparison" treatment subsequently being designated as an EST itself. Such occurred in the TDCRP (Elkin et al., 1989). In this seminal study, CT for depression was compared to IPT (Klerman, Weissman, Rounsaville, & Chevron, 1984), along with other placebo and medication control conditions. Although some differences among the treatments were obtained, for the most part IPT and CT were shown to be similarly effective (Elkin et al., 1995). Subsequent studies also showed IPT to be effective in the treatment of depression in adults (DeRubeis & Crits-Christoph, 1998). As a result, IPT was designated as an EST (because it was equivalent to an already established treatment, CBT).

Recently, Watson and colleagues (Watson et al., 2003) similarly showed that process–experiential therapy (PET) produced outcomes similar to those for CBT in the treatment of depression. Clients' depression, self-esteem, general distress, and dysfunctional attitudes significantly improved in both groups. Earlier, Greenberg and Watson (1998) had shown that both PET and client-centered therapy were effective in treating depression with effect sizes comparable to those obtained with CBT. However, PET produced significantly greater improvement in clients' interpersonal problems and self-esteem than the client-centered ND. On the basis of these two RCTs, and the comparable effect sizes to CBT (an already established intervention), it is probable that PET should also receive EST status. Demonstration of the efficacy of PET in these two studies is welcome, and the list of effective interventions for the treatment of depression continues to expand.

RECOMMENDATIONS AND CONCLUSIONS

A number of studies have shown that ESTs are superior to TAU and at least some "other" bona fide treatments. In addition, some "other" treatments have been shown to be as effective as those previously identified as empirically supported, and they too have attained EST status. In our ongoing pursuit of ESTs, it will be important to compare ESTs to other treatments that have some "reasonable expectation" of altering the specific disorder under consideration. Our approach should not be to just compare treatments for the sake of comparing treatments. In our opinion, some treatments are more likely to work for specific disorders than others. As an analogy in the medical field, we would surely not expect an appendectomy to address the same dysfunction and serve the same treatment function as a tonsillectomy.

Recently, Woody and Ollendick (in press) suggested that viable treatment programs should rest on a sound theoretical rationale that addresses both the determinants of the disorder (i.e., its pathogenesis) and the purported mechanisms for bringing about desired therapeutic change. They have identified five specific and five general principles of change that might guide the treatment of anxiety disorders. Not all treatments possess these characteristics.

The specific principles that directly address the specific psychopathology of anxiety and its disorders, as well as potential mechanisms of change, include (a) challenge faulty misconceptions by discussing and explicitly questioning the evidence, (b) actively test the validity of erroneous and maladaptive ideas through behavioral experiments, (c) use repeated exposure to the feared situation to reduce the intensity of the fear response, (d) eliminate or at least greatly reduce avoidance of the feared situation, and (e) improve skills for handling the feared situation. Implicit within these five principles are strategies to address the primary modalities of responding in the anxiety disorders: cognition, affect, and behavior. In addition to these five specific principles, Woody and Ollendick articulated five general principles that cut across the ESTs for the anxiety disorders. The principles are (a) therapists should be directive, and the therapeutic process should be structured and action oriented, (b) treatment strategies should focus on facilitating behavior change (in contrast to insight), (c) treatment should be time limited and relatively intense, (d) effective treatments for anxiety disorders should use emotionally evocative procedures, and (e) EST for anxiety disorders should be focused on intrapersonal dimensions (in contrast to interpersonal ones). These principles map to certain therapies more readily than others, and direct comparisons should be made among those therapies that have some "realistic expectation" of working, not just any treatment.

In summary, considerable support exists for the assertions that ESTs perform significantly better than non-ESTs and that their promulgation and dissemination ought to continue, and we suggest, at an even greater pace. Although methodological concerns can always be raised, it is unlikely that the "perfect" study will ever be conducted and that critics will always find fault with the published studies. The corpus of research, however, supports their use. It seems to us that we now have a number of specific treatments that work for specific disorders. These treatments work in applied clinical settings, yielding effect sizes that approximate those obtained in research setting. Moreover, although limited studies are currently available, they perform better than TAU in clinical settings, and they are superior to "other" bona fide therapies, especially when these other therapies are not variants of the designated EST and when bona fide disorders, rather than less severe problems, are treated. Although these treatments have produced beneficial outcomes, it is important to determine how these efficacious treatments can be enhanced to produce even greater gains in the clients we serve. Of course, we must also continue to develop and explore "other" treatments to determine if they might produce even greater effects than the currently established ones. In doing so, the currently designated ESTs, and the specific and general principles of intervention that underlie them, might serve as benchmarks to which these new and experimental treatments are compared.

Dialogue: Convergence and Contention

Bruce E. Wampold

I am in agreement with two fundamental points made by Ollendick and King. First, the contention of Eysenck that psychotherapy does not produce outcomes differentiable from the natural history of the disorder is incontrovertibly erroneous. The scientific evidence strongly suggests that psychotherapy is a healing practice that benefits clients. Second, we all agree that the development of specific change principles that address particular psychopathology is a useful way to proceed. It would seem that every therapist treating a depressed person (e.g., behavioral activation) or an avoidant patient (e.g., exposure) should imbed certain actions in treatment.

At the same time, we dramatically disagree about the evidence and its practice implications. Fundamentally, I am not convinced in the very least that evidence supports the contention that ESTs are consistently superior to any other treatments that are based on generally accepted psychological theory and that are delivered by competent therapists who have allegiance to the therapy. Arguments to the contrary rely on fallacious logic or flawed interpretations of the evidence.

A first error involves the construction of a system that can only confirm the conclusion for which it was designed to support. Nothing in the criteria mentions identifying an EST that requires an EST to be superior to another bona fide treatment, as I discussed in my position paper. The typical comparison group involves a treatment without psychological basis and is delivered by therapists who know it is a sham. Moreover, the criteria, imbedded in a medical model, were promulgated in ways that favored cognitive and behavioral treatments (e.g., treatments with manuals) and ignored factors that influence outcomes other than the treatment (e.g., alliance or the therapist). To say that, using these criteria, it is "patently and resoundingly obvious" that ESTs are more effective than other treatments displays a belief in a system (viz., the EST criteria and the process by which treatments are so designated) that is unwarranted scientifically.

A second error is that the studies cited by Ollendick and King actually tend to support the conclusion that ESTs are not superior to other treatments. In a way, they have been hoisted on their own petard. Hundreds of studies have compared treatments intended to be therapeutic; that Ollendick and King cited only a few showing the superiority of one treatment over another is exactly what one might expect by chance if indeed the null hypothesis of no differences among treatments were true. It is not permissible scientifically to cull the literature to find instances in which a hypothesis was supported and ignore those that were unsupportive. After all, it was Gene Glass who successfully defeated Eysenck's demoralizing statements about psychotherapy by including all studies bearing on this question, rather than relying on biased selection of studies.

The studies selected by Ollendick and King are, furthermore, not supportive of their conclusion that an EST is superior to treatments intended to be therapeutic. The preponderance of the studies cited (Borkovec et al., 1987; Borkovec & Costello, 1993; Craske et al., 1995; Kazdin et al., 1987) involved comparisons of cognitive or behavioral treatments to nondirective interventions, which, despite Ollendick and King's contention that they were "not sham treatments," did not meet anyone's criteria for a fair comparison. Researchers who conducted these studies had an allegiance to the behavioral or cognitive treatment and, as we know, allegiance has a profound biasing effect (Luborksy et al., 1999; Wampold, 2001). Moreover, the nondirective treatments were not instances of any known treatment for the disorders in question; they were not representative of modern process–experiential treatments as offered by, say, Leslie Greenberg. Finally, the nondirective therapists in each of these trials were quite aware that they were delivering a less desirable form of treatment.

The comparison of an EST to TAU constituted a major tenet of Ollendick and King's argument. Westen and colleagues (2004) discussed many of the problems with TAU as a comparison to ESTs and concluded that the validity of the comparison is suspect. These problems are quite apparent in the Addis et al. (2004) study cited prominently by Ollendick and King. First, the "superior" outcomes of the cognitive–behavioral treatment for panic were not dramatically more effective than the TAU. For the intent-to-treat sample, CBT outperformed TAU on only 2 of the 5 dependent measures at the most immediate posttest period; the mean effect size for the difference between CBT and TAU was about .14, which is extremely small; and for intent-to-treat, as well as the more complete sample, no significant differences occurred in the percentage of clients demonstrating clinically significant change. Second, the comparison between CBT and TAU was patently unfair. The primarily master's-level therapists, with no particular expertise in the treatment of panic disorder, were for the most part randomly assigned to CBT or TAU, which is a commendable design feature. However, the CBT therapists received a 2-day training workshop on panic disorder, feedback on training cases, and optional supervision by an expert in panic who was also the principal investigator, whereas the TAU therapists had no special training, feedback, or supervision. It is unclear whether the TAU therapists, given workshops on panic disorder and principles of treatment for the disorder, would not have achieved outcomes equivalent to the CBT therapists. This study suggests that additional training in a specific treatment for a specific disorder may produce marginally better outcomes, but it does not establish the superiority of CBT. The other two EST versus TAU studies cited by Ollendick and King (Teasdale et al., 1984; Linehan et al., 1991) suffered from similar problems. Clients in the EST condition received significantly more therapy from specially trained therapists and displayed more benefits only on some measures and only at limited time periods (e.g., in the Teasdale study, clients showed no differences at 3-month follow-up).

Some important studies, not cited by Ollendick and King, would dispute their contentions. Ollendick and King cite Crits-Christoph's criticism of Wampold et al. (1997) related to the use of follow-up assessments, the severity of disorders treated, targeted versus global measures, and the preponderance of cognitive–behavioral studies. They failed, however, to cite a reanalysis of these data designed to address these criticisms that found that assessment time, the severity of the disorder, and the specificity of measures did not mitigate the findings of no differences among treatments intended to be therapeutic (Wampold, Mondin, Moody, & Ahn, 1997). The idea that a cognitive treatment is generally more effective than other treatments belies the results of recent meta-analyses that demonstrate that psychodynamic therapy produces comparable effects for specific psychiatric disorders, including personality disorders (Leichsenring & Leibing, 2003; Leichsenring, Rabung, & Leibing, 2004).

To reject the null hypothesis that ESTs and non-ESTs are equivalent, sufficient evidence must be presented to contend that the null is false; I presented rigorous criteria for such a rejection in my position paper. The evidence presented by Ollendick and King, in my view, falls so short that rejection should not even be considered. Nevertheless, the hypothesis that principles of change for specific disorders is viable; efforts should be devoted to determine whether these principles are essential to producing benefits to patients with these disorders.

Thomas H. Ollendick and Neville J. King

We agree with Wampold's position on certain items but vigorously disagree on others. Not unlike the phenomenon of researchers' allegiance in treatment outcome studies, we suspect that many of our differences reflect worldviews about evidence-based practice (EBP) and its relevance to the clinical enterprise. Both Wampold and we are looking at the same proverbial elephant but from different vantage points, and we arrive at different conclusions. We maintain we must move beyond allegiance and "perceptual" differences and let the empirical evidence speak. To achieve true EBP (i.e., "the integration of best research evidence with clinical expertise and patient values," Sackett, Rosenberg, Muir-Gray, Haynes, & Richardson, 1996, p. 71), we must identify the treatments that work so that they can be "integrated" into routine clinical practice.

We agree with Wampold that because a psychological treatment for a particular disorder has not been shown to be empirically supported does not mean the treatment is either inefficacious or not as efficacious as an EST. As he notes, and as we comment as well, the treatment may simply not yet have been subjected to the test required for EST status. We differ greatly, however, on what action we would recommend on the basis of our shared conclusion. Wampold would have us undertake two RCTs in which allegiance is actively controlled or in which one trial is conducted by an advocate of an existing EST, the other by an advocate of an aspiring EST, and therapist effects are considered in the design and analysis of the experiment. Moreover, both trials would need to favor the existing EST using a multivariate test that models therapist effects and shows that the size of the difference is clinically significant.

It seems to us that Wampold puts the cart before the horse here. The burden of proof that a treatment enjoys the "privileged" (Wampold's descriptor) status of an EST falls squarely on the shoulders of the aspiring EST, not the existing one. That is, it is not required that advocates of ESTs undertake a series of studies to show that non-ESTs in current practice do not possess empirical support. Regulatory boards, including the Food and Drug Administration (FDA), would surely wince at such a suggestion. Basically, Wampold suggests that we submit a myriad of "bona fide" treatments (literally dozens, if not more) to such experimental scrutiny. Such a recommendation flies in the face of considerable research that indicates treatments that are based on certain principles of change for certain forms of psychopathology are more likely to produce change over other mismatched treatments (cf. Beutler & Castonguay, in press).

Barlow (2004) proposed three overriding principles to be used in evaluating candidate interventions: (a) match the intervention to the psychological or physical disorder or problem, (b) match the treatment to patient and therapist characteristics, and (c) match the treatment to actual settings in which the treatments are to be provided. The first recommendation is apropos to our discussion here. We need to ask whether the candidate treatment is theoretically designed and equipped to address the problems or psychopathology evident in the disorders we are treating before we undertake experimental evaluations of them. As noted recently by Edwards, Dattilio, and Bromley (2004, p. 590), "it would be wasteful to commit the considerable expense and effort involved in running RCTs to treatments for which there was not already a strong body of evidence regarding effectiveness." We concur with this appraisal, and in our position paper we stated, by analogy to the field of medicine, that we would not expect a treatment designed to address appendicitis to be useful with tonsillitis. Stated simply, some treatments are designed to address specific psychopathologies more than others (Woody & Ollendick, in press). It does not make good sense to us to submit all the various bona fide treatments to such experimental scrutiny. This would be a never-ending process for any one disorder, let alone the multiplicity of disorders with which we work.

Do therapies designated as ESTs for some of these specific disorders produce outcomes that are superior to non-EST therapies? In our position paper, we suggested that they "typically do," whereas Wampold asserted that there was not a "scintilla of evidence" to support such a conclusion. Quite obviously, we disagree greatly here. To support our position, we reviewed evidence for the superiority of ESTs over TAU in the clinical setting and the limited but emerging evidence for the superiority of ESTs over some non-ESTs for both children and adults. Wampold did not review the TAU literature, and he claimed that all or most of the studies that show ESTs are superior to non-ESTs were methodologically flawed. Nor did Wampold review the child and adolescent treatment literature as did we. As we noted, the bulk of the evidence from the child and adult literature supports ESTs as superior to TAUs and to those non-ESTs that have been evaluated. We lamented the fact that many non-ESTs have simply not been examined to date. However, as we note previously, the burden of proof falls on the non-ESTs, not the ESTs, to show such evidentiary support.

Elsewhere (Ollendick & Davis, 2004), we have raised the question as to how long we should continue to use non-ESTs in the absence of evidentiary support. Will we be using the same unsupported and perhaps even harmful (see review by Weisz et al., 1995) interventions 10 years from now? Although we readily acknowledge that we do not have sufficient evidence for the efficacy of psychosocial interventions for some psychological disorders, in our opinion we must move forward and establish treatments that do work, whatever their theoretical orientation.

Recently, the Institute of Medicine's Committee on Quality of Health Care in America concluded that the gap between the care that patients could receive and the care they do receive is greater than a shortfall; it is a chasm (Institute of Medicine, 2001). A similar report issued by the President's New Freedom Commission on Mental Health (2003) identified shortcomings in our health system including the underuse of proven treatments, the overuse of treatments for which little evidentiary support exists, and the misuse of even those treatments that have been found to be effective. For many psychological problems, we already know what treatments are likely to work; for other problems, considerable work remains to be done. Still, Levitt (1957) and Eysenck (1952) would likely need to qualify their conclusions about the efficacy of psychological interventions for children and adults: These days some treatments do work better than the simple passage of time, and some do work better than others.

REFERENCES

Addis, M. E. (1997). Evaluating the treatment manual as a means of disseminating empirically validated psychotherapies. *Clinical Psychology: Science and Practice, 4*, 1–11.

Addis, M. E., Hatgis, C., Bourne, L., Krasnow, A. D., Jacob, K., & Mansfield, A. (2004). Effectiveness of cognitive–behavioral treatment for panic disorder versus treatment as usual in a managed care setting. *Journal of Consulting and Clinical Psychology, 72*, 625–635.

Bandura, A., Blanchard, E. B., & Ritter, B. (1969). Relative efficacy of desensitization and modeling approaches for inducing behavioral, affective, and attitudinal change. *Journal of Personality and Social Psychology, 13*, 173–199.

Barlow, D. H. (2004). Psychological treatments. *American Psychologist, 59*, 869–878.

Barlow, D. H., Craske, M. G., Cerny, J. A., & Klosko, J. S. (1989). Behavioral treatment of panic disorder. *Behavior Therapy, 20*, 261–282.

Barlow, D. H., Gorman, J. M., Shear, M. K., & Woods, S. W. (2000). Cognitive–behavioral therapy, imipramine, or their combination for panic disorder: A randomized controlled trial. *Journal of the American Medical Association, 283*, 2529–2536.

Basham, R. B. (1986). Scientific and practical advantages of comparative design in psychotherapy outcome research. *Journal of Consulting and Clinical Psychology, 54*, 88–94.

Baskin, T. W., Tierney, S. C., Minami, T., & Wampold, B. E. (2003). Establishing specificity in psychotherapy: A meta-analysis of structural equivalence of placebo controls. *Journal of Consulting and Clinical Psychology, 71*, 973–979.

Berman, J. S., Miller, C., & Massman, P. J. (1985). Cognitive therapy versus systematic desensitization: Is one treatment superior? *Psychological Bulletin, 97*, 451–461.

Beutler, L. E., & Castonguay, L. G. (in press). *Principles of change in effective psychotherapies.* New York: Oxford University Press.

Borkovec, T. D., & Costello, E. (1993). Efficacy of applied relaxation and cognitive behavioral therapy in the treatment of generalized anxiety disorder. *Journal of Consulting and Clinical Psychology, 61*, 611–619.

Borkovec, T. D., Mathews, K. M., Chambers, A., Ebrahimi, S., Lytle, R., & Nelson, R. (1987). The effects of relaxation training with cognitive or nondirective therapy and the role of relaxation-induced anxiety in the treatment of generalized anxiety. *Journal of Consulting and Clinical Psychology, 55,* 883–888.

Borkovec, T. D., & Nau, S. D. (1972). Credibility of analogue therapy rationales. *Journal of Behavior Therapy and Experimental Psychiatry, 3,* 257–260.

Brody, N. (1980). *Placebos and the philosophy of medicine: Clinical, conceptual, and ethical issues.* Chicago: The University of Chicago Press.

Butler, G., Fennell, M., Robson, P., & Gelder, M. (1991). Comparison of behavior therapy and cognitive behavior therapy in the treatment of generalized anxiety disorder. *Journal of Consulting and Clinical Psychology, 59,* 137–175.

Chambless, D. L., Baker, M. J., Baucom, D. H., Beutler, L. E., Calhoun, K. S., Daiuto, A., et al. (1998). Update on empirically validated therapies, II. *The Clinical Psychologist, 51,* 3–16.

Chambless, D. L., & Hollon, S. D. (1998). Defining empirically supported treatments. *Journal of Consulting and Clinical Psychology, 66,* 7–18.

Chambless, D. L., & Ollendick, T. H. (2001). Empirically supported psychological interventions: Controversies and evidence. *Annual Review of Psychology, 52,* 685–716.

Clark, D. M., Salkovskis, P. M., Hackmann, A., Middleton, H., Anastasiades, P., & Gelder, M. (1994). A comparison of cognitive therapy, applied relaxation, and imipramine in the treatment of panic disorder. *British Journal of Psychiatry, 164,* 759–769.

Craske, M. G., Maidenberg, E., & Bystritsky, A. (1995). Brief cognitive–behavioral versus nondirective therapy for panic disorder. *Journal of Behavior Therapy and Experimental Psychiatry, 26,* 113–120.

Craske, M. G., Roy-Byrne, P., Stein, M. B., Donald-Sherbourne, C., Bystritsky, A., Katon, W., et al. (2002). Treating panic disorder in primary care: A collaborative care intervention. *General Hospital Psychiatry, 24,* 148–155.

Crits-Christoph, P. (1997). Limitations of the Dodo Bird Verdict and the role of clinical trials in psychotherapy research: Comment on Wampold et al. (1997). *Psychological Bulletin, 122,* 216–220.

Crits-Christoph, P., & Mintz, J. (1991). Implications of therapist effects for the design and analysis of comparative studies of psychotherapies. *Journal of Consulting and Clinical Psychology, 59,* 20–26.

DeRubeis, R. J., & Crits-Christoph, P. (1998). Empirically supported individual and group psychological treatments for adult mental disorders. *Journal of Consulting and Clinical Psychology, 66,* 37–52.

DiMascio, A., Weissman, M. M., Prusoff, B. A., Neu, C., Zwilling, M., & Klerman, G. L. (1979). Differential symptom reduction by drugs and psychotherapy in acute depression. *Archives of General Psychiatry, 36,* 1450–1456.

Dobson, K. S. (1989). A meta-analysis of the efficacy of cognitive therapy for depression. *Journal of Consulting and Clinical Psychology, 57,* 414–419.

Durham, R. C., Murphy, T., Allan, T., Richard, K., Treliving, L. R., & Fenton, G. W. (1994). Cognitive therapy, analytic therapy and anxiety management training for generalised anxiety disorder. *British Journal of Psychiatry, 165*, 315–323.

Edwards, D. J. A., Dattilio, F. M., & Bromley, D. B. (2004). Developing evidence-based practice: The role of case-based research. *Professional Psychology Research and Practice, 35*, 589–597.

Elkin, I., Gibbons, R. D., Shea, M. T., Sotsky, S. M., Watkins, J. T., Pilkonis, P. A., et al. (1995). Initial severity and differential treatment outcome in the NIMH Treatment of Depression Collaborative Research Program. *Journal of Consulting and Clinical Psychology, 63*, 841–847.

Elkin, I., Shea, T., Watkins, J. T., Imber, S. D., Sotsky, S. M., Collins, J. F., et al. (1989). National Institute of Mental Health Treatment of Depression Collaborative Research Program: General effectiveness of treatments. *Archives of General Psychiatry, 46*, 971–982.

Elliott, R., Greenberg, L. S., & Lietaer, G. (2004). Research on experiential psychotherapies. In M. J. Lambert (Ed.), *Bergin and Garfield's handbook of psychotherapy and behavior change* (5th ed., pp. 493–539). New York: Wiley.

Emmelkamp, P. M. G. (2004). Behavior therapy with adults. In M. J. Lambert (Ed.), *Bergin and Garfield's handbook of psychotherapy and behavior change* (5th ed., pp. 393–446). New York: Wiley.

Eysenck, H. J. (1952). The effects of psychotherapy: An evaluation. *Journal of Consulting Psychology, 16*, 319–324.

Gaffan, E. A., Tsaousis, I., & Kemp-Wheeler, S. M. (1995). Researcher allegiance and meta-analysis: The case of cognitive therapy for depression. *Journal of Consulting and Clinical Psychology, 63*, 966–980.

Gloaguen, V., Cottraux, J., Cucherat, M., & Blackburn, I. (1998). A meta-analysis of the effects of cognitive therapy in depressed patients. *Journal of Affective Disorders, 49*, 59–72.

Greenberg, L. S., & Watson, J. C. (1998). Experiential therapy of depression: Differential effects of client-centered relationship conditions and process experiential interventions. *Psychotherapy Research, 8*, 210–224.

Grissom, R. J. (1996). The magical number .7 $\pm$ .2: Meta-meta-analysis of the probability of superior outcome in comparisons involving therapy, placebo, and control. *Journal of Consulting and Clinical Psychology, 64*, 973–982.

Haaga, D. A. F. (2004). A healthy dose of criticism for randomized trials: Comment on Westen, Novotny, and Thompson-Brenner (2004). *Psychological Bulletin, 130*, 674–676.

Henry, W. P. (1998). Science, politics, and the politics of science: The use and misuse of empirically validated treatments. *Psychotherapy Research, 8*, 126–140.

Horvath, P. (1988). Placebos and common factors in two decades of psychotherapy research. *Psychological Bulletin, 104*, 214–225.

Institute of Medicine. (2001). *Crossing the quality chasm: A new health system for the 21st century*. Washington, DC: National Academy Press.

Jacobson, N. S., Dobson, K. S., Truax, P. A., Addis, M. E., Koerner, K., Gollan, J. K., et al. (1996). A component analysis of cognitive–behavioral treatment for depression. *Journal of Consulting and Clinical Psychology, 64,* 295–304.

Kazdin, A. E., Esveldt-Dawson, K., French, N. H., & Unis, A. S. (1987). Problem-solving skills training and relationship therapy in the treatment of antisocial child behavior. *Journal of Consulting and Clinical Psychology, 55,* 76–85.

Kim, D. M., Wampold, B. E., & Bolt, D. M. (in press). Therapist effects in psychotherapy: A random effects modeling of the NIMH TDCRP data. *Psychotherapy Research.*

Klerman, G. L., Weissman, M. M., Rounsaville, B. J., & Chevron, E. S. (1984). *Interpersonal psychotherapy of depression.* New York: Basic Books.

Leichsenring, F., & Leibing, E. (2003). The effectiveness of psychodynamic therapy and cognitive behavior therapy in the treatment of personality disorders: A meta-analysis. *American Journal of Psychiatry, 160,* 1223–1231.

Leichsenring, F., Rabung, S., & Leibing, E. (2004). The efficacy of short-term psychodynamic psychotherapy in specific psychiatric disorders. *Archives of General Psychiatry, 61,* 1208–1216.

Levitt, E. E. (1957). The results of psychotherapy with children: An evaluation. *Journal of Consulting and Clinical Psychology, 21,* 189–196.

Linehan, M. M., Armstrong, H. E., Suarez, A., Allmon, D., & Heard, H. L. (1991). Cognitive–behavioral treatment of chronically parasuicidal borderline patients. *Archives of General Psychiatry, 48,* 1060–1064.

Luborsky, L., Diguer, L., Seligman, D. A., Rosenthal, R., Krause, E. D., Johnson, S., et al. (1999). The researcher's own therapy allegiances: A "wild card" in comparisons of treatment efficacy. *Clinical Psychology Science and Practice, 6,* 95–106.

McLean, P. D., & Hakstian, A. R. (1979). Clinical depression: Comparative efficacy of outpatient treatments. *Journal of Consulting and Clinical Psychology, 47,* 818–836.

Merrill, K. A., Tolbert, V. E., & Wade, W. A. (2003). Effectiveness of cognitive therapy for depression in a community mental health center: A benchmarking study. *Journal of Consulting and Clinical Psychology, 71,* 404–409.

Moerbeek, M. (2004). The consequences of ignoring a level of nesting in multilevel analysis. *Multivariate Behavioral Research, 39,* 129–149.

O'Leary, K. D., & Borkovec, T. D. (1978). Conceptual, methodological, and ethical problems of placebo groups in psychotherapy research. *American Psychologist, 33,* 821–830.

Ollendick, T. H., & Davis, T. E., III. (2004). Empirically supported treatments for children and adolescents: Where to from here? *Clinical Psychology: Science and Practice, 11,* 289–294.

Ollendick, T. H., & King, N. J. (2004). Empirically supported treatments for children and adolescents: Advances toward evidence-based practice. In P. M. Barrett & T. H. Ollendick (Eds.), *Handbook of interventions that work with children and adolescents: Prevention and treatment* (pp. 3–26). New York: Wiley.

Öst, L. G., Salkovskis, P. M., & Hellstrom, K. (1991). One-session therapist-directed exposure vs. self-exposure in the treatment of spider phobia. *Behavior Therapy, 22*, 407–422.

Öst, L. G., & Westling, B. E. (1995). Applied relaxation vs. cognitive behavior therapy in the treatment of panic disorder. *Behaviour Research and Therapy, 33*, 145–158.

Öst, L. G., Westling, B. E., & Hellstrom, B. (1993). Applied relaxation, exposure in vivo and cognitive methods in the treatment of panic disorder with agoraphobia. *Behaviour Research and Therapy, 31*, 383–394.

Persons, J. B., Bostrom, A., & Bertagnolli, A. (1999). Results of a randomized controlled trial of cognitive therapy for depression generalized to private practice. *Cognitive Therapy and Research, 23*, 535–548.

Peterson, A. L., & Halstead, T. S. (1998). Group cognitive behavior therapy for depression in a community setting: A clinical replication series. *Behavior Therapy, 29*, 3–18.

President's New Freedom Commission on Mental Health. (2003). *Achieving the promise: Transforming mental health care in America* (Final report). Washington, DC: Author.

Robinson, L. A., Berman, J. S., & Neimeyer, R. A. (1990). Psychotherapy for the treatment of depression: A comprehensive review of controlled outcome research. *Psychological Bulletin, 108*, 30–49.

Rosenzweig, S. (1936). Some implicit common factors in diverse methods of psychotherapy: "At last the Dodo said, 'Everybody has won and all must have prizes.'" *American Journal of Orthopsychiatry, 6*, 412–415.

Sackett, D. L., Rosenberg, W. M. C., Muir-Gray, J. A., Haynes, R. B., & Richardson, W. S. (1996). Evidence based medicine: What it is and what it isn't. *British Medical Journal, 312*, 71–72.

Saunders, T., Driskell, J. E., Hall, J., & Salas, E. (1996). The effect of stress inoculation training on anxiety and performance. *Journal of Occupational Health, 1*, 170–186.

Shapiro, D. A., & Shapiro, D. (1982). Meta-analysis of comparative therapy outcome studies: A replication and refinement. *Psychological Bulletin, 92*, 581–604.

Shepherd, M. (1993). The placebo: From specificity to the non-specific and back. *Psychological Medicine, 23*, 569–578.

Sherman, J. J. (1998). Effects of psychotherapeutic treatments for PTSD: A meta-analysis of controlled clinical trials. *Journal of Traumatic Stress, 11*, 413–435.

Smith, M. L., & Glass, G. V. (1977). Meta-analysis of psychotherapy outcome studies. *American Psychologist, 32*, 752–760.

Smith, M. L., Glass, G. V, & Miller, T. I. (1980). *The benefits of psychotherapy.* Baltimore: The Johns Hopkins University Press.

Stark, K., Rouse, L., & Livingston, R. (1991). Treatment of depression during childhood and adolescence: Cognitive–behavioral procedures for the individual and family. In P. C. Kendall (Ed.), *Child and Adolescent Therapy* (pp.165–206). New York: Guilford Press.

Stuart, G. L., Treat, T. A., & Wade, W. A. (2000). Effectiveness of an empirically based treatment for panic disorder delivered in a service clinic setting: 1-year follow-up. *Journal of Consulting and Clinical Psychology, 68*, 506–512.

Task Force on Promotion and Dissemination of Psychological Procedures. (1995). Training in and dissemination of empirically-validated psychological treatment: Report and recommendations. *The Clinical Psychologist, 48*, 2–23.

Taylor, S. (1996). Meta-analysis of cognitive–behavioral treatments for social phobia. *Journal of Behaviour Therapy and Experimental Psychiatry, 27*, 1–9.

Taylor, T. K., Schmidt, F., Pepler, D., & Hodgins, C. (1998). A comparison of eclectic treatment with Webster–Stratton's Parents and Children Series in a children's mental health center: A randomized controlled trial. *Behavior Therapy, 29*, 221–240.

Teasdale, J. D., Fennell, M. J. V., Hibbert, G. A., & Amies, P. L. (1984). Cognitive therapy for major depressive disorder in primary care. *British Journal of Psychiatry, 144*, 400–406.

Trull, T. J., Nietzel, M. T., & Main, A. (1988). The use of meta-analysis to assess the clinical significance of behavior therapy for agoraphobia. *Behavior Therapy, 19*, 257–538.

Tynan, W. D., Schuman, W., & Lampert, N. (1999). Concurrent parent and child therapy groups for externalizing disorders: From the laboratory to the world of managed care. *Cognitive and Behavioral Practice, 6*, 3–9.

Van Balkom, A. J. L. M., van Oppen, P., Vermeulen, A. W. A., van Dyck, R., Nauta, M. C. E., & Vorst, H. C. M. (1994). A meta-analysis on the treatment of obsessive compulsive disorder: A comparison of antidepressants, behavior, and cognitive therapy. *Clinical Psychology Review, 14*, 359–381.

Wade, W. A., Treat, T. A., & Stuart, G. L. (1998). Transporting an empirically supported treatment for panic disorder to a service clinic setting: A benchmarking strategy. *Journal of Consulting and Clinical Psychology, 66*, 231–239.

Wampold, B. E. (1997). Methodological problems in identifying efficacious psychotherapies. *Psychotherapy Research, 7*, 21–43.

Wampold, B. E. (2001). *The great psychotherapy debate: Model, methods, and findings.* Mahwah, NJ: Erlbaum.

Wampold, B. E., & Bhati, K. S. (2004). Attending to the omissions: A historical examination of the evidenced-based practice movement. *Professional Psychology: Research and Practice, 35*, 563–570.

Wampold, B. E., Minami, T., Baskin, T. W., & Tierney, S. C. (2002). A meta-(re)analysis of the effects of cognitive therapy versus "other therapies" for depression. *Journal of Affective Disorders, 68*, 159–165.

Wampold, B. E., Mondin, G. W., Moody, M., & Ahn, H. (1997). The flat earth as a metaphor for the evidence for uniform efficacy of bona fide psychotherapies: Reply to Crits-Christoph (1997) and Howard et al. (1997). *Psychological Bulletin, 122*, 226–230.

Wampold, B. E., Mondin, G. W., Moody, M., Stich, F., Benson, K., & Ahn, H. N. (1997). A meta-analysis of outcome studies comparing bona fide psychotherapies: Empirically, "All must have prizes." *Psychological Bulletin, 122,* 203–215.

Wampold, B. E., & Serlin, R. C. (2000). The consequences of ignoring a nested factor on measures of effect size in analysis of variance. *Psychological Methods, 5,* 425–433.

Watson, J. C., Gordon, L. B., Stermac, L., Kalogerakos, F., & Steckley, P. (2003). Comparing the effectiveness of process–experiential with cognitive–behavioral psychotherapy in the treatment of depression. *Journal of Consulting and Clinical Psychology, 71,* 773–781.

Weersing, V. R., & Weisz, J. R. (2002). Community clinic treatment of depressed youth: Benchmarking usual care against CBT clinical trials. *Journal of Consulting and Clinical Psychology, 70,* 299–310.

Weisz, J. R., Donenberg, G. R., Han, S. S., & Kauneckis, D. (1995). Child and adolescent psychotherapy outcomes in experiments versus clinics: Why the disparity? *Journal of Abnormal Child Psychology, 23,* 83–106.

Weisz, J. R., Huey, S. M., & Weersing, V. R. (1998). Psychotherapy outcome research with children and adolescents: The state of the art. In T. H. Ollendick & R. J. Prinz (Eds.), *Advances in clinical child psychology* (Vol. 20, pp. 49–92). New York: Plenum Press.

Weisz, J. R., & Weiss, B. (1989). Assessing the effects of clinic-based psychotherapy with children and adolescents. *Journal of Consulting and Clinical Psychology, 57,* 741–746.

Westen, D., Novotny, C. M., & Thompson-Brenner, H. (2004). The empirical status of empirically supported psychotherapies: Assumptions, findings, and reporting in controlled clinical trials. *Psychological Bulletin, 130,* 631–663.

Woody, S. R., & Ollendick, T. H. (in press). Principles of effective psychosocial interventions with anxiety and its disorders. In L. E. Beutler & L. G. Castonguay (Eds.), *Principles of change in effective psychotherapies.* New York: Oxford University Press.

8

HOW WELL DO BOTH EVIDENCE-BASED PRACTICES AND TREATMENT AS USUAL SATISFACTORILY ADDRESS THE VARIOUS DIMENSIONS OF DIVERSITY?

Ethnic Minority Populations Have Been Neglected by Evidence-Based Practices

Stanley Sue and Nolan Zane

From the time of the 1978 President's Commission on Mental Health to the Surgeon General's (2001) and the President's New Freedom Commission (2003) reports, ethnic disparities in mental health have been nationally publicized. The disparities concerned the unmet mental health needs of members of ethnic minority groups (i.e., African Americans, American Indians, Asian Americans, and Latino[a]s). The reports concluded that the disparities were not so much due to racial and ethnic differences in rates of psychopathology but were due to inaccessible and ineffective treatment. Ethnic minority clients often saw psychotherapists or were administered treatments that did not consider the clients' lifestyles, cultural and linguistic backgrounds, and life circumstances. Thus, one critical task is to improve therapeutic effectiveness and quality of care for these clients.

The evidence-based practice (EBP) movement promises to reduce disparities by using those treatments that are effective according to controlled research studies. It uses research to provide the best evidence of what works and then directly applies those findings to treatment selection. How can anyone disagree with such a movement?

In this position paper, we examine the extent to which EBPs have been helpful in reducing disparities and in improving treatment effectiveness. In many ways, we do not have the luxury of debating controversies identified by others (Beutler, 2004; Levant, 2004), such as whether research priority should be directed to treatment or context, whether external validity should be sacrificed for internal validity, or whether efficacy or effectiveness research is more valuable. Rather, we need to emphasize that more ethnic research must be conducted.

From the outset, our position is that psychological treatment should be guided by research evidence. However, we believe that EBPs have not been very helpful in reducing treatment disparities or improving effectiveness for minorities, primarily for three reasons. First, little research has been conducted on EBPs with clients from ethnic minority groups. Second, a need exists to broaden the current definition of "evidence." Third, research that tests if existing interventions are effective is limiting. Research into culturally competent interventions is needed, and this kind of research is relatively new. Consequently, the conclusions regarding mental health disparities reached by the President's Commission on Mental Health in 1978 have not changed a quarter of a century later (President's New Freedom Commission, 2003; U.S. Surgeon General, 2001).

LACK OF RESEARCH

One major problem in trying to use the EBP model to guide treatments with ethnic minority clients is that relatively little research has been conducted on these clients, especially research that satisfies rigorous research criteria such as those involved in randomized clinical trials (RCTs) or empirically supported treatments (ESTs). Both attempt to convincingly demonstrate via scientific methods the effects of an intervention so that alternative explanations for treatment effects can be eliminated. RCTs involve random assignment of clients to an intervention of interest or to a control group of some kind. Because of random assignment, systematic differences between clients are minimized so that outcome differences can be attributed to treatment differences. In the case of ESTs (formerly named as EVTs or empirically validated treatments), Chambless and associates (1996) could not find a single rigorous study that examined the efficacy of treatment for any ethnic minority population. Others have also observed a lack of ESTs for ethnic minority populations (Bernal & Scharrón-Del Río, 2001; Zane, Hall, Sue, Young, & Nunez, 2003).

The U.S. Surgeon General (2001) reported that the gap between research and practice is particularly acute for racial and ethnic minorities. Research involving controlled clinical trials used to generate professional treatment guidelines did not conduct specific analyses for any minority group. Since 1986, about 10,000 participants have been included in RCTs evaluating the efficacy of treatments for certain disorders. For nearly half of these participants ($N = 4,991$), no information on race or ethnicity was given. For another 7% of participants ($N = 656$), studies only reported the general designation "non-white." For the remaining 47% of participants ($N = 4,335$), very few minorities were included; not a single study analyzed the efficacy of the treatment by ethnicity or race.

This sad state of affairs reveals the past history of ethnic mental health research. What portends for the future? Here we have mixed developments. On the one hand, disparities are being recognized, and funding agencies such as the National Institute of Mental Health (NIMH) and the Substance Abuse and Mental Health Services Administration are encouraging ethnic research or requiring research to include diverse groups.

On the other hand, ethnic research has been lacking because of systemic reasons. First, such research is often costly because of population sizes and difficulties in recruiting research participants. For example, African Americans and Latinos each represent less than 15% of the U.S. population, with Asian Americans at 5% and American Indians at 1%. Sampling ethnic clients from mental clinics and hospitals often yields samples that are too small to analyze, many ethnic clients may not want to participate, and convenience rather than representative samples often have to be used. Time for the research may have to be extended or special incentives may have to be given to secure participation. Second, the research is difficult to conduct. In addition to finding adequate clinical samples, tasks such as devising culturally valid measures, selecting appropriate samples that represent a particular ethnic group, deciding on whether to use interethnic versus intraethnic comparison designs, reducing cultural response sets, ensuring adequate English proficiency or translations for participants with limited English proficiency, controlling for potential confounds with ethnicity or cultural variables, and so on are daunting tasks. Third, psychology traditionally has been interested in achieving internal validity. It strives to make causal inferences so that rigorous experimental studies are the gold standard. In such a situation, external validity, or the extent to which research findings can be generalized to other populations or situations, is of secondary interest. The overwhelming majority of research has been conducted on mainstream Americans. Therefore, if empirical support for the effectiveness of a treatment is found, there seems to be little interest in determining the extent to which the findings can be generalized to other populations (Sue, 1999). Finally, ethnic research is often controversial. Because much of the research touches on topics such as disparities, inequities, differential treatment, prejudice, and values, investigators may be uncomfortable in initiating studies that systematically examine important ethnic and cultural variations. These problems involving sampling, research difficulties, deemphasis on external validity, and focus on controversial topics reveal both the major challenges to conducting such research and the complexities in achieving rigorous research designs.

TWO QUESTIONS

The paucity of ethnic treatment outcome research has raised two important questions: (a) If so little research has been done, particularly research that is rigorously conducted, how can we be sure that disparities in treatment actually exist? (b) If treatment effectiveness and efficacy have not gained empirical support with these populations, should we refrain from using ESTs when they have not been studied in ethnic populations?

In regard to the first question, ample evidence of treatment disparities shows that the quality of care for ethnic minority clients has often been inferior. Although few rigorous outcome studies have been done, the preponderance of research of varying degrees of rigor has pointed to service disparities. With respect to the second question, the U.S. Surgeon General (2001) emphasized that ethnic clients with mental health problems should seek treatment and be given treatments that are generally found to be effective. That is, treatments should be administered on the basis of the best available evidence. This position assumes that the best course of action is to rely on research findings, even if research has been conducted on mainstream populations rather than ethnic populations. One can assume the generality of treatment outcomes, unless proven otherwise by research. However, this is hardly "good science" where assumptions should not be made; rather, they must be tested.

The problem we see is that assuming generalization reduces the pressure to conduct research on ethnic minority populations and to study the external validity and generality of research findings. In other words, the assumption of generalization is made for convenience and necessity rather than for science and client welfare, which would demand that treatment outcomes be studied for all major populations. Guyll and Madon (2000) noted that it is practically impossible to study all groups to see if findings can be generalized. This may be true, but science and skepticism demand that generality be convincingly demonstrated in some manner. Furthermore, that treatment practices show differential validities for different populations has been demonstrated by findings showing, for example, that recommended dosages for psychotropic medications vary according to ethnicity. Asians who are given psychotropic medication at dosage levels found to be clinically effective for Caucasians may be overdosed, even after controlling for body weight (Lin, Cheung, Smith, & Poland, 1997).

RESEARCH METHODOLOGY

In ethnic minority issues, it is easy to complain or to engage in social criticism because of the history of inequities. We wish to turn now to a discussion of what can be done to increase the value of the EBP movement to ethnic minority groups. We offer some suggestions as to research in general and cultural competency in particular.

The criteria to establish ESTs are rigorous and experimental, strongly intended to allow causal inferences to be made. They help to establish the extent to which treatments work. On the other hand, EBPs are a broader class of research, treatments, and practices. ESTs are one type of EBP.

The important question is the intent of the research. In the long term, the goal is to identify and implement the use of effective treatments. EST criteria are especially helpful in testing the efficacy or outcome of identified treatments. However, the value of EST criteria is more limited in the absence of identified treatments to test. That is, in situations where one does not have a clear intervention or is uncertain about treatment processes, an intermediate goal of research may be to examine psychotherapeutic processes and phenomena. Bernal and Scharrón-Del Río (2001) called this discovery-oriented research. This type of research is not intended to test hypotheses or well-developed treatments. Rather, discovery-oriented research attempts to understand the dynamics of the treatment process to identify important variables that may lead to the formulation of treatment strategies to test. Discovery research can be conducted using all types of methodology, ranging from quantitative to qualitative approaches, experimental to correlations studies, and laboratory to naturalistic settings. This is important particularly in ethnic research where the interest is not only in whether certain treatments used with mainstream Americans work with ethnic clients but also in whether certain culture variables should be taken into consideration.

Hall (2001) made a similar observation in distinguishing between ESTs and culturally sensitive therapies (CSTs). He defined CSTs as involving the tailoring of psychotherapy to specific cultural contexts. People from one cultural group may require a form of psychotherapy that differs from psychotherapy for another cultural group (in addition to cultural variations among people within a cultural group that require additional modification). In fact, it can be argued that currently identified ESTs are really CSTs for mainstream Americans because they work for mainstream populations and have been largely untested for ethnic minority populations. There is, of course, no intrinsic reason why ESTs and CSTs cannot be the same.

This immediate discussion also shows why the simple inclusion of ethnic minorities as research subjects is inadequate. A 1994 National Institute of Health (NIH) policy required researchers to include ethnic minorities in their samples. Minority groups are defined by NIH as American Indian—Alaska Native, Asian—Pacific Islander, Black—African American not of Hispanic origin, and Hispanic (Hohmann & Parron, 1996). The exclusion of ethnic minority groups must be justified on scientific grounds. Only recruiting and including ethnic minorities in a research sample would fulfill the letter of the NIH policy and enable us to find out if research findings generalize from one group to another. But simple inclusion does not necessarily lead to new knowledge about ethnic minority populations (Hall, 2001). Thus, we believe that the full array of research methodologies and philosophies should be brought to bear in research on ethnic minority populations. Otherwise, research will not be of much benefit in responding to the observed ethnic disparities in mental health.

Furthermore, we should not be oblivious to the fact that research may not lead to improvements because policies and programs are influenced by political considerations. One disconcerting example of political influence and the manipulation of science findings occurred over a report entitled "Unequal Treatment: Confronting Racial and Ethnic Disparities in Health Care" (Smedley, Stith, & Nelson, 2003). The report documented racial and ethnic disparities in health care and presented recommendations made by the National Institute of Medicine to reduce these disparities. However, before the report was released, some staff at the Department of Health and Human Services (HHS) attempted to modify the conclusions of the report to downplay the extent of disparities. For example, one draft conclusion was that significant inequalities were found in health care in the United States and health care disparities constituted national problems. After the modifications by HHS staff, none of these conclusions appeared. Protests were made over the modifications made by HHS staff and over the Bush Administration's attempt to "whitewash" and hide disparities uncovered by scientists:

> "Just like a tumor cannot be healed by covering it with a bandage, healthcare disparities cannot be eliminated with misrepresented facts," said Rep. Elijah E. Cummings, Chair of the Congressional Black Caucus. "I urge the Bush Administration to stand by its commitment to eliminating racially-defined healthcare disparities by 2010. Disparities do not disappear by concealing information."
>
> "Instead of leading the fight against healthcare disparities, HHS is downplaying the serious inequities faced by racial and ethnic minorities," said Rep. Michael M. Honda, Chair of the Congressional Asian Pacific American Caucus. "By tampering with the conclusions of its own scien-

tists, HHS is placing politics before social justice." (Press release concerning letter sent to Tommy G. Thompson, U.S. Secretary of Health and Human Services by Waxman et al., 2004)

Only after such protests were sent to HHS Secretary Tommy Thompson did he say that his department had erred in rewriting the report on racial and socioeconomic health disparities and that he planned to release the report as originally written. This incident involving HHS as well as others altering research conclusions for political purposes, political litmus tests for grant reviewers, and ignoring scientific findings contrary to certain political thoughts (House Committee on Political Reform, 2004; Sluzki, 2003) should be of serious concern to psychological scientists. Manipulations of the scientific process and of research conclusions to achieve political ends are of great threat to science and society.

CULTURAL COMPETENCY RESEARCH

Cultural competency can be defined as having the cultural knowledge or skills to deliver effective interventions to members of a particular culture. At times, some skills may be effectively applied to many different cultures; at other times, some skills may be effective only with particular cultures. What are these skills? Are traditional treatments universally effective? Do traditional treatments need modification to be culturally competent? Can culturally competent skills be scripted and manualized? Do treatment processes differ according to ethnicity? What kind of cultural competency research should be conducted?

Four points are important to consider. First, culture is important in all phases of research and the treatment process. In terms of research, cultural considerations must be taken into account from the formulation of hypotheses, the selection of measures, the collection of data, and the analysis of data to the interpretation of findings. Second, at this stage in our research progress, most of the questions raised earlier cannot be meaningfully answered. We simply have a paucity of research. Third, in trying to ascertain the effectiveness of interventions on the outcomes of ethnic clients, serious complications exist that may impact the intervention used. The therapist may subtly and without awareness change the intervention to accommodate the ethnic client. For example, a therapist who is conducting therapy in English may not interpret literally what a limited English-speaking client is saying or may try to verify what the client is trying to convey. A therapist may engage in a "mental shift" in assessing a client from a different culture and be more cautious about making inferences. All these changes may occur without awareness. These may also help to increase cultural competency, but the intervention may be altered in important ways that are undetected in the research. Thus, if researchers are interested in studying whether psychodynamic approaches are effective with ethnic minority clients, care must be taken to control for, or consider, subtle changes in the intervention.

Fourth, in studying cultural competency, we often attempt to see if a type of treatment is effective. Such an approach focuses on the intervention and not on the context of the intervention. Norcross and Goldfried (1992) found that therapist and relationship factors accounted for 30% of the improvement in psychotherapy patients, whereas client, family, and other environmental factors accounted for 40%. Specific treatment techniques, when combined with the expectancy factors commonly associated with placebo effects, accounted for the other 30% of improvement. The emphasis on ESTs has often led to calls for standardizing these treatments to minimize "procedural slippage" on the part of the therapist or client. However, this effort to optimize the effect of ESTs tends to cancel out important therapist and client variations, and it does not capitalize on the major patterns found in outcome research. In view of the substantial amount of outcome variance accounted for by therapist and client factors, it seems wise instead to account systematically for and examine these sources of variation to determine how they can moderate the effects of evidence-based interventions. Attempts to see if different types of treatment are effective or to operationally define cultural competency simply as a technique cannot provide a meaningful test of treatment impact. Norcross (2003) argued that decision rules to determine evidence-based psychotherapies neglect three essential elements of psychotherapy: the therapist, the therapy relationship, and the client's nondiagnostic characteristics. Likewise, cultural competency depends on contextual factors such as client characteristics, therapist characteristics, the type of intervention or treatment, and the treatment setting. To study and understand cultural competency, we need to deconstruct the treatment process into various components.

Client factors such as the level of acculturation are crucial. For example, in empirically testing the value of ethnic match between therapist and client, the client's acculturation level interacts with the match. Ethnic match was particularly valuable for Mexican American and Asian American clients who were low in acculturation (Sue, 1998). This means that culture-specific interventions may or may not need to be used, depending on certain client factors. *Therapist factors*, including experience in working with members of a particular ethnic group and a proficiency in the ethnic language, may be very important to consider in cultural competency. After all, if therapists and clients are unable to communicate or must do so with an interpreter, treatment may be seriously affected. Very critical are the racial attitudes and biases that therapists may have. The vast majority of therapists are non-Hispanic Whites. Many may hold stereotypic views of ethnic minority clients or fail to appreciate the "White privilege" that they possess. These attitudes and beliefs can detrimentally influence their perceptions of and interactions with individuals who are ethnically and racially different from themselves (American Psychological Association, 2003b).

Treatment factors should also be examined. For instance, one criticism often made about treatment is that the interventions do not take culture into account or therapists interact with clients using stereotypes or inappropriate statements. Some intervention strategies may be less susceptible to these problems. Finally, *treatment setting* is likely to influence the use of cultural interventions. An Asian American client who has a great deal of shame and stigma over psychotherapy may not require much initial attention over them if the treatment is conducted in a prevention or educational setting rather than in a mental clinic or hospital. These factors help to determine whether certain cultural interventions are necessary; they also point to the complicated task of operationally defining and measuring cultural competency.

More recently, some attention has turned to another source of outcome variance: the treatment itself (e.g., Bracero, 1994; Chen, 1995; Yi, 1995). For example, Yi (1995) argued that psychoanalytic treatments often were ineffective with Asian clients because of the indiscriminate application of psychoanalytic concepts such as individuation separation. She recommended that therapists reconceptualize such concepts to accommodate nonindividualistic worldviews and use a sustained empathic–introspective approach to better access the experiential events of these clients. These conceptual advances notwithstanding, no sustained research effort has investigated how the life experiences of ethnic minority clients and their families, the attitudes and behaviors of their care providers, and the features of the treatment approaches affect the effectiveness of the intervention. As a result, we still have a rudimentary understanding of how mental health services can effectively respond to the needs of the severely mentally ill in ethnic minority communities.

CONCLUSIONS

EBPs can be of great benefit in cultural competency. However, the problem is that researchers and funding agencies have not paid much attention to ethnic and cultural research that determines if these treatments are effective, in other words, culturally competent. The conclusions reached by the President's Commission on Mental Health in the late 1970s are echoed today, some 35 years later, in the U.S. Surgeon General's supplement (2001) and the President's New Freedom Commission (2003). Research is needed that is inclusive of ethnic minority populations but also explanatory in nature about the effects of cultural variables. In particular, we point to the need to use a variety of methodologies, to examine the complexities in achieving cultural competency, and to resist political intrusions into science that undermine the significance of ethnic and cultural variations when the research indicates these should be considered.

Gender Is Neglected by Both Evidence-Based Practices and Treatment as Usual

Ronald F. Levant and Louise B. Silverstein

Gender as a dimension of diversity is not adequately addressed in either empirically supported therapies (such as those catalogued by the American Psychological Association [APA] Society of Clinical Psychology [Division 12], 1995; Chambless et al., 1996, 1998), nor in psychotherapy as usually practiced in the community. As we will show in this section, most practices within the mental health professions, including psychology, largely ignore gender as they do the other dimensions of diversity: race, ethnicity, nationality, immigration status, sexual orientation, age, religion, social class, and disability status. We hope this will begin to change, especially because the APA (2003b) has now adopted their Guidelines on Multicultural Education, Training, Research, Practice and Organizational Change for Psychologists. Although that document deals only with racial, ethnic, and national dimensions of diversity, other APA policy statements address additional dimensions of diversity in regard to mental health services (e.g., sexual orientation, APA, 2000; aging, APA, 2003a).

In this position paper, we begin by acknowledging our conceptual framework and social location. We then turn to an analysis of the field of gender studies and discuss the theoretical shift that has taken place over the past 25 years. This shift has moved away from understanding gender as an individual, biologically based trait (the Gender Role Identity Paradigm) to understanding it as socially constructed by the culture within which an individual is socialized (the Gender Role Strain Paradigm). Unfortunately, the psychotherapy research and practice communities have not yet made this conceptual shift, despite substantial evidence supporting the Strain Paradigm. We present an explanation of gender role strain in the hope that it can infuse mainstream psychotherapy, and that a body of psychotherapy research and a set of practices that do adequately address gender will be forthcoming.

OUR CONCEPTUAL FRAMEWORK AND SOCIAL LOCATION

First, we want to address why it is important for mental health professionals to be culturally competent. At the most basic level, APA's (2003, p. 377) multicultural guidelines point out that "all individuals exist in social, political, historical and economic contexts, and psychologists are increasingly called upon to understand the influence of these contexts on an individual's behavior." This is certainly important but in our view does not go far enough. The contexts that mental health professionals need to understand are the political, economic, historical, social, and psychological facts of oppression, prejudice, discrimination, stigmatization, and marginalization of minority groups. Oppression's impact on psychotherapy clients is often mediated by the fact that the majority of mental health service providers come from positions of relative power and privilege. These contrasting socio–political–economic perspectives too often render mental health service providers unaware of their power and privilege relative to their clients, and of how much their conscious beliefs and unconscious assumptions are influenced by oppressive ideologies, such as racism, sexism, heterosexism, and ageism. It is in this context that mental health service providers can commit dangerous errors. Examples of such errors include psychoanalytic theory's assertion that women were "naturally" masochistic and mainstream psychology's historical "approaches that have viewed cultural differences [between racial groups] as deficits" (APA, 2003, p. 382).

Second, we want to acknowledge our privileged social location. We are White, middle class, heterosexual, and able bodied. We also acknowledge the mentoring we have received over the years from esteemed colleagues from racial, ethnic, and sexual minority groups, which has helped us overcome some of our perceptual limitations that have resulted from our social location.

Third, we want to note the problematic nature of discussing only one dimension of diversity in isolation from the others. Although necessary for a brief position paper, it is artificial and can even lead to a biased perspective. Reid (2002) observed that the practice of looking at either gender or ethnicity but not both was true of both early feminist writings that ignored race and ethnicity, and multicultural literature, which has, for the most part, ignored gender.

Silverstein (2004) searched books, chapters, and journal articles in PsycINFO for the years 1990–2004, using the keywords race, ethnicity, gender, racism, and feminism. She found that only about one third (range of 32%–36%) of the multicultural publications included women–girls–gender. Even more discouraging, only about 5% of the publications on gender and feminism included race or ethnicity. Thus, Reid's (2002) observation that mainstream psychology focuses on a single domain of identity receives additional support.

Levant (2003) and others called for the development of a General Role Strain Paradigm, which would systematically attend to the multiple dimensions of multicultural diversity. Role strain refers to the process whereby social roles, imbedded in power hierarchies and communicated by ideologies, create stress and strain for oppressed and marginalized groups within our society. This approach is consistent with the concept of "minority stress" recently discussed with regard to sexual minorities (Meyer, 2003). Hence, a General Role Strain Paradigm might have the following components:

- Gender role strain exists because of the inequalities of power and opportunity in patriarchal society (even one partially mitigated by feminism).

- Race and ethnicity strain exist because of the inequalities of power and opportunity in a racist society (even one partially mitigated by the civil rights movement and its heirs).
- Sexual orientation strain exists because of the inequalities of power and opportunity in a heterosexist society (even one partially mitigated by the Gay, Lesbian, Bisexual, Transgendered [GLBT] movements).
- Class strain exists because of the inequalities of power and opportunity in a classist society (even one partially mitigated by democratic movements).
- Age strain exists because of the inequalities of power and opportunity in an agist society (even one partially mitigated by the grey panther movement).
- Disability strain exists because of the inequalities of power and opportunity in an ablebodyist society (even one partially mitigated by the disability movements).
- And so on . . .

These strains interact with and intensify one another.

In summary, our conceptual framework is inclusive of multiple domains of identity and eschews a focus on individual gender and cultural differences in favor of an awareness of systems of oppression. For the purposes of this position paper, we discuss gender in isolation solely because of space limitations.

GENDER STUDIES

The field of gender studies had its origins within the individual differences tradition in psychology, when investigators in the 1930s began to focus on what was then termed "sex differences" in personality (Terman & Miles, 1936) and later in cognitive and perceptual attributes (see Anastasi, 1958, for an early review). The field began with a focus on traits thought to reside in the individual, what Deaux (1984, p. 105) termed the "sex as a subject variable" approach. This approach dominated the field for over 50 years.

In the 1980s, gender studies began to view gender as the result of the interaction among people in a social context, in which gender-related beliefs and ideologies embedded in power hierarchies play an important role (Deaux, 1984; Pleck, 1981). Neither the psychotherapy research nor the practice communities have yet made this critical shift in perspective.

Although ESTs exist for disorders that are either more common in girls and women (e.g., anxiety, depression, eating disorders) or boys and men (e.g. substance abuse, conduct disorder, attention-deficit/hyperactivity disorder [ADHD]), none of the therapies that have made the various EST lists are feminist or pro-feminist in nature (Chambless & Ollendick, 2001). Furthermore, the few psychotherapy research studies that do assess gender variables operationalize them as personality traits, reflecting the older trait perspective. Similarly, the practice (treatment as usual [TAU]) community continues to understand gender as attributes of individuals. The failure of the research and practice communities to incorporate this theoretical shift may reflect, in part, the lag time in the diffusion of newer perspectives. However, it may also reflect a sexist bias.

The sexist nature of psychotherapy practice was first documented in 1975 (APA, 1975). Although the most overt forms of sexism have disappeared from the mental health professions in the ensuing four decades, covert sexism is alive and well in the helping professions, as it is in society at large. A draft set of guidelines for psychological practice with girls and women sponsored jointly by APA Divisions 17 (Society of Counseling Psychology) and 35 (Society for the Psychology of Women) reported that "scrutiny of a variety of theories of psychotherapy has found them to be based on non-inclusive versions of mental health" (APA Divisions 17 and 35, 2004, p. 40). This review included both the empirically supported therapies, such as cognitive–behavioral, as well as treatments usually practiced in the community, such as psychodynamic. The report goes on to catalogue the subtle bias found in these therapies:

> (a) overvaluing individualism and autonomy and undervaluing relational qualities, (b) overvaluing rationality instead of viewing mental health from a holistic perspective, (c) paying inadequate attention to context and external influences on girls' and women's lives, and (d) basing definitions of positive mental health on behaviors that are most consistent with "masculine" stereotypes of the lives of privileged men. (p. 40)

The draft guidelines also found gender bias within diagnostic criteria: "For example, women's and girls' gender role socialization may contribute to over-diagnosis of certain disorders such as histrionic and borderline personality disorder, depression, dissociative disorders, somatization disorder, premenstrual dysphoric syndrome, and agoraphobia" (APA Divisions 17 and 35, 2004, p. 2).

So far we have been talking about sexism as it affects girls and women. What about boys and men? It is our view that patriarchy stresses men, but we would not agree that it oppresses men. Attempting to conform to the norms of traditional masculinity limits boys' and men's psychological development and constrains their behavior. However, patriarchy is a political and social system that confers power and privilege on boys and men. With that in mind, how does the sexist bias in mental health practice serve boys and men? By uncritically accepting gender role stereotypes, mental health practitioners do not serve boys and men well. To illustrate this point with regard to both treatment and diagnosis, we offer the following: By overvaluing autonomy and undervaluing connections, therapists may fail to recognize that many boys and men are limited in their ability to form mature attachments and need help in becoming comfortable with intimacy.

By accepting the stereotype that boys and men are "naturally" unemotional, therapists may fail to recognize that many boys and men suffer from mild alexithymia and are unable to experience and express large parts of their emotional life. As a consequence, they tend to deal with stress in less healthy ways, such as somatizing, drinking, taking risks, being violent, isolating from others, and engaging in nonrelational sex.

By boys and men accepting the stereotype that they do not show vulnerability, they are probably reluctant to seek mental health treatment (Addis & Mahalik, 2003) and may be underdiagnosed for internalizing disorders. On the other hand, boys' and men's tendencies to externalize emotional distress may result in their greater likelihood of being diagnosed with antisocial and substance abuse disorders.

Unfortunately, the sophisticated analyses developed by feminist psychologists into the nature of covert sexism have not exerted much influence on mainstream psychotherapy research and practice. Nor has guidance on how to provide gender-competent therapy developed by feminist therapists for treating women (e.g., Brown, 1994; Dutton, 1992; Hare-Mustin, 1978; Jordan, 1997; Nutt, 1992; Silverstein & Goodrich, 2003; Walker, 1994; Worell & Johnson, 1997; Worell & Remer, 2003) and by pro-feminist therapists for treating men (e.g., Andronico, 1996; Brooks, 1998; Brooks & Good, 2001; Levant & Pollack, 1995; Pollack & Levant, 1998; Rabinowitz & Cochran, 2002; Scher, Stevens, Good, & Eichenfield, 1987).

In an effort to facilitate EBPs that address gender, we thought it might be useful to introduce an accessible, empirically supported perspective on gender that we have found quite useful, namely, the Gender Role Strain Paradigm.

GENDER ROLE STRAIN PARADIGM

The Gender Role Strain Paradigm is a social constructionist perspective that views gender roles not as biological or even social "givens" but rather as psychologically and socially constructed entities that bring certain advantages and disadvantages, and, most importantly, that can change. This perspective acknowledges the biological differences between men and women but argues that it is not biological differences that construct "masculinity" and "femininity."

The Gender Role Strain Paradigm, originally formulated by Joseph Pleck (1981), stands in contrast to the older trait approach, which he termed the Gender Role Identity Paradigm. The Identity Paradigm assumed that people have an inherent psychological need to have a sex-typed gender role identity, and that optimal personality development hinged on its formation. The extent to which this "inherent" need is met is determined by how completely a person embraces his or her traditional gender role. From such a perspective, the development of appropriate gender role identity is anxiously sought by parents, teachers, and physicians, and failure is dreaded. Failure for men to achieve a masculine gender role identity was thought to result in homosexuality, negative attitudes towards women, or defensive hypermasculinity. For women, faulty gender role socialization was thought to be manifested in a failure to marry and have children, a dislike of men, or lesbianism. In an exhaustive review of the personality development research literature, Pleck (1981) showed that the empirical data do not support the Gender Role Identity Paradigm, nor the notion that developing a sex-typed gender role identity was essential for normal personal development.

By contrast, the Gender Role Strain Paradigm proposes that gender roles are determined by the prevailing cultural gender ideology (which can be assessed through an empirical investigation of gender role stereotypes and norms). These roles are unwittingly imposed on the developing child by parents, teachers, physicians, and peers, the cultural transmitters who subscribe to the prevailing gender ideology. The imposition of gender roles results in gender role strain because gender roles are inevitably contradictory and inconsistent, and certain prescribed gender role traits (such as man aggression) are often dysfunctional. Therefore, the proportion of people who violate gender roles is high. The violation of gender roles leads to condemnation and negative psychological consequences.

Gender ideology is the central construct in the Strain Paradigm. It is very different from the older notion of gender role orientation (or sex role orientation). Gender role orientation "presumes that masculinity [or femininity] is rooted in actual differences between men and women" (Thompson & Pleck, 1995, p. 130). This approach has attempted to assess the personality traits more often associated with men or women, using such instruments as the Bem Sex Role Inventory (Bem, 1974) and the Personal Attributes Questionnaire (Spence & Helmreich, 1978).

In contrast, studies of gender ideology take a normative approach, in which masculinity and femininity are viewed as socially constructed gender ideals for men and women. Whereas the "masculine" man in the orientation–trait approach is one who possesses particular personality traits, the traditional man in the ideology–normative approach "is one who endorses the ideology that men should have sex specific characteristics (and women should not have these characteristics)" (Thompson & Pleck, 1995, p. 131). Thompson and Pleck cited evidence that gender role orientation and gender ideologies are independent constructs and have different correlates.

In an update on the Gender Role Strain Paradigm, Pleck (1995) pointed out that the original formulation of the paradigm stimulated research on three varieties of gender role strain, which he termed discrepancy strain, dysfunction strain, and trauma strain. Discrepancy strain results when one fails to live up to one's internalized gender ideal and can result in lowered self-esteem and other sequelae. A measure of Gender Role Conflict, a form of discrepancy strain, has been found to be associated with a host of psychological problems in men (O'Neil, Good, & Holmes, 1995). Dysfunction strain results even when one fulfills the requirements of the gender code, because many of the characteristics viewed as desirable in men and women can have negative side effects on them. Examples would be overaggressive behavior or alexithymia in men and the unhealthy pursuit of thinness (including eating disorders) in women. Trauma strain can result from many sources, the most important of which is the ordeal of the gender role socialization process. This process is now regarded as inherently traumatic because of its effects in truncating the emotionality of boys and men and the limiting the aggression of girls and women. One can see that using the lens of gender role strain in the diagnostic process could serve to correct some of the biases mentioned previously.

In summary, the Identity Paradigm views psychological health as predicated on conforming to traditional gender role norms, whereas the Strain Paradigm asserts that conforming to traditional gender role norms generates psychological stress and strain rather than well-being. Over 20 years of empirical research supports the strain paradigm (Eagly & Wood, 1999; French, 1985; Levant & Pollack, 1995; Levant & Richmond, 2004; Pleck, 1981, 1995; Silverstein & Goodrich, 2003; Worell & Johnson, 1997).

EBP AND GENDER

What, then, are the ideal relations of gender and EBP in mental health? First and foremost, we would advocate passionately for the development of greater gender competence in the mental health field. This would include not only accurate information but also self-awareness so that practitioners become aware of the effects of power and privilege in rendering sexism invisible.

Second, following the lead of the draft guidelines for psychological practice with girls and women (APA Divisions 17 and 35, 2004), we would recommend that therapists use interventions that have been demonstrated to be effective for treating those disorders that have higher prevalence among girls and women: depression, anxiety, and eating disorders. We make the same recommendation for those disorders that have higher prevalence among boys and men: pervasive developmental disorders, ADHD, conduct disorders, antisocial personality disorders, impulse control disorders, substance-related disorders, sexual paraphilias, and behaviors such as battering and sexual offending. However, we would note that sadly only a few of these disorders (ADHD, substance abuse, and conduct disorders) have treatments that are empirically supported.

Third, we recommend that the feminist and pro-feminist therapies be included in psychotherapy outcome research. These therapies will not easily lend themselves to manualization. However, the effort to evaluate them should begin. On a related note, the gender role strain paradigm should be integrated into the psychotherapy outcome research endeavor. That is, gender should be conceptualized as a social construction on the basis of power relations between the sexes, and interventions and outcomes should be defined accordingly. For example, Levant and Silverstein (2001) described the treatment of a "postmodern couple" at an impasse, where their previously egalitarian relationship had shifted dramatically to a traditional homemaker–breadwinner model following the birth of their first child. This shift resulted in the wife losing power because of her homemaker status. We described an approach to therapy that integrated gender and family systems theory.

Finally, following the APA Division 29 (Psychotherapy) Task Force (Norcross, 2001), we would note that the therapeutic relationship has consistently been an important contributor to outcome in the now extensive research on psychotherapy. EBPs should emphasize the use of such empirically supported relationship (ESR) factors as the therapeutic alliance empathy and goal consensus. These relationship qualities create a therapeutic environment in which women and men can feel accepted and understood, preconditions to their being able to tell their stories and rework the narratives of their lives.

CONCLUSION

Evidence-based approaches should be evaluated in terms of their effectiveness in addressing a client's cultural context, including gender. To do so effectively, a commitment to analyzing systems of power and privilege is necessary. Effective treatment must include a commitment on the part of therapists to acknowledge their own biases and prejudices, and the systems of power and privilege within which they are embedded. Many psychotherapy paradigms have required that therapists examine aspects of their intrapsychic life and their family relationships. Cultural variables must now be added to this list.

In order for evidence-based treatments to effectively address gender, feminism must be moved from the margins to the center of psychological practice. This change requires a paradigm shift in mainstream psychology. Although the discipline of psychology now acknowledges the relevance of cultural variables such as gender, it is still considered a specialty, taught and practiced primarily by feminists. As feminism gradually becomes defined as part of the core of mainstream psychology, evidence-based treatments will lose their sexist biases and become more fully human and helpful.

The Neglect of Lesbian, Gay, Bisexual, and Transgendered Clients

Laura S. Brown

The movement for evidence-based and empirically supported treatments has done an admirable job of compiling lists of interventions that are proven to be helpful in the treatment of specific disorders. However, if the client in front of us is seen not as the manifestation of a diagnostic category but rather as a complicated human being whose distress exists within a particular social context, then it becomes necessary to question the adequacy of a strictly evidence-based approach to psychotherapy. Bernal and Scharrón-Del Río (2001) initiated the discussion of whether the presence of empirical support for a given intervention should always be the first decision rule when choosing therapy with clients of color. What follows extends their argument to another at-risk population, lesbian, gay, bisexual, and transgendered people.

There is probably no group of people for whom these questions of therapeutic efficacy are more salient than clients who are gender atypical or members of sexual minorities. Lesbian, gay, bisexual, and transgendered (LGBT) clients constitute a diverse group within themselves, representing all variations of age, ethnicity, social class, and gender. There is no typical LGBT client, given the wide variations within these populations. Although the bulk of the literature informing the current discussion does not refer to transgendered individuals, in this position paper transgendered people will be considered part of the population under discussion, because the experience of being gender atypical leads to social and psychological consequences very similar to those common to being lesbian, gay, or bisexual.

Despite the heterogeneity of this group, what binds LGBT clients together is the experience of discrimination and stigma. Sexual minority and gender atypical people are daily subjected to assaults, frequently psychological and at times physical, on their worth and dignity as human beings, based entirely on their sexual or gender orientations. As this paper is being written, the President of the United States and his political allies are attempting to amend the Constitution so as to permanently deny marriage to lesbians and gay men. Across the United States, LGBT people continue to be fired from jobs or lose access to children simply because of their sexuality. Military service is closed to openly gay and lesbian individuals. Gender-atypical people are at a particularly high risk for being targets of violent and sometimes deadly hate crimes. Even in places considered friendly to LGBT people, violence targeted against this population continues. Discrimination and bias create the foundation of the social context in which all LGBT people live.

This shared experience of stigma and discrimination as the backdrop to psychotherapy raises serious questions of what makes psychotherapy efficacious for these clients. Two related factors inform the urgency of the discussion. First, this is a group that uses psychotherapy at rates double or higher than the heterosexual population (Perez, DeBord, & Bieschke, 2000). As frequent and often sophisticated consumers of psychotherapy services who see psychotherapy as having intrinsic value, LGBT clients may be more aware than most of questions of empirical support for what their therapists are doing. Additionally, as frequent users, LGBT clients are more at risk for harm from ineffective therapies. As a vulnerable population, LGBT clients have an enhanced need to receive psychotherapies that are effective and empowering.

Second, the available data from population-based rather than patient studies strongly suggest that lesbians and gay men are more likely than heterosexual counterparts to suffer from anxiety, depression, and substance abuse disorders than their heterosexual counterparts (Cochran & Mays, 2000; Cochran, Sullivan, & Mays, 2003). Lesbians and gay men are also more likely than heterosexual people to have a history of sexual and physical victimization; gay men, in particular, have suffered strikingly higher rates of adult sexual assault experiences than heterosexual men (Balsam, Rothblum, & Beauchaine, 2005). One might reasonably extrapolate from these last data that LGBT people may thus have higher rates of posttraumatic stress disorder (PTSD) and other disorders associated with a history of childhood maltreatment or adult sexual assault. A logical inference is that because so many of the ESTs have been developed specifically for the treatment of anxiety, depression, and, more recently, PTSD, this is a group that would particularly benefit from access to ESTs for their disorders, and conversely, be potentially more harmed when evidence-based treatments are not being used.

This is the argument pursued by Martell, Safren, and Prince (2003) in their volume on cognitive–behavioral therapies (CBTs) for LGB clients. However, while arguing for the effectiveness of CBTs, many of which are empirically supported, these authors also comment that "there are few clinicians with expertise in both LGB-affirmative psychotherapy and CBT" (p. xi). They go on to note that "most training programs that focus on CBT do not have adequate course work in LGB issues" (p. xi).

Therein lies the crux of the question regarding whether empirical support for the treatment is, or should be, the primary consideration when working with an LGBT client. I will argue here that, although empiricism is of value in the choice of interventions, LGBT clients also require therapists who are culturally competent in the realities and social contexts informing the lives of their clients. This cultural competence, to be described later, is not inherent in any of the treatments that have to date been empirically found to be useful in the treatment of specific disorders. The degree to which the social context informs the development of distress and the inner and outer resources available to an LGBT client is not taken into account by the ESTs. The successful outcome of psychotherapy with LGBT clients may consequently rely less on empirically supported interventions and more heavily on the ESR variables present in the therapy process (Norcross, 2000), many of which lend themselves to enhanced cultural competence. The absence of cultural competence may lead to treatment failures with LGBT clients even when the diagnosis and treatment of the client's presenting problems fall squarely within the realm of an EST.

TREATMENT AS USUAL: GOOD ENOUGH?

Treatmane as usual (TAU) for LGBT clients has been as wildly varying in its cultural competence as the ESTs. The construct of "affirmative psychotherapies" for LGBT clients, first advanced by Malyon (1982) and other writers, argued for a departure from the usual treatment of LGBT clients as inherently sick and for the integration into the therapy process of the active affirmation of the client's sexual minority identity. When an affirmative stance is absent, TAU, irrespective of a therapist's theoretical orientation, may be at best neutral and at worst harmful because of the therapist's inability to prize the client fully as a lesbian, gay, bisexual, or transgendered individual. The anecdotal and autobiographical literature of the LGBT rights movements is replete with stories of failed treatments as usual, in which therapists alternately ignored a client's sexual minority status as irrelevant, or treated it as the disorder to be eradicated (Duberman, 1992; Scholinski, 1997).

Affirmative TAU represents an integrative stance in which the therapist melds an affirmative stance with her or his theoretical orientation. No specific outcome research exists on this approach, but the information on its perceived helpfulness by LGBT clients appears to be consistent (Perez, DeBord, & Bieschke). The affirmative stance appears to implicitly rely on the quality of the relationship with the client and on respect held by the therapist for the paradox that being an LGBT person is both unique and yet ordinary, and that the pain of an LGBT client is human pain, yet pain informed and flavored to some unpredictable degree by the experience of the sexual minority status.

An affirmative stance requires that any therapist working with LGBT clients needs to be attentive to issues of the therapy relationship and to ESR processes (Norcross, 2000). Sexual minority and gender atypical people have historically fared poorly at the hands of cultural authorities. The psychotherapy professions have barely begun in the last three decades to undo the harm perpetrated on LGBT individuals in the previous 70 years. Positive regard and empathy are the core and foundation of working with LGBT clients. This is a proactive stance that says, "I value you, not despite your homosexuality, bisexuality, or gender atypicality, but, because you are human and your gender and sexuality are components of your humanity, because of it."

CULTURAL COMPETENCE WITH LGBT CLIENTS

In 2000, the APA adopted their *Guidelines for Psychotherapy With Lesbian, Gay, and Bisexual Clients*. These guidelines, while aspirational rather than prescriptive, delineate the universe of capacities that a therapist should bring to working with LGB clients (transgendered people are not specifically addressed by this document and will again be subsumed in the discussion of LGB individuals). My view is that this document outlines the basics of culturally competent practices with this population, as well as with gender atypical people, and I will use the *Guidelines* as a framework for discussing the primacy of ESRs over empirically supported techniques in working with LGBT clients.

Central to effective psychotherapy with LGBT clients is a view of these clients as being variations on the human norm, rather than pathological per se because of their sexual or gender orientation. Guideline One states, "Psychologists understand that homosexuality and bisexuality are not indicative of mental illness." Higher rates of depression and anxiety in this population are not evidence of the pathology of nonheterosexuality but rather of the deleterious effects of living in cultural contexts that are discriminatory and sometimes dangerous. The narrative accompanying the first section of the *Guidelines*, "Attitudes toward homosexuality and bisexuality," underscores the essential and core importance of the therapist's affirmative stance toward LGBT clients.

Such an affirmative stance cannot be assumed. Homosexuality was removed from the diagnostic manual in the early 1970s, within the professional and training lifetime of many therapists; the diagnosis of "Ego dystonic homosexuality" remained in the *Diagnostic and Statistical Manual of Mental Disorders, Fourth Edition* (DSM–IV; American Psychiatric Association, 1994) until the middle 1980s, and homosexuality can still be covertly diagnosed as a mental disorder via the use of Sexual Disorder Not Otherwise Specified. Transgendered people are still constructed in the *DSM–IV–TR* as experiencing a pathology, Gender Identity Disorder, the diagnosis of which is required before a transsexual person is eligible for gender reassignment surgery. Many psychotherapists continue to hold covertly homophobic or heterosexist attitudes, irrespective of the official pronouncements of professional organizations, and psychotherapies that claim to reorient clients from homosexual to heterosexual are on the upsurge (Haldeman, 2002). Because of the infrequency with which training programs for psychologists have addressed psychotherapists' own heterosexism and homophobia (Fassinger, 2000; Phillips, 2000), it is inevitable that many psychotherapists will have covertly biased attitudes toward their LGBT clients.

To effectively work with LGBT clients, a therapist must be able to avoid making the client's sexual or gender orientation the problem and rather focus on the distress that brings the client into treatment; at the same time, the therapist must not ignore the salience of the client's LGBT identity. The therapist must thus be able to demonstrate and experience positive regard for the LGBT client. Rogers's (1957, p. 101) original definition of this phenomenon describes elegantly the stance necessary for successful work with an LGBT client: "A warm acceptance of each aspect of the client's experience as being a part of that client . . . there are no conditions of acceptance . . . it means a 'prizing' of the person . . . it means a caring for the client as a separate person."

Farber and Lane's (2002) recent meta-analysis suggested that positive regard is a significant factor in determining treatment outcome, regardless of the therapist's theoretical orientation. I would suggest that for LGBT clients the therapist's capacity for the genuine demonstration of affirmation will be a larger factor contributing to the outcome of the psychotherapy process, simply because the therapist then makes the therapy room and process a place safe from stigma, bias, and discrimination.

Effective psychotherapy with LGBT clients also requires the therapist's awareness of her or his own heterosexist biases, which are more likely to creep into the therapy process than overt homophobia. Heterosexism is defined as "the ideological system that denies, denigrates, and stigmatizes any non-heterosexual form of behavior, identity, relationship or community" (Herek, 1995, p. 157). The *Guidelines* comment that "Heterosexism pervades the language, theories, and psychotherapeutic interventions of psychology" (Anderson, 1996; Brown, 1989). Heterosexism can manifest in something as simple as the intake form on which common relational denominators (married, single, divorced) exclude the experiences of most LGBT clients. As Guideline Seven notes, "Psychologists recognize that the families of lesbian, gay, and bisexual people may include people who are not legally or biologically related." The culturally competent therapist is aware of how heterosexism pervades the culture and will take seriously and with respect the powerful meanings of small things that resist heterosexist norms.

Heterosexism manifests itself as well in "sexual orientation blindness," in which the therapist, striving for an impossible neutrality, ignores or dismisses the unique experiences, histories, and social contexts of LGBT clients, insisting that such contextual variables make no difference to diagnosis and treatment. This form of apparently benign heterosexism, in which the therapist fails to prize the client's uniqueness as an LGBT person, can leave clients with the impression that a therapist lacks empathy for their personal realities as members of a sexual minority group and is indeed falling back on a cookie-cutter approach from a manual, even when the therapist does nothing overtly biased or discriminatory.

Heterosexual therapists may also be unaware of the power and privilege inherent in their majority sexual orientation and thus be blind to the effects of the absence of this power and privilege in the lives of LGBT clients (or colleagues, for that matter). Heterosexual people in Western cultures take for granted that they may marry, participate fully in the religious faith of their choice, receive survivor benefits when a spouse dies, and in general be treated as sexually acceptable on the basis of the gender of their sexual object choice. Although LGBT people have made tremendous strides in securing some of the rights once denied, many do not have access to these rights, and those who have them must constantly be engaged in protecting them. The extra psychic effort required to live in society as an LGBT person is something frequently invisible and unknowable to members of the heterosexual majority. Well-meaning heterosexual therapists may abuse their privilege and power by dismissing the impact of continual exposure to discrimination, and they should acknowledge explicitly how their privilege may create an empathic void from time to time with LGBT clients.

The client's experience of being the recipient of accurate empathy has been shown empirically to be a powerful determinant in psychotherapy outcome, accounting for an average of 9% to 10% of the variance according to a recent meta-analytic review (Bohart, Elliott, Greenberg, & Watson, 2002). Perhaps a large yet unstated reason why LGBT clients frequently express a preference for therapists of their own sexual orientation (Liddle, 1996) is the expectation (not always accurate) that a therapist who has shared the experience of a sexual minority status will be less heterosexist and more accurately empathetic. Culturally competent therapists are more likely to display accurate empathy with an LGBT client because such therapists are attuned to the social and contextual realities of clients' lives.

Some aspects of cultural competence with LGBT clients are not addressed directly by the literature on empirically supported psychotherapy relationships but can be inferred as being synchronous. For instance, Guideline Three states, "Psychologists strive to understand the ways in which social stigmatization (i.e., prejudice, discrimination, and violence) poses risks to the mental health and well-being of lesbian, gay, and bisexual clients." Concretely, this means that the culturally competent therapist can differentiate between a reasonable response to external context and a diagnosable disorder, or between internalized homophobia or heterosexism and a diagnosable disorder. Additionally, because a disorder and oppression can and frequently do cooccur, a culturally competent therapist must know how to diagnose and respond to both within the context of treatment. A manualized approach to psychotherapy, which has been advocated by some of the developers of ESTs, does not allow the therapist the flexibility or clinical judgment necessary to make this sort of determination. Depression is depression, and anxiety is anxiety; the presence or absence of cooccurring social environment factors that might aggravate or moderate the distress are not taken into account. In the absence of accurate empathy for the realities of the client's context as an LGBT person, ineffective psychotherapy with an EST may ensue.

Imagine, for a moment, the hypothetical LGBT client who is seeking treatment for agoraphobia. The not very culturally competent therapist is proceeding in an empirically supported fashion, but the client's symptoms do not ameliorate and in fact seem to worsen. Now imagine that during the third week of therapy a gay man has been gay-bashed while leaving a local gay establishment, and that his attackers have yet to be found. The not very culturally competent therapist may be unaware of this event and, even if apprised of it by the client, may fail to see its relevance to therapy.

A culturally competent therapist would be aware of cultural and social factors that might affect LGBT clients and so would have known of the attack because of remaining current with issues affecting the LGBT communities. He or she would have deviated from the EST at this juncture and instead begun to address the real-world situation that is aggravating the client's agoraphobic symptoms. For this client, the world is, in fact, dangerous; the client has been handed potent evidence to that effect. The culturally competent therapist would acknowledge and validate that reality, and perhaps reconsider the diagnosis. Is this agoraphobia, or a posttraumatic agoraphobic response, brought on by repeated witnessing other assaults on LGBT people? The culturally competent therapist would be aware of the construct of insidious traumatization (Root, 1992), which posits that members of oppressed target groups may develop PTSD solely through indirect but repeated exposure to the knowledge of harm to others in their reference group.

A core assumption of treatment for agoraphobia is that no danger exists in leaving one's home. By contrast, a core assumption of culturally competent treatment with an apparently agoraphobic LGBT client is that the world is indisputably potentially dangerous. There may be other strategies for coping with that danger than not leaving home and other ways to address the presenting symptoms than standard therapies for agoraphobia. Culturally competent treatment in this instance might include referring the client to a self-defense class, consistent with Guideline Sixteen, which states, "Psychologists make reasonable efforts to familiarize themselves with relevant mental health, educational, and community resources for lesbian, gay, and bisexual people."

This hypothetical case highlights Guideline Two, which states, "Psychologists are encouraged to recognize how their attitudes and knowledge about lesbian, gay, and bisexual issues may be relevant to assessment and treatment and seek consultation or make appropriate referrals when indicated." In this case, a therapist who lacks knowledge of LGBT issues may make an inaccurate assessment and inappropriately apply a treatment primarily because of the apparent match between the client's symptoms and the psychotherapy research findings. Assessments in the EST literature typically focus on accurate assessments of the client's DSM–IV diagnosis; this literature, aside from the work of Martell, Safren, and Prince (2003), fails almost entirely to take into account sexual orientation or gender atypicality. Culturally competent assessments of LGBT clients examine not only the clients' DSM–IV diagnosis but their relationship to their LGBT identity and the interaction between identity development, distress, and coping strategies (Morrow, 2000).

Finally, research on therapy relationships indicates that self-disclosure can, when accurately used, be a component of effective treatment (Hill & Knox, 2002). Although not all LGBT clients will want a therapist of similar sexual or gender orientation, many express feeling more comfortable in the therapy process when they are aware of the therapist's orientation (Liddle, 1996). Culturally competent therapists will also use self-disclosure as a strategy for letting LGBT clients know that they are familiar with LGBT lives and realities outside the therapy office.

BOTH TAU AND EBP

Does this mean that affirmative psychotherapy with LGBT clients should eschew the use of empirically supported psychotherapies? Clearly, this is not the case; as Martell, Safren, and Prince (2003) demonstrated, it is possible to practice culturally competent and empirically supported psychotherapy simultaneously. One does not preclude the other in any way. However, in both assessment and intervention, the therapist who chooses an EST will need to actively interweave an LGBT affirmative mindset into the treatment process. A therapist whose strong point is cultural competence, conversely, may want to be aware of the possible efficacy of an EST.

Researchers need to turn their attention to the specific needs of LGBT clients. We need to begin the process of teasing out the etiologies of higher depression and anxiety rates, and better understand what it means when an LGBT person presents to therapy with the symptoms of depression or anxiety. Trauma as a factor in the lives of LGBT people (Brown, 2003) needs to be better taken into account in an assessment prior to psychotherapy research, as well as in the development of ESTs. LGBT clients need both: culturally competent, empathic therapists and the most effective treatments for their distress. We cannot pretend that we know yet what constitutes the latter, but we can and certainly do know how to implement the former.

Evidence-Based Practices Have Ignored People With Disabilities

Rhoda Olkin and Greg Taliaferro

We have been unable to locate any published materials on EBPs and people with disabilities (Taliaferro, 2004). This absence in the literature mirrors the relative invisibility of disability issues in metal health and fuels our concern that EBP will develop without due consideration of this minority group. Thus, we are pleased that this book includes a section on the interface of EBP and people with disabilities.

Addressing the treatment of people with disabilities immediately raises the problem of the tremendous heterogeneity among individuals with disabilities. Relevant factors include age of onset of the disability, functional abilities, the visibility of the disability, the course of the disability, the effects on life expectancy, and the presence of other disabilities. These disability-specific factors are in addition to the *and* factor: disability *and* gender, age, sexual orientation, or race–ethnicity. Further compounding the difficulty is the differential degree of stigma associated with various disabilities. And, of course, people with disabilities come to treatment with their own unique personal histories and personalities.

Before discussing the relationship between disabilities and EBPs, an important question must be raised: Are people with disabilities any more likely to be in need of treatment than those without disabilities? We know a little about this question, but there is much more we do not know. Even if we focus only on *DSM–IV* diagnostic categories, there cannot be a blanket answer to this question. A review of the prevalence of depression in disabilities (Olkin, 2004) underscores the necessity of examining rates of depression for specific disabilities. Rates may be higher than in the general population for some disabilities (e.g., multiple sclerosis or spinal cord injury), but rates are not higher for other disabilities (early onset blindness). Although several studies found higher rates of PTSD among people with spinal cord injury, as might be expected for a disability often associated with traumatic onset (Boyer, Knolls, Kafkalas, Tollen, & Swartz, 2000; Kennedy & Duff, 2001; Radnitz et al., 1998), another study found the rate the same as for the general population (Stougaard-Nielsen, 2004). (Note, however, that there were important differences in age of onset of the injury and populations studied across this research.) A literature search finds no data on the prevalence rates of bipolar disorder or schizophrenia among people with disabilities.

We have no reason to believe that people with disabilities have less need for mental health treatment than their nondisabled peers, though they may have less insurance and less private means to obtain such treatment. However, large-scale, community-sample studies of the mental health needs of people with disabilities are relatively absent. Few epidemiological studies have investigated the incidence and prevalence rates of *DSM–IV* categories in children and adults with disabilities. Such studies are needed to allocate services and inform social and public policy. These studies would help researchers of evidence-based treatments direct their time and resources in adapting evidence-based treatments to people with disabilities.

Addressing disability in the context of EBPs should be done for several good reasons. One of the strengths of evidence-based treatments is their demonstrated efficacy in controlled studies, yet there has been little research indicating the efficacy of evidence-based treatments for people with disabilities. Further, some incompatibility may exist between the assumptions underlying evidence-based treatment and those of the disability community.

The three main models of disability (Priestley, 2001) are the moral model (disability is a manifestation of flaws in character or morality), the medical model (disability resides in the individual and is a defect in a bodily function or system), and the social model (disability is socially constructed and reflects problems in society). The social model of disability provides an important perspective on the experience of living with a disability and is the framework underlying disability studies. Some evidence suggests that the model of disability would affect the intervention method that was seen as appropriate (Williams, Hershenson, & Fabian, 2000). The social model is mostly inconsistent with a medical model and the assumptions underlying evidence-based treatment (e.g., pathology resides in the client); the former would seek to remove social and political barriers and the latter seeks to resolve intrapersonal symptoms. People with disabilities may seek treatment for issues that are not addressed by EBPs. Disabilities are associated with known risk factors such as sexual and physical abuse, neglect, unemployment, poverty and economic disadvantage, social ostracization, stigma, and discrimination, as well as barriers to jobs, housing, and social and recreational opportunities. Although EBPs may focus on the person's response to these environmental factors, such as depression, it is not designed to address social and political factors that may contribute to depression in people with disabilities.

In the absence of EBPs for people with disabilities, what is the current practice? Therapy as usual? Outside of rehabilitation, there is a remarkable paucity of literature on general therapy with people with disabilities (Olkin, 1999; Taliaferro, 2004). Disability culture and issues are mostly unknown to practitioners without direct ties to the disability community, and thus culturally competent practice with regard to people with disabilities is not the norm. Although Domain D of APA's accreditation guidelines (APA, 1995) focuses on diversity, disability often is not included in such training (Leigh, Powers, Vash, & Nettles, 2004; Olkin, 2002a). In APA-accredited programs, the modal number of required courses on disability is zero, and only 11% of programs have at least one course on disability (Olkin & Pledger, 2003). Despite a lack of training and low levels of perceived competence in this area, respondents in one study of graduates of clinical and counseling programs were providing services to clients with disabilities (Allison, Crawford, Echemendia, Robinson, & Knepp, 1994). Another study indicates that 70% of child custody evaluators have performed assessments on parents with physical disabilities, despite the fact that over 84% of the respondents received no training at all with regard to performing such evaluations with people with physical disabilities (Breeden, 2004). Consumers and disability advocates perceive mental health professionals' knowledge and skills regarding severe disabilities as a barrier to treatment (Pelletier, Rogers, & Dellario, 1985). Our concern is that practitioners do not perceive the need for specialized knowledge, supervision, or consultation when working with clients with disabilities.

In the absence of disability training, clinicians may not understand how case formulation and treatment are affected by a disability. For example, no RCTs of treatment exist for depression among persons with spinal cord injuries, leading the authors to speculate whether this absence reflects a lack of interest "in examining the effects of different interventions for depression among persons with spinal cord injury" (Elliott & Kennedy, 2004, p. 137). Two factors may foster this lack of interest. One factor is that depression, which is a treatable disorder, gets confused with disability, which may be immutable. The other factor is the pervasive myth that people with disabilities should be depressed, and the corollary view that depression is a necessary stage of adaptation (Gething, 1997; Langer, 1994; Livneh & Sherwood, 1991). Although rehabilitation psychologists may be familiar with this "requirement of mourning" (Wright, 1983, p. 78), practitioners in general may equate disability with loss, and having done so the "fundamental connection between loss and depression leads to a natural conceptual bridge" (Langer, 1994, pp. 181–182). But depression (a) is not the modal response to disability, (b) complicates recovery, and (c) predicts further episodes of depression.

Without specialized training, practitioners encountering clients with disabilities are prone to mistakes. DeLoach and Greer (1981) outlined four common mistakes we think are still pervasive. One mistake is interpreting as abnormal behaviors by people with disabilities that are considered normal for others (for example, labeling anger over daily hassles and discrimination as maladjustment or a chip on the shoulder). A second mistake is overemphasizing the effects of disability on adjustment (such as assuming a woman's marital problems are because of her disability). A third mistake is underestimating the potential of clients with disabilities (for example, thinking a man with significant cerebral palsy will not be in a romantic relationship). A fourth mistake is treating clients in terms of the disability with little regard to other personal characteristics (such as ignoring ethnicity, gender, and personality). Whether the therapist focuses almost exclusively on the disability or conversely minimizes the disability's role and impact (Esten & Willmott, 1993), the disability is not appropriately contextualized within the larger case formulation. Without disability-specific training or supervised experience, and in the absence of rich clinical literature and research on clients with disabilities, therapy as usual cannot attain the sophistication necessary for cultural competence.

EBPS AND DISABILITY

EBPs rest on valid assessments and diagnoses, and on evidence of treatment efficacy on the basis of group studies. Pitfalls occur in both of these steps regarding people with disabilities. Assessment measures can be misapplied to people with disabilities through several errors. Measures typically do not have norms for people with disabilities. Some measures contain items that have different meanings within a disability context, and the endorsement of such items may inflate scores. For example, a statement on the Minnesota Multiphasic Personality Inventory—II (MMPI–II) about difficulty with standing or walking may be endorsed because of a physical disability. Further, measures may not assess stressors germane to people with disabilities (e.g., disability-specific hassles or effects of discrimination) or the skills necessary to living with a disability (e.g., self-advocacy or negotiation with medical service provider systems). So a first step toward a valid application of EBP with people with disabilities is to develop assessment measures and practices appropriate for and normed on people with disabilities.

Regarding evidence of treatment efficacy on the basis of group studies, which are then applied to clients with disabilities, several notable problems exist. First, the research may use assessment measures that have the difficulties outlined previously. Second, the research itself may not be accessible to people with disabilities. Methods of outreach, eligibility screening, data collection, assessment, and intervention may all inadvertently preclude people with visual, hearing, mobility, cognitive, or other disabilities. For example, publicity in print form (e.g., newspapers, magazines, and flyers) may not reach people with visual impairments. Data collection may be conducted in a setting not readily accessibly by public transportation. Measures may not be easily understood by those who are deaf or people with cognitive impairments (see Olkin, 2002b, for a discussion of accessible research). Third, group-based studies may not allow for the flexibility needed to tailor intervention to the needs of specific disabilities (e.g., those with intellectual impairments). At the very least, we argue that all therapy outcome studies collect and report on information about the disability status of participants.

Although people with disabilities might have the same range of problems as others, they also are likely to face unique challenges not typically addressed by EBP. The pervasive prejudice, stigma, and discrimination that people with disabilities encounter in every sphere—housing, restaurants, transportation, employment, health care, recreational sites and activities, social and intimate interactions—means that many problems are external to the person. Additionally, the sequela of some disabilities—pain, uncertainty, fatigue, weakness, daily hassles, misunderstanding by others, and a lack of empathy for the disability experience—carry psychological ramifications that might need addressing. Relationship factors also can be affected by a disability; dating, sexuality, partnering, and even separation–divorce (Olkin, 2003), as well as friendship patterns (and the possible loss of friendships after disability onset) involve a disability to varying degrees. Thus, good intentions coupled with knowledge of EBP are not enough to know how best to address the mental health needs of people with disabilities.

The therapeutic relationship is a critical variable in treatment outcomes (Lambert & Barlay, 2001), and the alliance is no less central with clients with disabilities. But much is unknown about the effects of disability on the therapeutic alliance. The issue of countertransference is paramount, as attitudes toward disabilities are still predominantly negative, and therapists are no exception to this. Therapists' attitudes, feelings, and personal experiences will likely influence their work with their clients with disabilities. If therapists hold negative beliefs or experience emotional reactions to clients with disabilities that they do not acknowledge, the therapeutic relationship and process will be adversely impacted.

The meaning of behaviors in the context of a disability can differ, such that the relationship may be affected by variables of which the therapist is unaware. For example, simple acts such as holding the door open, rearranging chairs to accommodate a wheelchair, having (or not) a large-print copy of a treatment contract, or writing something down for the client to remember can all resonate differently for people with disabilities. People with disabilities often are helped by family members, friends, and strangers, and sometimes this is useful and other times intrusive and demeaning. Thus, simple therapist behaviors can convey relationship messages that will be perceived differently by people with disabilities. And therapists may have more difficulty drawing clear guidelines for themselves when it comes to assisting someone put on a coat, calling to obtain a paratransit application, getting an informational brochure from a national disability organization, or filling out forms. How does one decide which is useful and appropriate versus caretaking or being countertherapeutic? These disability relationship issues must be better articulated in evidence-based research.

Disability research and theory have made much of the three models of disability and, more recently, empowerment models of treatment (Condeluci, 1989; Fawcett et al., 1994; Kosciulek & Wheaton, 2003). However, disability models have not been well articulated or applied clinically (for exceptions, see Blotzer & Ruth, 1995; Olkin, 1999). We do not know if models of disability impact mental health outcomes. These are important clinical questions for clients with disabilities and ones not addressed by current EBPs. The social model places most of the problems faced by people with disabilities in the social, political, legal, and economic arenas. Therefore, interventions are aimed at helping clients work with and perhaps change these external problems. However, a person with a disability might still have a depressive disorder that may be related to internal psychological variables (e.g., cognitive distortions). How do we interface these two frameworks for intervention, the social model and EBPs? Our point is not that EBPs should not inform the treatment. Rather, it is that problems should be viewed and treated simultaneously from both perspectives. Conceptualizing clinical issues only from the viewpoint of evidence-based treatments misses half the picture. Perpetuating the view that the problems of people with disabilities are related to their adjustment (or maladjustment) to a disability makes therapy risk recapitulating the often painful experiences faced by people with disabilities in their interactions with others and in larger society.

EBPs are attractive to insurance companies, who may exert financial pressure to use them and who consider them the standard of care even before they are shown to be effective with people with disabilities. We cannot ignore the pressures of funding in the treatment of people with disabilities. Already incentives exist for nursing care over home-based care. However, as one practice demonstrates effectiveness, the inverse is not necessarily true, that unexamined practices are not effective. But when defining the desired outcomes of therapy, "who defines a 'good' outcome, and is there a risk here that, in the defining, some stakeholder group will be passed by?" (Nemec, 2004, p. 134).

Psychotherapy should not duplicate the ostracization experienced by people with disabilities. When they are excluded from important outcome research, when the information about their disability status is not seen as important to be collected or reported, when the research is inaccessible to them, and when results normed on people without disabilities are assumed to apply to people with disabilities, this replicates the world in which they live, in which people with disabilities are outsiders.

SUMMARY

We do not argue that EBPs are inapplicable to people with disabilities, but rather that, with our current state of knowledge, we do not know. We are not advocating for specific ways that EBPs should be modified or how these modifications would differ for specific disabilities, because we do not know. We are proposing that people with disabilities be incorporated into the investigation—as researchers, as participants, and ultimately as beneficiaries.

Dialogue: Convergence and Contention

Stanley Sue and Nolan Zane

With respect to EBPs and the dimensions of diversity, our points of agreement with Levant and Silverstein, Brown, and Olkin and Taliaferro are striking. In fact, we want to examine the similarity of themes because they are not coincidental. Rather, they reveal underlying principles. We present five common themes and illustrate them with statements made by the respective authors.

First, there is a lack of research on general practice and EBPs in particular devoted to ethnic minorities, women, LGBT individuals, and people with disabilities. As one example, Olkin and Taliaferro note that, "We have been unable to locate any published materials on EBPs and people with disabilities" (p. 353). Olkin and Taliaferro also point to the sad state of research on people with disabilities:

> We do not argue that EBPs are inapplicable to people with disabilities, but rather that, with our current state of knowledge, we do not know. We are not advocating for specific ways that EBP should be modified or how these modifications would differ for specific disabilities, because we do not know. (p. 359)

Second, these diverse groups are oppressed in society. The oppression is revealed in many ways, through White privilege; the evolution of norms that define diversity as deviant, undesirable, or negative; the development of negative stereotypes; prejudice and discrimination; and a lack of attention and aid. As noted by Levant and Silverstein, society is largely "White, middle class, heterosexual, and able bodied" (p. 339) with the assumption that these are privileged characteristics. Brown argues that, "What binds LGBT clients together is the experience of discrimination and stigma" (p. 346). Indeed, these experiences bind all the diverse groups together. Research and practice are conducted in this setting.

Third, culture and context are important to consider. As we noted in our position paper, culture is important in all phases of the research and treatment process. Levant and Silverstein adopt "a social constructionist perspective that views gender roles not as biological or even social 'givens' but rather as psychologically and socially constructed entities that bring certain advantages and disadvantages, and, most importantly, that can change" (p. 342).

Fourth, traditional TAU and EBPs have been inadequate in meeting the needs of diverse populations. Brown criticizes TAU for "wildly varying in its cultural competence, as have the ESTs" (p. 348). We have criticized research in general for (a) sacrificing external validity in favor of internal validity and (b) generally ignoring the value of discovery-oriented research that attempts to understand the dynamics of the treatment process to identify important variables that may lead to the formulation of treatment strategies to test. Discovery research can be conducted using all types of methodology, ranging from quantitative to qualitative approaches, experimental to correlations studies, and laboratory to naturalistic settings. A mistaken notion exists that testing the validity of EBPs with minority and other diverse groups would lead the field into an endless series of effectiveness studies on these groups, as well as on certain subgroups of these groups. However, the approach to studying diverse clinical samples should be very consistent with a major principle underlying EBPs: These tests of effectiveness should be guided by the best available empirical evidence. In this case, we would make use of empirical evidence that points to certain groups as possibly being more at risk for poor responses to psychotherapy because of their cultural backgrounds and other factors. For example, convergent evidence (Zane, Hall, Sue, Young, & Nunez, 2003) shows that immigrant, unacculturated Asian American clients may not find psychotherapy credible and may not respond well to certain psychological treatments. Priority should be placed on validation studies for these clients, as well as for other client groups similarly identified by the research.

Fifth, new approaches to research and intervention are advocated by the contributors to this chapter. Levant and Silverstein recommend that feminist and pro-feminist therapies be included in psychotherapy outcome research while recognizing that these therapies will not easily lend themselves to manualization. Brown calls for affirmative treatment in which "the therapist melds an affirmative stance with her or his theoretical orientation. No specific outcome research exists on this approach, but the information on its perceived helpfulness by LGBT clients appears to be consistent" (p. 348). We called for therapists' cultural competency, which depends on contextual factors such as client characteristics, therapist characteristics, intervention types, and treatment setting. Thus, the various authors recognize the need for the establishment and evaluation of newer forms of treatment.

The four position papers in this chapter show these five themes. To be sure, the diverse groups examined also show important differences. One apparent difference is in the utilization of mental health services, which appears to be high among women and LGBT groups, but low among ethnic minorities. Nevertheless, that the general themes are so consistent points to the social–cultural dynamics in our society, dynamics that need to be studied and altered in the interest of society.

Ronald F. Levant and Louise B. Silverstein

First of all, we would like to say that we are honored to be included with such highly esteemed colleagues in this chapter. Second, we would like to note that, in reading the other position papers in this chapter, we are struck by the unanimity of the views expressed. It appears that all of the authors agree that neither EBPs nor TAU satisfactorily address the various dimensions of human diversity in mental health. Race–ethnicity, gender, sexual orientation, and disability status have largely been ignored to date. This is a powerful conclusion! It suggests that we must make diversity issues and multicultural competence a much higher priority in our field.

How can we do this? We don't claim to have all the answers, but we will sketch out a few thoughts. First and foremost, we need to develop greater multicultural competence in professional psychology, which not only includes multicultural information but also self-awareness exercises to help practitioners become aware of the effects of privilege in rendering various forms of oppression invisible. Effective treatment must include a commitment on the part of the therapist to acknowledge his or her own biases and prejudices, and the systems of power and privilege within which they are embedded.

This effort should begin with the academic training programs, which, despite the requirements of APA accreditation for promoting cultural competence for all dimensions of diversity, probably do not do a uniformly good job of helping students become culturally competent. We also need to build cultural and gender competence into continuing education programs and state licensure requirements for the continuing education of mental health professionals.

Second, we need to develop a research methodology that identifies effective treatment from a multicultural standpoint. We want to highlight the appropriateness of qualitative methodology in this regard. As Sue and Zane point out, very little research has been done on EBPs with ethnic minority clients. In a context in which very little is known about a phenomenon, qualitative research is often the methodology of choice because it is hypothesis generating rather than hypothesis testing. In this early stage of knowledge construction, qualitative evaluation, with its emphasis on the subjective experience of the participants, is especially useful in providing information about clients (e.g., the impact of race–ethnicity or immigrant status on identity formation), therapists (e.g., the presence of sexist or heterosexist attitudes or beliefs), and the relationship context (e.g., affirmative versus homophobic attitudes toward gender atypical clients or espousing a moral versus a social model of disability). Generating rich descriptions of local contexts is likely to represent the complexity of the interplay between both individual and cultural variables.

In the quantitative paradigm, in contrast, professionals who are from social locations significantly different from those of the population being studied define the research questions and design the measures. This cultural chasm has too often produced hypotheses that are irrelevant to the lived experiences of the participants or findings that pathologize their differences. To be truly effective in this endeavor, we need to engage the clinical scientists who conduct research on EBPs and the funding agencies who fund and thereby set the priorities for such research. These two groups are critical to the future of EBP and hold the key to the eventual empirical assessment of multiculturally competent assessment procedures and therapies.

Finally, we want to urge the development of a conceptual framework that is inclusive of multiple domains of identity and that eschews a focus on individual cultural differences in favor of an awareness of systems of oppression.

Laura S. Brown

It was a remarkable but not surprising experience for me to read the contributions of the authors in this section on diversity. Many of these writers are familiar to me; some of them are dear friends, and others are people whose work has inspired and informed my own. Together we represent the views of a community of thought within psychology that is frequently perceived as marginal to the "real work" of our field. Each of these position papers describes similar problems from the standpoint of the social locations of ethnicity, gender, sexual orientation, and disability. The message from all is that no matter where we stand, we see very similar problems: exclusion, invisibility, and the absence of culture competence among psychological researchers and practitioners. Each of us believes that all practice for all clients will be improved when cultural competence with target group clients becomes a norm for best practices.

I find myself, in consequence, simply wishing to shout "Amen" to my sister and brother authors, and then to pose a question. How is it possible that in the 21st century issues of social location and identity continue to be marginalized in the training and practice of psychologists? How is attention to gender, ethnicity, sexual orientation, and disability (along with the dimensions not addressed here, such as age, social class, immigrant or refugee status, religious identity, and heritage of colonization) ghettoized into the "diverse populations" class, literally and figuratively, rather than being mainstreamed into the norms for best practice?

This is a truly challenging dilemma. We have all been working diligently to change this state of affairs, some of us (like Stan Sue) doing so for upwards of 30 years now. How is it that our efforts continue to meet with only token success? Inattention to diversity is pervasive across graduate and undergraduate curricula in psychology. Diversity is bowed to in a perfunctory manner but rarely taken seriously as having meaning for everything that psychologists do. The majority (although not all) of my clinical psychology doctoral students arrive in my classes with the belief that diversity is of concern only to those officially deemed "diverse." Their attitudes are shaped and formed at the undergraduate level and are enabled by what they encounter in many of their practicum settings. My colleagues and I intensively educate these students in the centrality of diversity; these same students, now transformed, return to us in shock and distress after taking this training into practicum sites when they find that many psychologists whom they encounter in the "real world" outside of our campus see their diversity focus as odd or unnecessary. TAU and EBP both continue to be problematic for target group clients because of the ongoing marginalization of a diversity epistemology among psychologists who practice in either or both of these therapeutic frameworks.

Finally, a word for singularity in the midst of similarity in the service of our shared goals. Although our concerns about the neglect of our respective populations by psychology are similar, the needs of our populations are not. We all call for cultural competence in working with target populations. In the name of such competence I'd like to suggest that LGBT people (who all have a gender and an ethnicity, and some of whom are members of the disability community) have a particular set of therapeutic needs that differ meaningfully from those of people of dominant sexual orientations with whom they may share these other social markers and identities.

Women, people of color, and people with disabilities all have won at least legal equal rights in the United States. Although biased attitudes and unfair treatment persist, none of those inequitable experiences are supported or enabled today by laws. This is not the case for LGBT people. The laws of the United States do not protect us; they may, in some cases, endanger us. Since I wrote my initial contribution, the legal situation for LGBT people has worsened in the United States (although ironically has improved greatly in Canada, making what follows less relevant to Canadian readers). During fall 2004, 11 states passed constitutional amendments outlawing marriage for us; some of these laws even forbade domestic partner arrangements. The marriages of 3,000-plus lesbian and gay couples solemnized in San Francisco in 2004 have all been declared invalid, and those married in Portland, Oregon, find themselves in limbo in the wake of the new constitutional amendment that illegitimates such unions. LGBT people are currently under attack, and this attack is legitimized by laws that do not protect us.

So as all of us who are concerned with the integration of social justice into treatment join together to develop practices that will be the most efficacious for people with histories of discrimination and targeting, let us not forget to also develop treatment strategies for those clients whose legal discrimination is present and intensifying rather than lessening. In the field of trauma treatment where I have spent much of my professional life, my international colleagues speak of the reality that for many people there is no *post*-traumatic stress disorder, as the trauma is not past but ongoing. This is the reality of life for LGBT clients in the United States today. For LGBT clients, we must design therapies in which cultural competence includes an acknowledgement by the therapist that not only is the playing field not level, nor in the process of leveling, but that it is being actively tilted off balance by governmental and religious leaders. Perhaps in discovering practices that work well for clients in situations of such continuous risk we will also uncover principles of good and effective practices for all persons in distress.

Rhoda Olkin and Greg Taliaferro

We are impressed with the other position papers in this chapter, finding many areas of overlap and some critical differences. Strong agreement exists about the need for culturally competent therapists with skills and knowledge, enabling appropriate therapy with individuals from diverse populations. But culturally competent therapists must emerge from a culturally competent field of psychology, including culturally informed theories of psychopathology, personality, and psychotherapy. However, these are arenas in which disability has been framed as deviant, abnormal, and aberrant. Students and clinicians rarely have training opportunities in disability-competent assessments, case formulation, and treatments. We call for the field of psychology to become disability culturally competent such that therapists can be trained in cultural competence within a disability affirmative context.

An ongoing problem for minority groups is that diversity issues often are relegated to one or two classes, one chapter in a book, or one lecture in a series. This communicates that diversity is an add-on, an afterthought, and students and clinicians are not encouraged to integrate these topics into their work. Further, each diverse group is considered separately, decontextualized, as if the single minority status is the defining characteristic. Even within diversity, disability has been an add-on, making it even more marginalized. For example, a class on diversity may have one period devoted to disability. Unfortunately, this position of riding the coattails of diversity pits disability against other minorities, and time spent on disability is taken away from time spent on other areas of diversity. Similar to other minorities, all disabilities are lumped together despite enormous variations among disabilities, and critical intragroup differences are minimized.

All four position papers call for more research, but research must go beyond the inclusion of individuals from diverse populations into RCTs assessing EBP. The inclusion of people with disabilities means not only involving them as participants but as researchers as well. Disability factors must be included in all facets of the research, from the development of research questions and methods to understanding and interpreting data. We agree with the other authors who have noted the importance of ESRs in psychotherapy. We emphatically agree, but it is unknown how prejudice and discrimination are manifested in the therapeutic relationship. We need more research on the process variables of therapy with clients with disabilities and a better understanding of how therapists actually work with such clients. Three important areas for research are the effects of the disability status on therapists' empathy and relationship behaviors, how therapists handle disability content in the clinical interview, and how disability is incorporated into the case formulation.

We agree with Sue and Zane that there are practical reasons why minorities are excluded from research. Particularly for disabilities, methods of outreach, data collection, and measures have to be made accessible (e.g., in alternate formats or accessible venues). These methods can require extra funding, must be tailored to different types of disabilities, and may not be well understood by researchers without disability experience or training. As others have noted, it is not clear what to do in the meantime: how to understand outcome studies that have not included minorities. We probably should not assume generalizability and must consider the possibility that treatment proven on nondisabled populations could be harmful to clients with disabilities.

Other authors have noted the political aspects of minority status. Disability, too, is a social construct. We agree with Brown that in the face of a condition that encompasses political, economic, historical, social, and psychological factors, it is insufficient for therapy to address only the psychological. If people experience both psycho-emotional distress and oppression, we lack interventions that have been addressed by EBP. Disability-affirmative therapy does not imply any particular theory or intervention but a framework for therapy. The interface of this framework and EBP is not yet articulated.

We agree with Brown that therapy itself should not duplicate the oppression experienced by minorities. We cannot assume this for disability, when offices may not meet basic access requirements. We also agree that the daily hassles of minority status are often invisible to others. The therapy setting itself may impose such hassles (a lack of handicapped parking or an accessible bathroom, or paperwork not available in large print). And the hassles and oppression of other people with disabilities can profoundly affect the client with a disability: a blind parent whose child is removed at birth by child protective services, a man with quadriplegia who is denied coverage for home assistance but instead must live in a nursing home, or a conference speaker who finds the podium inaccessible. These reported or observed events have a differential impact on families with disabilities.

Foremost among the differences from other groups is that they have a rich clinical and theoretical literature from which to draw. Additionally, the APA governance approves guidelines and other reports that discuss culturally competent therapy with respective groups. These are notably lacking for disability. There is less research, theory, and practice defining cultural competence with people with disabilities, and no APA-sanctioned report or guidelines exist on the topic. We can begin by using examples from other groups to begin defining what constitutes cultural competence in disability.

Lastly, we take care to note that the section on disability was written by two authors with disabilities, as this is unusual. No other area of diversity is so dominated by people not of that minority as is disability. In contrast to other diverse groups, it is usually taught and practiced not by people with disabilities but those without disabilities. This both reflects and perpetuates the marginalization of disability, even amongst marginalized groups. Disability is still considered a specialty, relegated to a single area of psychology (rehabilitation psychology) and not incorporated into the mainstream of psychology. Disability benefits from the forerunners in diversity, but we want to stress that disability is still far behind other groups in terms of awareness, skill training, knowledge base, theory, and visibility within psychology.

REFERENCES

Addis, M. E., & Mahalik, J. R. (2003). Men, masculinity, and the contexts of help seeking. *American Psychologist, 58,* 5–14.

Allison, K., Crawford, I., Echemendia, R., Robinson, L., & Knepp, D. (1994). Human diversity and professional competence. *American Psychologist, 49,* 792–796.

American Psychiatric Association. (1994). *Diagnostic and statistical manual of mental disorders.* (4th ed.) Washington, DC: Author.

American Psychological Association. (1975). Report of the Task Force on Sex Bias and Sex-Role Stereotyping. *American Psychologist, 30,* 1169–1175.

American Psychological Association. (1995). *Guidelines and principles for accreditation of programs in professional psychology.* Washington, DC: Author.

American Psychological Association. (2000). *Guidelines for psychotherapy with lesbian, gay and bisexual clients.* Washington, DC: Author.

American Psychological Association. (2003a). *Guidelines for psychological practice with older adults.* Washington, DC: Author

American Psychological Association. (2003b). Guidelines on multicultural education, training, research, practice and organizational change for psychologists. *American Psychologist, 58,* 377–402.

American Psychological Association, Society of Clinical Psychology. (1995). Training in and dissemination of empirically-validated psychological treatments: Report and recommendations. *The Clinical Psychologist, 48,* 3–27.

American Psychological Association Divisions 17 and 35. (2004, June). *Draft guidelines for psychological practice with girls and women.* Washington, DC: Author.

Anastasi, A. (1958). *Differential psychology* (3rd ed.). New York: Macmillan.

Anderson, S. (1996). Addressing heterosexist bias in the treatment of lesbian couples with chemical dependency. In J. Laird & R. Green (Eds.), *Lesbians and gays in couples and families* (pp. 316–340). San Francisco, CA: Jossey-Bass.

Andronico, M. (Ed.). (1996). *Men in groups.* Washington, DC: American Psychological Association.

Balsam, K. F., Rothblum, E. D., & Beauchaine, T. P. (2005). *Victimization over the lifespan: A comparison of lesbian, gay, bisexual, and heterosexual siblings.* Manuscript in preparation.

Bem, S. L. (1974). The measurement of psychological androgyny. *Journal of Personality and Social Psychology, 42,* 155–162.

Bernal, G., & Scharrón-Del Río, M. R. (2001). Are empirically supported treatments valid for ethnic minorities? *Cultural Diversity and Ethnic Minority Psychology, 7,* 328–342.

Beutler, L. (2004). The empirically supported treatments movement: A scientist–practitioner's response. *Clinical Psychology: Science and Practice, 11,* 225–229.

Blotzer, M. A., & Ruth, R. (1995). *Sometimes you just want to feel like a human being: Case studies of empowering psychotherapy with people with disabilities.* Baltimore: Brookes Publishing.

Bohart, A. C., Elliott, R., Greenberg, L. S., & Watson, J. C. (2002). Empathy. In J. C. Norcross (Ed.), *Psychotherapy relationships that work: Therapist contributions and responsiveness to patients* (pp. 89–108). New York: Oxford University Press.

Boyer, B. A., Knolls, M. L., Kafkalas, C. M., Tollen, L. G., & Swartz, M. (2000). Prevalence and relationships of posttraumatic stress in families experiencing spinal cord injury. *Rehabilitation Psychology, 45,* 339–355.

Bracero, W. (1994). Developing culturally sensitive psychodynamic case formulations: The effects of Asian cultural elements on psychoanalytic control–mastery theory. *Psychotherapy, 31,* 525–532.

Breeden, C. (2004). *Child custody evaluations when one divorcing parent has a physical disability.* Unpublished doctoral dissertation, California School of Professional Psychology, San Francisco, CA.

Brooks, G. R. (1998). *A new psychotherapy for traditional men.* San Francisco: Jossey-Bass.

Brooks, G. R., & Good, G. E. (Eds.). (2001). *The new handbook of psychotherapy and counseling with men.* San Francisco: Jossey-Bass.

Brown, L. S. (1989). New voices, new visions: Toward a lesbian/gay paradigm for psychology. *Psychology of Women Quarterly, 13,* 445–458.

Brown, L. S. (1994). *Subversive dialogues: Theory in feminist therapy.* New York: Basic Books.

Brown, L. S. (2003). Sexuality, lies, and loss: Lesbian, gay, and bisexual perspectives on trauma. *Journal of Trauma Practice, 2,* 55–68.

Chambless, D. L., Baker, M. J., Baucom, D. H., Beutler, L. E., Calhoun, K. S., Daiuto, A., et al. (1998). Update on empirically validated therapies II. *The Clinical Psychologist, 51,* 3–16.

Chambless, D. L., & Ollendick, T. H. (2001). Empirically supported psychological interventions: Controversies and evidence. *Annual Review of Psychology, 5,* 685–716.

Chambless, D. L., Sanderson, W. C., Shoham, V., Bennett-Johnson, S., Pope, K. S., & Crits-Christoph, P. (1996). An update on empirically validated therapies. *The Clinical Psychologist, 49,* 5–18.

Chen, C. P. (1995). Counseling applications of RET in a Chinese cultural context. *Journal of Rational–Emotive and Cognitive Behavior Therapy, 13,* 117–129.

Cochran, S. D., & Mays, V. M. (2000). Relation between psychiatric syndromes and behaviorally defined sexual orientation in a sample of the U.S. population. *American Journal of Public Health, 92,* 516–523.

Cochran, S. D., Sullivan, J. G., & Mays, V. M. (2003). Prevalence of mental disorders, psychological distress and mental health services use among lesbian, gay and bisexual adults in the United States. *Journal of Consulting and Clinical Psychology, 71,* 53–61.

Condeluci, A. (1989). Empowering people with cerebral palsy. *Journal of Rehabilitation, 55,* 15–16.

Deaux, K. (1984). From individual differences to social categories: Analysis of a decade's research on gender. *American Psychologist, 39,* 105–116.

DeLoach, C., & Greer, B. G. (1981). *Adjustment to severe physical disability.* New York: McGraw–Hill.

Duberman, M. (1992). *Cures.* New York: Plume Press.

Dutton, M. A. (1992). *Healing the trauma of women battering: Assessment and intervention.* New York: Springer Press.

Eagly, A. H., & Wood, W. (1999). The origins of sex differences in human behavior: Evolved dispositions vs. social roles. *American Psychologist, 54,* 408–423.

Elliott, T. R., & Kennedy, P. (2004). Treatment of depression following spinal cord injury: An evidence-based review. *Rehabilitation Psychology, 49,* 134–139.

Esten, G., & Willmott, L. (1993). Double bind messages: The effects of attitude toward disability on therapy. *Women and Therapy, 14,* 29–41.

Farber, B. A., & Lane, J. S. (2002). Positive regard. In J. C. Norcross (Ed.), *Psychotherapy relationships that work: Therapist contributions and responsiveness to patients* (pp. 175–194). New York: Oxford University Press.

Fassinger, R. E. (2000). Applying counseling theories to lesbian, gay and bisexual clients: Pitfalls and possibilities. In R. M. Perez, K. A. DeBord, & K. J. Bieschke (Eds.), *Handbook of counseling and psychotherapy with lesbian, gay and bisexual clients* (pp. 107–131). Washington, DC: American Psychological Association.

Fawcett, S. B., White, G. W., Balcazar, F. E., Suarez-Balcazar, Y., Mathews, R. M., Paine-Andrews, A., et al. (1994). A contextual–behavioral model of empowerment: Case studies involving people with physical disabilities. *American Journal of Community Psychology, 22,* 471–496.

French, M. (1985). *Beyond power: On women, men and morals.* New York: Ballantine Press.

Gething, L. (1997). *Person to person: A guide for professionals working with people with disabilities* (3rd ed.). Baltimore: Brookes Publishing.

Guyll, M., & Madon, S. (2000). Ethnicity research and theoretical conservatism. *American Psychologist, 55,* 1509–1510.

Haldeman, D. C. (2002). Gay rights, patient rights: The implications of sexual orientation conversion therapy. *Professional Psychology: Research and Practice, 33,* 260–264.

Hall, G. N. (2001). Psychotherapy research with ethnic minorities: Empirical, ethical, and conceptual issues. *Journal of Consulting and Clinical Psychology, 69,* 502–510.

Hare-Mustin, R.T. (1978). A feminist approach to family therapy. *Family Process, 17,* 181–194.

Herek, G. (1995). Psychological heterosexism in the United States. In A. D'Augelli & C. Patterson (Eds.), *Lesbian, gay, and bisexual identities over the lifespan: Psychological perspectives* (pp. 157–164). New York: Oxford University Press.

Hill, C. E., & Knox, S. (2002). Self-disclosure. In J. C. Norcross (Ed.), *Psychotherapy relationships that work: Therapist contributions and responsiveness to patients* (pp. 255–266). New York: Oxford University Press.

Hohmann, A. A., & Parron, D. L. (1996). How the new NIH guidelines on inclusion of women and minorities apply: Efficacy trials, effectiveness trials, and validity. *Journal of Consulting and Clinical Psychology, 64,* 851–855.

House Committee on Political Reform. (2004). *Politics and science.* Retrieved July 3, 2004, from http://www.house.gov/reform/min/politicsandscience

Jordan, J. V. (Ed.). (1997). *Women's growth in diversity: More writing from the Stone Center.* New York: Guilford Press.

Kennedy, P., & Duff, J. (2001). Post-traumatic stress disorder and spinal cord injuries. *Spinal Cord, 39,* 1–10.

Kosciulek, J. F., & Wheaton, J. E. (2003). Rehabilitation counseling with individuals with disabilities: An empowerment framework. *Rehabilitation Education, 17,* 207–214.

Lambert, M. I., & Barlay, D. E. (2001). Research summary on the therapeutic relationship and psychotherapy outcome. *Psychotherapy, 38,* 357–361.

Langer, K. G. (1994). Depression and denial in psychotherapy of persons with disabilities. *American Journal of Psychotherapy, 48,* 181–194.

Leigh, I. W., Powers, L., Vash, C., & Nettles, R. (2004). Survey of psychological services to clients with disabilities: The need for awareness. *Rehabilitation Psychology, 49,* 48–54.

Levant, R. F. (2003, January). *The new psychology of men and masculinities.* Presentation at the National Multicultural Conference and Summit, Hollywood, California.

Levant, R. F. (2004). The empirically validated treatments movement: A practitioner/educator perspective. *Clinical Psychology: Science and Practice, 11,* 219–224.

Levant, R. F., & Pollack, W. S. (Eds.). (1995). *A new psychology of men.* New York: Basic Books.

Levant, R. F., & Richmond, K. (2004). *Fifteen years of research on masculinity and femininity ideologies.* Manuscript submitted for publication.

Levant, R., & Silverstein, L. (2001). Integrating gender and family systems theories: The "both/and" approach to treating a postmodern couple. In D. Lusterman, S. McDaniel, & C. Philpot (Eds.), *Casebook for integrating family therapy* (pp. 245–252). Washington, DC: American Psychological Association.

Liddle, B. J. (1996). Therapist sexual orientation, gender, and counseling practices as they related to ratings on helpfulness by gay and lesbian clients. *Journal of Counseling Psychology, 43*, 394–401.

Lin, K. M., Cheung, F., Smith, M., & Poland, R. E. (1997). The use of psychotropic medications in working with Asian patients. In E. Lee (Ed.), *Working with Asian Americans: A guide for clinicians* (pp. 388–399). New York: Guilford Press.

Livneh, H., & Sherwood, A. (1991). Application of personality theories and counseling strategies to clients with physical disabilities. *Journal of Counseling and Development, 69*, 525–538.

Malyon, A. (1982). Psychotherapeutic implications of internalized homophobia in gay men. In J. Gonsiorek (Ed.), *Homosexuality and psychotherapy: A practitioner's handbook of affirmative models* (pp. 59–69). New York: Haworth Press.

Martell, C. R., Safren, S. A., & Prince, S. E. (2003). *Cognitive–behavioral therapies with lesbian, gay and bisexual clients.* New York: Guilford Press.

Morrow, S. L. (2000). First do no harm: Therapist issues in psychotherapy with lesbian, gay and bisexual clients. In R. M. Perez, K. A. DeBord, & K. J. Bieschke (Eds.), *Handbook of counseling and psychotherapy with lesbian, gay and bisexual clients* (pp. 137–156). Washington, DC: American Psychological Association.

Meyer, I. H. (2003). Prejudice, social stress, and mental health in lesbian, gay, and bisexual populations: Conceptual issues and research evidence. *Psychological Bulletin, 129*, 674–697.

Nemec, P. B. (2004). Evidence-based practice: Bandwagon or handbasket? *Rehabilitation Education, 18*, 133–135.

Norcross, J. C. (Ed.). (2000). *Psychotherapy relationships that work: Therapist contributions and responsiveness to patients.* New York: Oxford University Press.

Norcross, J. C. (2001). Purposes, processes, and products of the Task Force on Empirically Supported Therapy Relationships. *Psychotherapy, 38*, 345–356.

Norcross, J. C. (2003). Empirically supported psychotherapy relationships. *International Clinical Psychologist, 6*, 10.

Norcross, J. C., & Goldfried, M. R. (1992). *Handbook of psychotherapy integration.* New York: Basic Books.

Nutt, R. L. (1992). Feminist family therapy: A review of the literature. *Topics in Family Psychology and Counseling, 1*, 13–23.

Olkin, R. (1999). *What psychotherapists should know about disability.* New York: Guilford Press.

Olkin, R. (2002a). Could you hold the door for me? Including disability in diversity. *Cultural Diversity and Ethnic Minority Psychology, 8*, 130–137.

Olkin, R. (2002b). Making research accessible to participants with disabilities. *Journal of Multicultural Counseling and Development, 32*, 332–343.

Olkin, R. (2003). Women with physical disabilities who want to leave their partners: A feminist and disability–affirmative perspective. *Women and Therapy, 26*, 237–246.

Olkin, R. (2004). Disability and depression. In S. L. Welner & F. Haseltine (Eds.), *Welner's guide to the care of women with disabilities*. Philadelphia: Lippincott Williams & Wilkins.

Olkin, R., & Pledger, C. (2003). Can disability studies and psychology join hands? *American Psychologist, 58*, 296–304.

O'Neil, J. M., Good, G. E., & Holmes, S. (1995). Fifteen years of theory and research on men's gender role conflict: New paradigms for empirical research. In R. F. Levant & W. S. Pollack (Eds.), *A new psychology of men*. New York: Basic Books.

Pelletier, J. R., Rogers, E. S., & Dellario, D. J. (1985). Barriers to the provision of mental health services to individuals with severe physical disability. *Journal of Counseling Psychology, 32*, 422–430.

Perez, R. M., DeBord, K. A., & Bieschke, K. J. (Eds.). (2000). *Handbook of counseling and psychotherapy with lesbian, gay and bisexual clients*. Washington, DC: American Psychological Association.

Phillips, J. C. (2000). Training issues. In R. M. Perez, K. A. DeBord, & K. J. Bieschke (Eds.), *Handbook of counseling and psychotherapy with lesbian, gay and bisexual clients* (pp. 337–358). Washington, DC: American Psychological Association.

Pleck, J. H. (1981). *The myth of masculinity*. Cambridge, MA: MIT Press.

Pleck, J. H. (1995). The gender role strain paradigm: An update. In R. F. Levant & W. S. Pollack (Eds.), *A new psychology of men* (pp. 1–32). New York: Basic Books.

Pollack, W. S., & Levant, R. F. (Eds.). (1998). *New psychotherapy for men*. New York: Wiley.

President's Commission on Mental Health. (1978). *Report to the President*. Washington, DC: U.S. Government Printing Office.

President's New Freedom Commission on Mental Health. (2003). *Achieving the promise: Transforming mental health care in America. Report of the President's New Freedom Commission on Mental Health*. Rockville, MD: Author.

Priestley, M. (2001). *Disability and the life course: Global perspectives*. New York: Cambridge University Press.

Rabinowitz, F. E., & Cochran, S. V. (2002). *Deepening psychotherapy with men*. Washington, DC: American Psychological Association.

Radnitz, C. L., Hsu, L., Tirch, D. D., Willard, M., Lillian, L. B., Walczak, S., et al. (1998). A comparison of posttraumatic stress disorder in veterans with and without spinal cord injury. *Journal of Abnormal Psychology, 107*, 676–680.

Reid, P. T. (2002). Multicultural psychology: Bringing together gender and ethnicity. *Cultural Diversity and Ethnic Minority psychology, 8*, 103–114.

Rogers, C. R. (1957). The necessary and sufficient conditions of therapeutic personality change. *Journal of Consulting Psychology, 21*, 95–103.

Root, M. P. P. (1992). Reconstructing the impact of trauma on personality. In L. S. Brown & M. Ballou (Eds.), *Personality and psychopathology: Feminist reappraisals* (pp. 229–265). New York: Guilford Press.

Scher, M., Stevens, M., Good, G., & Eichenfield, G. A. (Eds.). (1987). *Handbook of counseling and psychotherapy with men.* Newbury Park, CA: Sage Press.

Scholinski, D. (1997). *The last time I wore a dress: A memoir.* New York: Riverhead Books.

Silverstein, L. B. (2004, July). Teaching feminism in a multicultural world. In P. Arredondo (Chair), *Implementing the APA multicultural guidelines.* Symposium presented at the annual meeting of the American Psychological Association, Honolulu, Hawaii.

Silverstein, L. B., & Goodrich, T. J. (Eds.). (2003). *Feminist family therapy: Empowerment in context.* Washington, DC: American Psychological Association.

Sluzki, C. (2003). Censorship looming. *American Journal of Orthopsychiatry, 73,* 131–132.

Smedley, B. D., Stith, A. Y., & Nelson, A. R. (2003). *Unequal treatment: Confronting racial and ethnic disparities in health care.* Washington, DC: National Academies Press.

Spence, J. T., & Helmreich, R. L. (1978). *Masculinity and femininity: Their psychological dimensions, correlates, and antecedents.* Austin, TX: University of Texas Press.

Stougaard-Nislon, M. (2004). Prevalance of posttraumatic stress disorder in persons with spinal cord injuries: The mediating effect of social support. *Rehabilitation Psychology, 48,* 289–295.

Sue, S. (1998). In search of cultural competence in psychotherapy and counseling. *American Psychologist, 53,* 440–448.

Sue, S. (1999). Science, ethnicity, and bias: Where have we gone wrong? *American Psychologist, 54,* 1070–1077.

Taliaferro, G. (2004). *Empirically supported treatments and disability.* Manuscript submitted for publication.

Terman, L., & Miles, C. (1936). *Sex and personality.* New York: McGraw-Hill.

Thompson, E. H., & Pleck, J. H. (1995). Masculinity ideology: A review of research instrumentation on men and masculinities. In R. F. Levant & W. S. Pollack (Eds.), *A new psychology of men* (pp. 129–163). New York: Basic Books.

U.S. Surgeon General. (2001). *Mental health: Culture, race, and ethnicity—A supplement to mental health: A report of the Surgeon General.* Rockville, MD: U.S. Department of Health and Human Services.

Walker, L. E. A. (1994). *Abused women and survivor therapy.* Washington, DC: American Psychological Association.

Waxman, H. A., Cummings, E. E., Rodriguez, C. D., Honda, M. M., Christensen, D. M., Solis, H. L., et al. (2004, January 13). Press release concerning letter to Tommy G. Thompson, U.S. Secretary of Health and Human Services.

Williams, D. T., Hershenson, D. B., & Fabian, E. S. (2000). Causal attributions of disabilities and the choice of rehabilitation approach. *Rehabilitation Counseling Bulletin, 43*, 106–112.

Worell, J., & Johnson, N. G. (1997). *Shaping the future of feminist psychology: Education, research and practice.* Washington, DC: American Psychological Association.

Worell, J., & Remer, P. (2003). *Feminist perspectives in therapy: Empowering diverse women.* New York: Wiley.

Wright, B. (1983). *Physical disability: A psychosocial approach* (2nd ed.). New York: Harper & Row.

Yi, K. (1995). Psychoanalytic psychotherapy with Asian clients: Transference and therapeutic considerations. *Psychotherapy, 32*, 308–316.

Zane, N., Hall, G. N., Sue, S., Young, K., & Nunez, J. (2003). Research on psychotherapy with culturally diverse populations. In M. J. Lambert (Ed.), *Bergin and Garfield's handbook of psychotherapy and behavior change* (5th ed., pp. 767–804). New York: Wiley.

9

ARE EFFICACIOUS LABORATORY-VALIDATED TREATMENTS READILY TRANSPORTABLE TO CLINICAL PRACTICE?

Efficacious Laboratory-Validated Treatments Are Generally Transportable to Clinical Practice

Martin E. Franklin and Robert J. DeRubeis

The spirited and ongoing debate about the relevance of randomized clinical (or controlled) trial (RCT) findings to clinical practice has had at least one very positive outcome: It has brought concerns about the external validity of RCT findings to the forefront. A shift in emphasis on generalizability is already evident in the field. Indeed, journals such as the *Journal of the American Medical Association* have taken a more active role in requiring that investigators report data on sample characteristics as they pertain to screening patients and postrandomization retention. Investigators themselves have also begun to report on sample characteristics and on generalizability both in primary outcome articles (e.g., Pediatric OCD Treatment Study

Team, 2004) and in secondary reports (e.g., Hofmann et al., 1998; Huppert, Franklin, Foa, & Davidson, 2003), and by testing empirically validated treatments outside the context of the expert clinics in which they were developed (e.g., Wade, Treat, & Stuart, 1998; Weersing & Weisz, 2002). These are welcome advances, because determining the transportability of empirically validated treatment to a wider variety of clinical settings is of paramount importance in making effective treatments more available for consumers of mental health services.

In this position paper, we argue that the transportability of laboratory-validated treatments to clinical practice is an important empirical question that warrants answers driven by data. Our interpretation of the extant data is that such treatments generally transport well to other practice settings. We review the data on obsessive–compulsive disorder (OCD) and depression in particular to support this position, but also comment briefly on effectiveness studies on other disorders across the developmental spectrum that are relevant to the issues being discussed here.

The ultimate clinical utility of empirically supported treatments (ESTs) has been questioned for a number of reasons. First, from a sampling perspective, some have purported that, because of the use of exclusion criteria and the willingness to accept randomization, patients who are able and willing to enter such studies are not representative of the complex patients seen in clinical settings (Silberschatz in Persons & Silberschatz, 1998); that issue is addressed specifically by Stirman and DeRubeis in this volume. Second, from a procedural perspective, treatments tested in RCTs are said to be designed to emphasize internal validity, ignore comorbidity if it is present, and deliver the treatment rather inflexibly as if it is an experimental manipulation and not in response to the particular patient's needs, as would be the case in clinical settings (e.g., Westen, Novotny, & Thompson-Brenner, 2004a). However, research on the transportability of empirically validated treatments to clinical settings has only just begun.

In many ways this reflects the current stage in the developmental progression of psychotherapy research. Treatment validation typically begins with small case studies in which patient response and feedback can be used to further inform the treatment development, followed by larger open studies. Then RCTs compare the treatment of interest to a credible control, and perhaps larger RCTs compare the now validated treatment to alternative treatments, opening up the sampling frame to be more inclusive, or this is followed by dismantling studies designed to identify the active ingredients of the protocol. With the most common mental health problems, a good deal of this initial work has been done with at least some forms of psychotherapy. Fortunately, data are also now available to inform the field on the use of ESTs in clinical practice settings; this constitutes the next stage of treatment development in most contemporary models of psychotherapy outcome research.

TRANSPORTABILITY OF OCD TREATMENTS

Strong empirical support has been garnered in the last 25 years for the efficacy of exposure and response (ritual) prevention (EX–RP) in the treatment of OCD in adults (Franklin & Foa, 2002). Consistent with the research progression described previously, the development of EX–RP began with open trials of initial protocols (e.g., Meyer, 1966) followed by open trials of modified protocols (e.g., Foa & Goldstein, 1978). Then RCTs compared EX–RP to other treatments, such as relaxation (e.g., Marks, Hodgson, & Rachman, 1975), anxiety management training (e.g., Lindsay, Crino, & Andrews, 1997), and pill placebo (e.g., Foa et al., in press). EX–RP has been compared in RCTs to active pharmacotherapy (e.g., Cottraux et al., 1990) and psychotherapy (e.g., McLean et al., 2001). EX–RP findings have also been extended from individual to group treatment (e.g., Fals-Stewart, Marks, & Schafer, 1993), as well as from intensive (daily) treatment to twice-weekly treatment (Abramowitz, Foa, & Franklin, 2003). Along the way, studies have also been conducted to determine the active ingredients of treatment (e.g., Foa, Steketee, Grayson, Turner, & Latimer, 1984) to extend the findings to patients with significant psychiatric comorbidity (e.g., Foa, Kozak, Steketee, & McCarthy, 1992) and, in open trials, to various subtypes of OCD (e.g., Abramowitz, Franklin, Schwartz, & Furr, 2003) and to pediatric patients (e.g., Franklin et al., 1998). Thus, the efficacy of EX–RP has been clearly established, and the groundwork has now been laid with respect to examining EX–RP's effectiveness. This work sets the stage for a broader examination of EX–RP's transportability to the very settings in which most OCD patients can receive clinical services.

The main study in our EX–RP effectiveness research involved a benchmark comparison of outcomes achieved with EX–RP in the context of the Center for the Treatment and Study of Anxiety's (CTSA) outpatient clinic against those found in RCTs (Franklin, Abramowitz, Kozak, Levitt, & Foa, 2000). This study was conducted specifically to bridge what we viewed as a growing chasm between controlled treatment outcome research and clinical practice. Outcome data were collected from 110 adults with OCD who received fee-for-service EX–RP treatment in our outpatient OCD clinic. Notably, the EX–RP treatment delivered in this context was very similar to that validated in RCTs, which allowed us to focus on the contribution to the outcome of sampling differences. In comparison to typical RCT samples, our fee-for-service patients were more representative of the broader population of patients with OCD in that they also suffered from comorbid conditions (e.g., major depression), they were unwilling to discontinue ongoing pharmacotherapy or to risk randomization to inactive treatment, and they chose their own therapy. Moreover, as was the case in other generalizability studies of anxiety disorder treatments (e.g., panic disorder; Wade et al., 1998), no adult patient was excluded from participation because of age, secondary comorbid diagnoses, medical problems, treatment history, the use of concomitant medication, or Axis II disorders.

We found considerable similarities between the CTSA and the RCT samples. The pretreatment OCD severity of the CTSA sample was comparable to that reported in three studies (Kozak, Liebowitz, & Foa, 2000; Lindsay et al., 1997; van Balkom et al., 1998), and somewhat greater than that of one study (Fals-Stewart et al., 1993). In terms of treatment outcome, the mean reduction on the Yale–Brown Obsessive Compulsive Scale (Y-BOCS) at posttreatment for the outpatient clinic group was 60%. This was comparable to the result reported in two studies (54%, Kozak et al., 2000; 62%, Lindsay et al., 1997) yet apparently larger than that found in two other studies (40%, Fals-Stewart et al., 1993; 32%, van Balkom et al., 1998). Within-subject Y-BOCS effect sizes of 3.26, 3.88, 2.31, 0.93, and 1.00 were found for the five samples, respectively. In terms of treatment retention, 10 of 110 patients (9%) dropped out in the CTSA sample, which is almost identical to that reported in one study (9%, Fals-Stewart et al., 1993) and lower than that reported for EX–RP in two studies (15%, van Balkom et al., 1998; 28%, Kozak et al. 2000).

Collectively, our results suggest that the EX–RP results from RCTs may very well be representative of what can be achieved with "real" patients being seen outside research trials. Although outcome was determined using a reliable and valid interview conducted by trained clinicians not otherwise involved in the patient's care, the absence of independent evaluators blind to treatment conditions is a limitation that should be addressed in subsequent efforts of this kind. This caveat notwithstanding, our benchmarking study did set the stage for subsequent dissemination efforts that can expand beyond the research context in which EX–RP had been developed, modified, and empirically evaluated.

In any research endeavor, the nature of the question dictates design choices, and design choices come with implications both positive and negative. We were particularly interested in focusing on the effects of patient selection on EX–RP outcomes, which dictated that the study should be conducted using a similar EX–RP protocol delivered by therapists trained in much the same way as were those who provided treatment in the RCTs. Thus, conducting this study in our own outpatient EX–RP clinic filled these requirements and allowed us to address a somewhat focused question about sampling. However, that decision came at a cost with respect to determining the generalizability of EX–RP to other settings. Indeed, one of the most clever criticisms of our benchmarking study was that the study was limited in the extent to which the context and therapists were representative of "real-world" clinics. Hence, the transportability of EX–RP was not given a strong test because the travel distance from the specialty clinic was not great (Warren & Thomas, 2001). We agree wholeheartedly with that criticism, and we believe that our benchmarking study constituted a small link in a large chain, rather than a definitive answer to the question of EX–RP's effectiveness in clinical practice settings.

Importantly, Warren and Thomas (2001) went on in that same paper to examine EX–RP outcomes in an open trial conducted in a private practice setting headed by a highly competent and experienced therapist. Results from this study were quite encouraging, even with a weekly EX–RP protocol. Another report also demonstrated that EX–RP was effective for patients who completed the treatment in a different clinical context, although a lower than usual retention rate in that study suggested that setting differences may influence dropouts (Rothbaum & Shahar, 2000). Unfortunately, our original benchmarking study and these trials did not include a comparison condition or long-term follow-up data.

The three studies that have explored the effectiveness of EX–RP in less restrictive samples (Franklin et al., 2000) and in clinical practice settings (Rothbuam & Shahar, 2000; Warren & Thomas, 2001) were conducted by EX–RP experts who either treated or closely supervised all the treatment. To address the question of the degree of prior expertise with EX–RP needed to produce good outcomes, a pediatric OCD effectiveness study was recently completed in Norway (Valderhaug, Gotestam, Larsson, & Piacentini, 2004). This study is notably different from the previous three EX–RP effectiveness studies in that access to the pediatric EX–RP expert was much more limited, the model included a training of supervisors element, and the treatment was conducted by therapists who were not highly experienced in implementing EX–RP protocols with children and adolescents. The preliminary outcomes of EX–RP with 24 children and adolescents who completed open treatment were very encouraging and appeared comparable to those achieved in open trials conducted in expert clinics (e.g., Franklin et al., 1998; March, Mulle, & Herbel, 1994; Piacentini, Bergman, Jacobs, McCracken, & Kretchman, 2002; Wever & Rey, 1997), to RCT findings (de Haan, Hoogduin, Buitelaar, & Keijsers, 1998; Pediatric OCD Treatment Study Team, 2004), and with adult OCD patients (e.g., Foa et al., in press). The study by Valderhaug and colleagues constitutes an important next step in determining the extent to which EX–RP can be taught and then implemented in representative clinical settings.

One of the primary complaints leveled against manualized treatments is that they require therapists to implement the protocols in a "cookbook" fashion, carefully following prespecified steps to avoid compromising the internal validity of the experimental manipulation. Taking such an approach would inevitably restrict the generalizability of such protocols to real-world settings, where no such rigorous requirements would be in place. Moreover, it is likely that this level of inflexibility would also limit clinicians' effectiveness as well. On the putative inflexibility of manualized treatments, we concur that most (but not all) manuals do include session-by-session checklists of material to be covered, but we believe that most RCTs do not actually restrict clinical flexibility in such a way as to interfere with real-world applicability. Kendall, Chu, Gifford, Hayes, and Nauta (1998) wrote eloquently about this common misconception, correctly pointing out that manuals are best thought of as guides that are theoretically informed yet still clinically flexible, requiring creativity and clinical skill to be used optimally. A recent issue of *Cognitive and Behavioral Practice* was devoted to "Going Beyond the Manual" (Huppert & Abramowitz, 2003), and the papers published in that special issue collectively underscored the importance of the clinician's ability to grasp the core theoretical concepts that drive the intervention to best tailor treatment to the particular needs of specific patients. As summarized by Kendall and associates (1998),

> Perhaps it goes without saying that a manual requires implementation with good clinical skills . . . the rampant misunderstanding of treatment manuals, along with the overzealous assumptions about the potency of manuals, combined to reaffirm the need to explicitly state that a manual operationalizes the treatment but practitioners must be able to breathe life into a manual. (p. 197)

TRANSPORTABILITY OF DEPRESSION TREATMENTS

A related issue concerns the fate of manualized treatments when clinicians already functioning within other theoretical systems test the effectiveness of such treatments. Research is needed on this question, but a case study can illustrate what is possible.

In 1977, Steven D. Hollon arrived in Minnesota after he had played a key role in the landmark Rush, Beck, Kovacs, and Hollon (1977) comparison of cognitive therapy (CT) versus antidepressant medications for depression. That study was the first to show that a psychotherapy could match the effectiveness of antidepressant medications in the reduction of depressive symptoms in patients diagnosed with unipolar depression.

Hollon wished to continue his investigations of CT's effectiveness relative to antidepressant medications in a new environment that had few of the structures in place for conducting such research. The Rush et al. (1977) study had been conducted at the Center for Cognitive Therapy at the University of Pennsylvania, the birthplace of CT. The founder of CT, Aaron T. Beck, had trained the cognitive therapists, who clearly were committed to this new form of therapy. Patients in the Rush et al. study were referrals, or self-referrals, to a research clinic in an academic psychiatry department. When Hollon arrived in Minnesota, there were no cognitive therapists to be found there. Indeed, few clinicians had heard much, if anything, about Beck or his therapy. Patient participants were to be drawn from a county community mental health center (CMHC).

What ensued was a study that in many ways presaged and anticipated, mostly of necessity, the "effectiveness" movement in psychotherapy research.

The therapists, who ranged in experience from 8 to 20 years, began their CT training with a variety of theoretical orientations; they used Gestalt, client-centered, psychodynamic, rational–emotive, and reality therapy methods. Training consisted of a series of workshops, conducted by eventual study authors Hollon, DeRubeis, and Evans. Weekly group supervision was used throughout the study, but after the first 6 months these therapists were largely helping each other to think about their cases, so supervision came to resemble a case conference over time. This last point is important, because although many clinical practices and public clinics do not support regular clinically oriented staff meetings, it is not difficult to imagine that such systems could be made cost effective.

The Hollon et al. (1992) study was in many ways a typical modern RCT. After meeting inclusion criteria and giving their informed consent, the patients with the diagnosis of major depressive disorder (MDD) were randomly assigned to receive CT, antidepressant medications (imipramine), or their combination. Outcome assessments were blind, and a 2-year naturalistic follow-up was conducted to test for relapse-prevention effects of acute treatment with CT and of continued medications (compared to the absence of acute-treatment CT and the cessation of medicines following acute treatment with medicines). Patients with borderline personality disorders, psychotic disorders, or active substance use disorders were excluded, but the study sample included those with anxiety disorder comorbidities, as well as Cluster C personality disorders.

Patients who were assigned to these newly trained cognitive therapists, who were anything but novice psychotherapists, evidenced symptom reduction as substantial on average as those who were given antidepressant medications, the standard of care for patients with a major depressive episode (MDE) diagnosis. Moreover, the relapse rate among those who received CT was lower than that observed in patients who were given short-term medication alone (Evans et al., 1992). The therapy, as well as its effects on symptom reduction and the prevention of relapse, mirrored very closely the therapy and findings from the seminal Rush et al. (1977) research, even though the clinic and its clinicians had little or no exposure to CT prior to Hollon and colleagues' dissemination effort. Thus, CT, one of the most complex manualized therapies, was successfully transported from a university research clinic in Philadelphia, Pennsylvania, to a county mental health facility in St. Paul, Minnesota.

Many questions are relevant to the issues discussed in this paper that the Hollon et al. (1992) study did not address. What results would these therapists have achieved if they had conducted their own brand of eclectic therapy, prior to learning manualized CT? How would other therapists from that setting have performed (i.e., how generalizable were the results to other therapists in that setting and in other settings)? These are questions that can be addressed by studies specifically designed to test rigorously the transportability of CT for depression.

OTHER TRANSPORTABILITY STUDIES

The studies on OCD and depression described previously provide illustrative examples from the burgeoning literature on the effectiveness of ESTs in a variety of clinical practice settings. Similarly encouraging outcomes have been found with cognitive–behavioral interventions for other disorders as well, including posttraumatic stress disorder (PTSD; Cahill, Hembree, & Foa, in press; Gillespie, Duffy, Hackmann, & Clark, 2002), social anxiety disorder (Blomhoff et al., 2001), and panic disorder (Wade et al., 1998) in adults, and depression (Weersing & Weisz, 2002) and oppositional–defiant disorder (Taylor, Schmidt, Pepler, & Hodgins, 1998) in children and adolescents. In all but one of these studies, manualized CBT protocols were delivered by mental health professionals who were not cognitive–behavior therapy (CBT) experts but were trained by those who were. Clearly, an important next line of effectiveness research will involve manipulating the amount of training and access to supervision to determine how much is needed to achieve outcomes that are comparable to the generally large and durable gains reported in RCTs. Notably, Blomhoff and colleagues (2001) found encouraging outcomes with exposure therapy for social anxiety disorder with general practice physicians who were trained by CBT experts. This perhaps affords another avenue to improving pharmacotherapy patient outcomes as well as disseminating ESTs. In light of recent safety concerns about the use of SSRIs in children and adolescents, this line of work would appear to be of particular public health relevance.

Collectively, the effectiveness studies published thus far are encouraging with respect to the transportability of CBT programs beyond the research context; little has been done thus far to examine the transportability of other forms of psychotherapy (e.g., interpersonal psychotherapy) or of validated pharmacotherapy protocols. Thus, it seems that there is reason for optimism that ESTs can be made more widely available, but improvements in research designs are needed to provide more definitive evidence about the ultimate clinical utility of ESTs. Although we agree with the cautionary words of Chambless and Ollendick (2001) that the practice of evidence-based psychotherapy is complex and that ESTs are only one piece of the puzzle, we also hold fast to the notion that the question of whether or not ESTs are effective in clinical practice settings is an empirical one that should be studied rather than simply debated.

SUMMARY

There is, of course, no single answer to the question, "Are efficacious laboratory-validated treatments readily transportable to clinical practice?" The answer will probably depend on the patient populations, treatments, and psychotherapists under consideration. However, in general, the extant research indicates that such treatments can transport to other practice settings. Moreover, we have yet to encounter data to the contrary.

In concluding, we speculate about patient, treatment, and therapist dimensions. Regarding patient populations, will ESTs for patients with more circumscribed disorders or problems travel especially well? The two examples given previously would seem to differ on this dimension; most clinicians would say that OCD is more circumscribed, even if often more disabling, than major depression. Another dimension that may become relevant is the age of patients. The field might discover that manualized treatments are more or less effective with children, adults, and elderly adults.

Regarding transporting treatments, one might imagine that more straightforward, technique-rich therapies would be easier to teach clinicians and therefore that these might be more readily embraced and adopted. In this view, EX–RP for OCD might be expected to transport more readily than CT for major depression, because the latter is driven more by general principles. Thus, CT for major depression may be more difficult to train clinicians to do, and it may prove more difficult to verify whether this treatment has been adequately implemented after it has been disseminated.

As psychotherapy researchers report more on the transportability and limits of their treatments, we should obtain a clearer picture as to which treatments, for which disorders, and to which kinds of clinics can laboratory-tested treatments enhance the care of patients who suffer from mental disorders. Given the available evidence, we are optimistic that a variety of efficacious treatments for a range of clinical problems will prove to be transportable, and that the quality of mental health care will improve as a consequence.

Transporting Laboratory-Validated Treatments to the Community Will Not Necessarily Produce Better Outcomes

Drew I. Westen

One of the major questions today in the EST debate is the question of transportability. To what extent can ESTs tested in the laboratory be "transported" (or, perhaps more aptly, transplanted) to everyday clinical settings? Will doing so generate outcomes similar to those obtained in RCTs? And will it generate better outcomes than currently obtained in private practice? In part, these questions depend on the representativeness of patients in RCTs (whether laboratory patient samples adequately generalize to patients in the community), an issue addressed elsewhere in this volume. In this position paper I address three questions central to the transportability of ESTs: (a) What are we transporting? (b) For what problems are we transporting? and (c) How clear are the data from studies explicitly intended to demonstrate transportability?

WHAT ARE WE TRANSPORTING?

The first question regards precisely what we hope to transport from the laboratory to everyday practice settings. On one end of the spectrum, one could consider the "unit" of transportation a treatment package, specified by a particular manual that has been supported in studies and replicated. Viewing the treatment package as the unit of transportation is perhaps the modal answer to this question in the EST literature. Thus, Stuart, Wade, and Treat (2000) transported Barlow's Panic Control Therapy (see Brown & Barlow, 1995) to a CMHC and found that close adherence to the manual led not only to strong initial outcomes but also to even better outcomes at follow-up than have been obtained in the laboratory. Franklin and colleagues (Franklin et al., 2000) applied exposure-based treatment for OCD patients to a group of patients previously excluded from RCTs at their site and similarly found considerable evidence for transportability. A variant of this unit of transportation is a manual adapted slightly to meet the demands of naturalistic settings, such as CBT for depression adapted for Latino immigrants, which is then tested in this new setting for its effectiveness (see Stirman, Crits-Christoph, & DeRubeis, 2004).

At the other end of the spectrum, the unit of transportation could be general principles, theory-driven technical strategies, or a general treatment approach (e.g., CBT). Thus, instead of taking Foa's (1999) eight-session treatment manual for PTSD into the community to apply to a group of polysymptomatic, low socioeconomic status (SES) inner-city patients in a county hospital who suffer from multiple traumas, one might extract the general principle that PTSD patients often respond to exposure to memories of traumatic events and apply this as appropriate to patients with trauma histories. Prior to the emergence of the EST movement in the mid-1990s, this version of "transportation" was the general goal of treatment researchers conducting RCTs.

Whether the goal is to transport manuals that will be administered faithfully by practitioners or to transport principles to be used in empirically informed psychotherapies is not academic. The latter goal would be unobjectionable to any clinician interested in making use of scientific data to guide interventions and is essential to bringing evidence-based practice (EBP) to psychology (see Beutler, 2000; Rosen & Davison, 2003). The former, however, is fraught with difficulties, including the following.

First, it is highly unlikely that a treatment developed for a specific Axis I condition (the usual target of ESTs) can be applied "as is" to the average patient in clinical practice, who is polysymptomatic and is likely to differ from the patients tested in RCTs in multiple respects. As described in this volume and elsewhere (Westen & Morrison, 2001), the average RCT excludes 30% to 70% of patients screened for inclusion to minimize within-condition variations. (Patients are not necessarily free from "secondary" disorders, but investigators choose their exclusion criteria carefully.) In clinical practice, in contrast, variability of presentation and symptomatology is the norm.

Second, if indeed patients in everyday practice differ from patients in RCTs in patterns of comorbidity, social class, ethnicity, and so forth, we would need an infinite number of manuals to address the various combinations and permutations (see Beutler, Moleiro, & Talebi, 2002; Weinberger, 2000). Consider manuals for depression. Unless we assume that all forms of comorbidity are independent (e.g., that a depressed patient with substance abuse and panic attacks is just a depressed person who happens to have the misfortune of having two other disorders), and that class and culture just require minor modifications to the manual, we would need manuals for uncomplicated depression, depression plus generalized anxiety disorder (GAD), depression plus GAD and panic, depression plus panic, depression plus GAD for low-SES Latinos, and so forth. And that is not even addressing different types of depression (e.g., dysthymic disorder, major depression, melancholic depression, self-critical depression, depression secondary to sexual abuse, etc.).

Third, it is difficult to imagine how we could test even a fraction of these interventions specialized for subpopulations. The first step might be to apply a manual to a new population with few alterations to see if it needs altering. But how much smaller should the effect be before we determine that the manual needs revision or is not useful for this population? And suppose we determine that it needs revision. How do we decide which ways to adapt it for the population under consideration? The usual situation is that the investigator makes an educated guess, and if that "works" (i.e., leads to what the investigator considers reasonable findings in an RCT), the new manual is now disseminated without any further study of alternative methods, which are considered empirically unsupported.

Fourth, treatment manuals are often deliberately constructed to be distinct from other manuals and to minimize common factors so that they can be compared in RCTs to other treatments or to treatments that purportedly control for common factors. However, such common factors produce much of the effect of brief psychotherapies for many disorders (Wampold, 2001). Thus, to make for clean experiments, the manuals tested in RCTs often exclude interventions that any good clinician would normally use. Clinicians are then exhorted to use the manuals as tested because only the tested version has the imprimatur of "empirical validation." Just as experimenters cannot afford the loss of statistical power that invariably follows from the implementation of impure treatments, clinicians cannot afford the loss of therapeutic power that follows from the implementation of pure treatments (Westen et al., 2004a).

TRANSPORT FOR WHAT PROBLEM?

A second question regards the problem, syndrome, or diagnosis for which we transport a treatment. The standard practice in EST research is to design treatments for specific disorders as defined by the *Diagnostic and Statistical Manual of Mental Disorders, Fourth Edition* (*DSM–IV*; American Psychiatric Association, 1994). In many respects, this is sensible, allowing standardization across sites and studies.

DSM–IV diagnosis is not, however, the only possible target of intervention. One alternative would be to design (and transport) treatments for functionally defined problems, such as peer rejection in children, avoidant attachment dynamics that interfere with intimacy in adults, or public speaking anxiety. Clinicians of virtually every orientation tend to think in functional rather than descriptive terms, rendering functionally defined problems particularly useful targets for intervention.

Alternatively, instead of testing and transporting manualized treatments for specific disorders such as major depression, we might develop treatments for spectrum disorders (e.g., depression in general), which could be applied to a much wider range of patients. Or we might develop treatments for broadband personality dimensions that constitute diathesis for multiple disorders, such as internalizing or externalizing pathology (Krueger & Piasecki, 2002). We could then transport general treatment strategies as well as strategies for addressing more specific disorders.

Although all potential targets have strengths and weaknesses, current thinking about transportation in the EST literature, which is tied to *DSM–IV* diagnosis, has a number of problems. First, we have little idea what brings most patients in for treatment in the community, but we know that most patients do not present with specific syndromes for which we have well-validated treatment manuals (Stirman, DeRubeis, Crits-Christoph, & Brody, 2003). Many patients, for example, receive a diagnosis of "adjustment disorder," for which manualization is unlikely because it is not a "real" diagnosis characterized by any specific features. Transporting manuals for specific disorders assumes that most patients can be treated as if they have a single disorder or, if they are polysymptomatic, that polysymptomatic presentations have no emergent properties. Without this assumption, one is confronted with the problem described previously, in which researchers need to develop treatments for major depression × panic, major depression panic × GAD, and so forth.

Although many treatment researchers would explicitly disavow an additive model of psychopathology, common notions of transportability or dissemination implicitly assume such a model. Consider, for example, the following statement about flexible implementation in a recent article on how to achieve successful dissemination of ESTs to community settings: "Alteration of protocols may . . . be necessary to accommodate culturally sensitive issues, as well as the needs of patients with comorbid substance abuse, history of trauma, language barriers," and so forth (Stirman et al., 2004, p. 352). The implication is that treating depression on a Hopi reservation is essentially the same as treating depression in middle-aged White patients in Philadelphia as long as the clinician shows some flexibility in applying the treatment to the two populations. This could be true, but it is just one of many possibilities. A history of oppression, parental neglect, childhood trauma, alcoholism, and cultural disintegration, not to mention different cultural norms about agency or control that might change the meaning of cognitive interventions, could have emergent properties that would require more than a slight alteration of protocols.

Second, the notion of transportation for specific disorders assumes that patients with a similar Axis I diagnosis require similar treatments. It may be that an adolescent who is depressed in response to a recent parental divorce requires the same interventions as an adolescent who is chronically self-critical or sensitive to rejection (or one whose depression reflects a strong biological diathesis), but this seems unlikely.

Third, although EST researchers test treatments for specific disorders, they often use much more generalized language when talking about transporting their treatments into everyday practice. Most meta-analyses and qualitative reviews of ESTs for major depression, for example, lapse into the language of "treatment of depression" without the qualifier of the specific disorder for which the treatments have been tested. To what extent such generalizations are appropriate is an empirical question.

A fourth problem pertains to the role of case formulation in transporting treatments. In psychotherapy research, the assessment is conducted prior to the treatment, usually by someone other than the therapist, and its primary purpose is to see whether the patient meets study criteria. The therapist does not conduct a systematic evaluation and hence usually knows nothing about the patient's personality, history, or comorbid problems. Case formulation is limited in brief, manualized treatments by the brevity of the treatment and the absence of sessions included for systematic assessment. It is also limited by a requisite of experimental method required for drawing causal inferences: To minimize within-condition variance, RCT therapists need to minimize potentially idiosyncratic formulations (Westen et al., 2004a). Instead, patients in RCTs for ESTs are typically given relatively generic formulations as part of psychoeducation about the factors that cause or maintain their symptoms.

The point here is that few studies of ESTs have actually tested a genuine, transportable psychotherapeutic encounter in which the clinician assesses the patient for the range of possible problems for which he or she may be seeking treatment, assesses personality and other contextual (e.g., family or cultural) variables, develops a comprehensive case formulation to make sense of the entire clinical picture, and then executes a treatment on the basis of this formulation. It may be that clinicians can transplant a set of manualized procedures into a treatment without much assessment of their problems. This, however, is an article of faith, and one that conceals serious problems with the "hard constraint" version of ESTs (i.e., that we should transport manuals, not principles). If comorbidity matters, then one cannot exclude it from RCTs and hope to generalize to patients in the community. If personality matters, then one cannot transport any manualized therapy for an Axis I disorder that does not begin with an assessment of personality and that does not systematically integrate the findings of that assessment into the treatment. The only ways around these problems are to assume that comorbidity and personality do not matter (an assumption that is empirically disconfirmed; see Westen et al., 2004a) or to adopt a "softer constraint" model of ESTs. In this latter model, what is transported is not a manual to be implemented by a paraprofessional but scientific data regarding principles or techniques of potential use to competent clinical decision-makers.

HOW CLEAR ARE THE DATA ON TRANSPORTABILITY?

A third question concerns the explosion of recent research designed to demonstrate the generalizability and transportability of ESTs to community settings. In response to critics about the unrepresentativeness of samples in RCTs, EST advocates have produced an array of studies purporting to show that the exclusion criteria they have used over the last 20 years really do not matter. This would indeed be a welcome finding, although it creates a conundrum: Why did researchers exclude most of the patients who walked in their doors for two decades, imposing exclusion criteria such as substance abuse or suicidal ideation in studies of patients with major depression? In fact, the whole point of creating manuals for specific *DSM–IV*-defined symptoms and syndromes reflected the assumption that the prior era of psychotherapy research, and the prior 70 years of practice, had failed to recognize that specific symptoms require specific techniques.

Under this assumption, it is certainly possible (and likely) that treating panic will have some impact on reducing GAD (and empirically that is the case; see Barlow, 2002). However, one cannot assume specificity of symptoms when it is convenient and generality of effects when it is not. Either we need to target specific symptoms, in which case we have to study and transport treatments for relatively pure patients, or we need to target broad symptom ranges or diathesis, allow clinicians and patients considerable latitude in selecting targets of change, and lengthen treatments accordingly. Ironically, treatments targeting these broader foci were the norm in psychotherapeutic practice until the EST movement asserted priority for brief, focal treatments readily tested in RCTs.

In prior publications, colleagues and I have examined the existing literature on transportability (Westen et al., 2004a; Westen, Novotny, & Thompson-Brenner, 2004b), but for every head we examine the hydra seems to sprout 10 more (e.g., Weisz, Weersing, & Hengeler, in press). Rather than address an additional set, we will describe a prominent study published in the *Journal of Consulting and Clinical Psychology* designed to test the hypothesis that CBT for depression in children and adolescents is superior to treatment for the same disorders in the community (Weersing & Weisz, 2002). We describe this study because the authors considered our prior description of it (which was condensed because of space constraints in *Psychological Bulletin*) a serious misrepresentation (Weisz, Weersing, & Henggeler, in press).

Weersing and Weisz (2002) compared treatment responses among patients from what appear to have been six inner-city CMHCs with the average response of children and adolescents with similar levels of depression treated in high-quality RCTs. Patients in RCTs showed much more rapid improvement, although outcome converged by 1-year follow-up. The authors concluded that the treatment trajectories of CMHC-treated youth "more closely resembled those of control condition youth than youth treated with CBT" in RCTs and drew implications about the transportability and benefits of manualized treatments relative to "the effectiveness of community psychotherapy for depressed youth" (p. 299). They noted that the "CMHC services were predominantly psychodynamic, whereas therapists in clinical trials provided a pure dose of CBT" and suggested that these treatment differences likely accounted for much of the difference in outcome.

The investigators compared a low-SES sample of children and adolescents, who can be presumed to have had a high likelihood of (unmeasured) exposure to poverty, violence, and trauma, to a benchmark sample that appears to have overlapped very little with the CMHC sample except in severity of depression. The investigators did not unfortunately report any data on SES of the CMHC sample, and they acknowledged that the benchmark samples typically did not provide data on ethnicity or comorbidity that would allow valid comparisons. They did indicate, however, that unlike the CMHC sample, the benchmark samples were primarily Caucasian (and presumably of higher SES, given the association in the United States between class and minority status).

Mood disorder diagnoses in the benchmark and CMHC samples did not differ substantially, nor did severity of depression, leading the investigators to consider the samples largely comparable. However, from what could be gleaned about comorbidity from data the authors reported in tabular form, the rates of conduct disorder and oppositional defiant disorder averaged 10.8% in benchmark studies that either reported or excluded these diagnoses versus 61.0% in the CMHC sample. The rates of anxiety disorders were 25.0% and 58.0%, respectively. Although the authors reported that comorbidity was not significantly correlated with the slope of outcome in the 34 CMHC patients whose data appeared to be the basis for this conclusion, they did not report the magnitude of the correlations, which would be important given that these analyses had minimal statistical power. It is difficult to imagine that a sample of depressed adolescents with significant externalizing pathology would be comparable in treatment response to a sample without this feature. Nor did the investigators distinguish what may well have been differences in the types of anxiety disorders in the two samples bearing on their equivalence (e.g., a likely higher prevalence of PTSD among inner-city youth). Ethnicity was a significant predictor of outcome, even with an N of 34, although the authors point out that Caucasian CMHC youth (presumably low SES) still showed slower recovery than benchmark subjects (of unknown SES).

What was perhaps most surprising about sample selection, however, was that the authors did not use a strategy for maximizing the similarity of samples that had been used in other studies aimed at assessing the generalizability of RCTs to clinical practice (e.g., Humphreys & Weisner, 2000; Mitchell, Maki, Adson, Ruskin, & Crow, 1997; Thompson-Brenner & Westen, in press): applying the same inclusion and exclusion criteria as used in RCTs to the community sample. Instead, they excluded patients only if they "were unable to complete study measures as a result of psychosis or developmental disability" (Weersing & Weisz, p. 301). We are not aware of any RCT for depression in either adults or adolescents with such lenient inclusion criteria. Although we appreciate the effort to maximize external validity, in this case doing so was discordant with the goal of the study, namely to compare outcome in two samples.

In light of these selection biases, it is difficult to see how any obtained results could bear on the question of transportability or of the relative outcome of treatment in RCTs to "treatment in the community" (equated with treatment in inner-city CMHCs). However, several data-analytic decisions rendered the findings even more difficult to interpret. For example, the investigators considered any CMHC patient who participated in at least one therapy hour as a "completer" (Weersing & Weisz, p. 301). As best as we could ascertain from the article, they then compared these patients to completers (rather than intent to treat patients) from their benchmarking sample. Doing so, however, would substantially inflate the relative success rates of RCTs, where completion is typically defined as finishing the intended course of treatment or some substantial portion of it. In fact, the authors did find a substantial dose-response relationship in the CMHC sample by splitting patients into those who had eight or more sessions and those who had less than eight. A more appropriate number of sessions for this analysis, however, would have been the mean in the benchmark studies (15.9 sessions) to control for number of sessions as an obvious confound, or perhaps the median, which was 11 for both the CMHC and benchmark samples.

In both the abstract and the discussion, the authors went even further than concluding that patients treated in RCTs do better than those treated in the community. They argued that the CMHC-treated patients looked more like patients in RCT control conditions. This conclusion rested on an extrapolation from the slope of change in RCT control groups from pretreatment to 3 months (because, for ethical reasons, no control groups lasted longer than that) to 12 months. It is worth noting that this extrapolation, which produced a return to normalcy for the average patient at 1 year, would dissolve all treatment effects ever documented at 1 year post-treatment for any EST for child or adult depression of which we are aware, and this extrapolation would produce strong negative effect sizes for the benchmark treatments relative to controls, had the investigators extrapolated the data to 2 years. The authors' explanation of the convergence in outcome between their CMHC and benchmark samples at one year, that this likely reflected the natural course of the illness, may well be true. However, this explanation is notably different from the conclusion typically drawn from the same finding when obtained in RCTs, where continued improvement after follow-up is usually considered a delayed treatment effect.

My point here is not to take issue with a particular study but to note the problems that can result when researchers, journal editors, and reviewers share a common agenda, namely to answer critics' concerns about generalizability, and hence fail to notice obvious problems in methodology or reporting. (This is a problem to which we are all prone, but it is compounded when editorial allegiance effects converge with investigator allegiance effects.)

At this point, the best way to deal with questions about generalizability and transportability would be to institute a moratorium on funding or publishing RCTs that impose exclusion criteria other than those a reasonable clinician would apply in everyday practice (e.g., reliably documented organic brain disease) or that are medically or ethically essential. If the goal is to generalize to the community, then samples should look like community samples, including private practice samples with doctoral-level clinicians. Indeed, I see no reason why investigators should first test their treatments with unrepresentative samples in efficacy studies and then move to community samples when they could start with patients in naturalistic settings in the first place. Patients do not tend to segregate their problems temporally so that clinicians can treat the set of symptoms they consider primary first using one manual and then sequentially apply other manuals on their own timetable. If we want studies to generalize, we should maximize the resemblance of samples to the intended targets of transportation.

This leads to a final point. I suspect a handful of experienced clinician–researchers can integrate the latest science (both basic and applied) with clinical horse sense to generate genuinely novel treatments. However, we would do well to consider psychotherapy in the community a natural laboratory for identifying treatments and techniques associated with positive outcomes. We should consider transportation a bidirectional process, using the practices of clinicians who empirically obtain the best results, along with novel interventions from the laboratory, to develop the next generation of treatment approaches to be tested in clinical trials (Westen et al., 2004a, 2004b). The laboratory is a wonderful venue for testing treatments, but in the history of our field the consulting room has been at least as important for developing them (e.g., cognitive therapy for depression). I suspect there is much to transport from one side of the great divide in our field to the other, but I have not yet seen convincing evidence that one side has a monopoly on precious cargo.

CONCLUSION: LOST IN TRANSPORTATION?

I conclude by returning to a point with which this position paper began. If we take the unit of transportation to be principles of treatment (operationalized using manuals in RCTs), no scientifically minded clinician could possibly argue that the data from such studies should not assume their place along with data from basic science, correlational studies, naturalistic designs, systematic case studies, and clinical experience in contributing to empirically informed therapies. Further, given the possibilities for causal inference that distinguish experimental methods, experimental data should take precedence over other forms of evidence when RCTs consistently demonstrate that ESTs genuinely outperform what clinicians are currently doing in the community. This is the case, for example, with some of the creative, multifaceted interventions researchers have tested for severe and persistent mental disorders such as schizophrenia (e.g., Drake, Mueser, Brunette, & McHugo, 2004), which consistently outperform treatment as usual (TAU) in the community. For these patients, however, TAU is malignant neglect: occasional sessions with a psychiatrist for medication management, often punctuated by long periods of homelessness.

We need to be much more careful, however, in specifying who the patients and clinicians are "in the community" whom we intend as the recipients of our scientific cargo. For the average middle-class patient entering outpatient psychotherapy in the community, and particularly for patients who can afford private treatment, we have no idea whether ESTs outperform or underperform TAU for most disorders. Until such time as researchers address this question, the justification for transportation of many treatments from the laboratory to the clinic will remain an article of faith. Rather than waging a war of attrition against experienced practitioners (e.g., hoping that managed care companies will induce them to "get with the program"), psychotherapy researchers would do well to join with them to compare experimental treatments with TAU for patients who can afford it. This would be in the interest of both researchers and clinicians, and most importantly it would be in the best interest of our patients, who are interested in the best care, not partisan turf battles.

Dialogue: Convergence and Contention

Martin E. Franklin and Robert J. DeRubeis

Like many of his recent publications, the position paper by Westen in this book serves a useful function for those of us who devote our careers to the development and empirical evaluation of treatments for psychiatric disorders: It articulates eloquently the views of some who look on the EST literature with skepticism. The invitation to wake up and smell this particular pot of coffee should be graciously accepted, and in the following paragraphs we hope to filter the brew from the grounds. Westen partitions his paper into three essential questions, and we will remain faithful to this division by responding to points of convergence and divergence within each category.

First Westen raises the question of what is being transported, where he duly notes (and we concur) that if different manuals were needed for every difference between RCT samples and clinical patients then the task of manualizing treatment in clinical settings would be untenable. He further suggests that if the end product of RCTs is a set of general principles or theory-driven techniques then most clinicians would find this unobjectionable, whereas if specific manuals are the product then it raises a nearly infinite number of unanswerable questions and devolves into chaos. What is missing from this dichotomous argument, however, is that manuals are comprised of theory-driven principles that must always be adapted to the specific needs of individual patients, even within the context of RCTs. Those of us who support their dissemination would suggest that they continue to be used in this way beyond the research context. As a brief clinical example, one of us (MEF) who served as a clinician on an adult OCD efficacy study was once asked by a study supervisor to clarify why much of a CBT maintenance session was apparently devoted to the discussion of defensive strategies in an upcoming football playoff game, at least according to the treatment fidelity rater. Reviewing the tape with the investigator, the therapist was able to clearly highlight that the conversation had to do with helping the patient anticipate what "OCD would do next," which was entirely within the stated session goals of discussing relapse prevention issues, and that the use of the football metaphor was simply a way to make the core principles more salient to a patient with interest in and great knowledge of that particular topic. Notably, on further review, the ruling on the field was overturned, and the session was deemed an appropriate use of the latitude inherent in conducting a clinically sensitive treatment outcome trial. Creativity was not punished, and blind adherence to rigid rules was not demanded. It may be that many clinicians have the same impression that Westen articulates about the rigidity of therapy conducted in clinical trials. In our experience, therapy in RCTs is clinically sensitive. It is incumbent on RCT researchers to articulate this critically important point more clearly than we have done in the past so that those who might use the RCT findings are fully informed.

Westen's second section deals with the target of the transportation, and he highlights the limitations of focusing strictly on *DSM–IV*-defined disorders and their associated symptoms. Indeed, it is important to allow for and to take clinical complexity and comorbidity into account; accordingly, many current RCTs are doing just that (e.g., Pediatric OCD Treatment Study Team, 2004). Moreover, published treatment manuals do exist for "functionally defined problems" such as school refusal behavior (e.g., Kearney & Albano, 2000), and such treatments are indeed viable candidates for study in RCTs despite the deviation from *DSM–IV* categories. The shift toward more inclusive sampling frames has much more to do with the progress made in the field in the last 20 years than a repudiation of the need to carefully consider study inclusion and exclusion criteria. These selections are based on the research questions at hand and are contextualized by what has been done in a given field at the time of trial conception: the less that is known about a given treatment for a given disorder, the more likely it is that the study inclusion bar will be set higher, which is in accordance with the goal of not stepping too far beyond the available data. One could, as Westen suggests, start treatment studies with highly complex cases in clinical practice settings, at the risk perhaps of generating null findings and having multiple, plausible explanations for why this was the case, none of which can be isolated using study data. Room exists for both approaches, and we would suggest that the approach chosen should be tethered to the existing knowledge base, rather than chosen as a matter of (a rigid) principle or, worse yet, investigator preference.

The third point, regarding how clear the data are, has already been addressed in our chapter: They are promising, but not unequivocal. We believe that a tremendous amount of clinically useful knowledge has been obtained from RCTs over the last several decades, as well as from more recent, successful attempts to transport ESTs into the clinic. The most prudent position is not one that demands perfect research before action is taken, as this would lead to the absence of (other than personal, idiosyncratic) standards and would result in a grave disservice to the patients whose lives we aim to make better. And we certainly cannot agree with Westen's implication that an alliance has existed among biased investigators, biased journal editors, and biased reviewers, the aim of which is "to answer critics' concerns about generalizability" (p. 391). We are concerned that such characterizations, as well as a focus on what is wrong with treatment research, rather than what it can teach us, distract from the (admittedly imperfect) contributions of science. We end with a quote from the 19th-century English writer William Hazlitt: "The surest hindrance of success is to have too high a standard of refinement in our own minds . . . He who is determined not to be satisfied with anything short of perfection will never do anything to please himself or others" (Hill, 2004).

Drew I. Westen

The position paper by Franklin and DeRubeis is well reasoned, well argued, and encouraging. I agree with their overall message: "the question of whether or not ESTs are effective in clinical practice settings is an empirical one that should be studied rather than simply debated" (p. 382); "manuals are best thought of as guides that are theoretically informed yet still clinically flexible, requiring creativity and clinical skill to be used optimally" (p. 380); and "As psychotherapy researchers report more on the transportability and limits of their treatments, we should obtain a clearer picture as to which treatments, for which disorders, and to which kinds of clinics can laboratory-tested treatments enhance the care of patients" (p. 383).

In these statements, Franklin and DeRubeis are taking what I described in my position paper as the "soft constraints" approach to RCTs. This model views manuals as ways of operationalizing principles or strategies, which constitute samples of the ways one could operationalize these constructs but are not constitutive of them. In this view, the goal of "transportation" is to inform clinicians about useful ways of thinking about and intervening with patients who have pathologies that resemble the patients treated in RCTs, not to prescribe that when they see a patient with a particular diagnosis they should faithfully follow a prefabricated set of procedures.

If this were the position taken by most EST advocates over the last decade, we would have had a very harmonious decade, but we would also have had no lists of approved (and by implication, no unapproved) treatments. We already knew, since Smith and Glass (1977), that the mélange of things clinicians do tends to be very helpful, and process–outcome studies have shown clear links between positive outcomes and variables, such as empathic attunement, focusing on interpersonal problems, fostering insight, exposure and response prevention, and focusing on the therapeutic relationship (e.g., Ablon & Jones, 2002; Greenberg & Malcolm, 2002; Hilsenroth, Ackerman, Blagys, Baity, & Mooney, 2003; Orlinsky, Ronnestad, & Willutzski, 2004; Wampold, 2001). All of these are empirically supported interventions. Even limiting our discussion to RCTs, we know that psychodynamic therapy (at least time-limited variants of it) is efficacious for many problems when administered in RCTs by clinicians who intend it as a bona fide treatment (see Hilsenroth et al., 2003; Luborsky & Crits-Christoph, 1990; Price, Hilsenroth, Callahan, Petretic-Jackson, & Bonge, in press; Strupp & Binder, 1984).

If this soft constraints model were the position of the EST movement, students would not be learning in virtually every introductory and abnormal psychology textbook that CBT is the treatment of choice for virtually every disorder (occasionally along with interpersonal therapy [IPT]); top-ranked clinical psychology programs would not be replacing training in "traditional" psychotherapy with training in manualized treatments; graduate students in many programs would not be learning that the way to treat patients is to make a DSM–IV diagnosis and then to search the literature for the appropriate manual; and site visitors would not be asking directors of graduate programs and internships about their coverage of manual-based treatments.

Indeed, if this were the position of the EST movement, there would be no EST movement, because the view Franklin and DeRubeis present is a reaffirmation of what psychotherapy researchers have believed for 50 years. What distinguished the EST movement from all prior approaches to psychotherapy research, and what has led to a decade of acrimony, are its methodological imperialism (ruling out-of-court data from all methods other than a very specific use of RCT methodology, namely the thumbs-up–thumbs-down evaluation of treatment packages for specific disorders) and its predication on a series of assumptions (e.g., that psychopathology comes in specific, discrete variants that require specific, discrete manuals or modules) that are clinically and empirically unsupportable (see Wampold, 2001; Westen et al., 2004a, 2004b, in press).

But perhaps I am picking a fight unnecessarily when we are now all in agreement. (If so, I hope the authors will suggest a good 12-session treatment for this aversive behavior.) I will conclude, however, with one complication. (Okay, 16 sessions.) If we abandon the hard constraints model of transportation, we also have to abandon an increasingly prevalent view of clinicians as technicians who faithfully (even if flexibly) apply empirically supported interventions.

Consider an example. Some time ago I treated a young woman with a complex symptom picture, including atypical major depression, several anxiety diagnoses, a substance use disorder, and a complex personality disorder. Early in treatment, my primary goal was to keep the patient, who was actively suicidal, alive. Over time (4 years), we moved through a range of issues, organized not by a set of prioritized *DSM–IV* diagnoses addressed sequentially but by issues on her mind and by my understanding of who she is and why she thought, felt, and behaved as she did (i.e., by a case formulation). At one point, we stumbled on some hoarding behavior that was interfering with a goal of the treatment at the time. My response, which may shock many readers, was to email Gail Steketee to ask her for her manual for hoarding. Although I could imagine ways to apply exposure principles, this was a symptom with which I had relatively little experience, and I thought it would make much more sense to find out, in as concrete detail as possible, how someone who had treated many such patients successfully had done so. (As it turned out, a manual was unavailable and TAU, which in this case was a blend of psychodynamic exploration and exposure, solved the problem within a few weeks.)

My point in describing this example is that I did not conceive of this patient as a major depressive, then a GAD patient, then a social phobic, then a substance abuser, then a hoarder, and so forth, and work my way through a dozen manuals. Rather, I tried to understand the common and specific processes that led to a wide-ranging set of symptoms and used everything I know about the mind, psychopathology, and psychotherapy, including what I have learned in 20-plus years of doing psychotherapy, and what I learned over time about her as an individual, to try to help her. That, to me, is EBP. Fallible, yes, but no more fallible, I suspect, than the design and interpretation of treatment research.

If patients came in neat packages, so could treatments. But everything we know suggests that they do not.

REFERENCES

Ablon, J. S., & Jones, E. E. (2002). Validity of controlled clinical trials of psychotherapy: Findings from the NIMH Treatment of Depression Collaborative Research Program. *American Journal of Psychiatry, 159,* 775–783.

Abramowitz, J. S, Foa, E. B., & Franklin, M. E. (2003). Exposure and ritual prevention for obsessive–compulsive disorder: Effects of intensive versus twice-weekly sessions. *Journal of Consulting and Clinical Psychology, 71,* 394–398.

Abramowitz, J. S., Franklin, M. E., Schwartz, S. A., & Furr, J. M. (2003). Symptom presentation and outcome of cognitive–behavior therapy for obsessive–compulsive disorder. *Journal of Consulting and Clinical Psychology, 71,* 1049–1057.

American Psychiatric Association. (1994). *Diagnostic and statistical manual of mental disorders* (4th ed.). Washington, DC: Author.

Barlow, D. (2002). *Anxiety and its disorders* (2nd ed.). New York: Guilford Press.

Beutler, L. E. (2000). David and Goliath: When empirical and clinical standards of practice meet. *American Psychologist, 55,* 997–1007.

Beutler, L. E., Moleiro, C., & Talebi, H. (2002). How practitioners can systematically use empirical evidence in treatment selection. *Journal of Clinical Psychology, 58,* 1199–1212.

Blomhoff, S., Haug, T. T., Hellstrom, K., Holme, I., Humble, M., & Wold, J. E. (2001). Randomised controlled general practice trial of sertraline, exposure therapy and combined treatment in generalised social phobia. *British Journal of Psychiatry, 179,* 23–30.

Brown, T. A., & Barlow, D. H. (1995). Long-term outcome in cognitive behavioral treatment of panic disorder: Clinical predictors and alternative strategies for assessment. *Journal of Consulting and Clinical Psychology, 63,* 754–765.

Cahill, S. P., Hembree, E. A., & Foa, E. B. (in press). Dissemination of prolonged exposure therapy for posttraumatic stress disorder: Successes and challenges. In Y. Neria, R. Gross, R. Marshall, & E. Susser (Eds.), *9/11: Public Health in the Wake of Terrorist Attacks.* Cambridge, England: Cambridge University Press.

Chambless, D. L., & Ollendick, T. H. (2001). Empirically supported psychological interventions: Controversies and evidence. *Annual Review of Psychology, 52,* 685–716.

Cottraux, J., Mollard, E., Bouvard, M., Marks, I., Sluys, M., Nury, A. M., et al. (1990). A controlled study of fluvoxamine and exposure in obsessive–compulsive disorder. *International Clinical Psychopharmacology, 5,* 17–30.

de Haan, E., Hoogduin, K. A., Buitelaar, J. K., & Keijsers, G. P. (1998). Behavior therapy versus clomipramine for the treatment of obsessive–compulsive disorder in children and adolescents. *Journal of the American Academy of Child and Adolescent Psychiatry, 37,* 1022–1029.

Drake, R. E., Mueser, K. T., Brunette, M. F., & McHugo, G. J. (2004). A review of treatments for people with severe mental illnesses and co-occurring substance use disorders. *Psychiatric Rehabilitation Journal, 27,* 360–374.

Evans, M. D., Hollon, S. D., DeRubeis, R. J., Piasecki, J. M., Garvey, M. J., Grove, W. M., et al. (1992). Differential relapse following cognitive therapy and pharmacotherapy for depression. *Archives of General Psychiatry, 49,* 802–808.

Fals-Stewart, W., Marks, A. P., & Schafer, J. (1993). A comparison of behavioral group therapy and individual behavior therapy in treating obsessive–compulsive disorder. *Journal of Nervous and Mental Disease, 181,* 189–193.

Foa, E. B., Dancu, C. V., Hembree, E. A., Jaycox, L. H., Meadows, E. A., & Street, G. P. (1999). A comparison of exposure therapy, stress inoculation training, and their combination for reducing posttraumatic stress disorder in female assault victims. *Journal of Consulting and Clinical Psychology, 67,* 194–200.

Foa, E. B., & Goldstein, A. (1978). Continuous exposure and complete response prevention in the treatment of obsessive–compulsive neurosis. *Behavior Therapy, 9,* 821–829.

Foa, E. B., Kozak, M. J., Steketee, G. S., & McCarthy, P. R. (1992). Treatment of depressive and obsessive–compulsive symptoms in OCD by imipramine and behavior therapy. *British Journal of Clinical Psychology, 31,* 279–292.

Foa, E. B., Liebowitz, M. R., Kozak, M. J., Davies, S. O., Campeas, R., Franklin, M. E., et al. (in press). Treatment of obsessive compulsive disorder by exposure and ritual prevention, clomipramine, and their combination: A randomized, placebo-controlled trial. *American Journal of Psychiatry.*

Foa, E. B., Steketee, G., Grayson, B., Turner, M., & Latimer, P. (1984). Deliberate exposure and blocking of obsessive–compulsive rituals: Immediate and long-term effects. *Behavior Therapy, 15,* 450–472.

Franklin, M. E., Abramowitz, J. S., Kozak, M. J., Levitt, J., & Foa, E. B. (2000). Effectiveness of exposure and ritual prevention for obsessive compulsive disorder: Randomized compared with non-randomized samples. *Journal of Consulting and Clinical Psychology, 68,* 594–602.

Franklin, M. E., & Foa, E. B. (2002). Cognitive–behavioral treatment of obsessive compulsive disorder. In P. Nathan & J. Gorman (Eds.), *A guide to treatments that work* (2nd ed., pp. 367–386). New York: Oxford University Press.

Franklin, M. E., Kozak, M. J., Cashman, L. A., Coles, M. E., Rheingold, A. A., & Foa, E. B. (1998). Cognitive–behavioral treatment of pediatric obsessive–compulsive disorder: An open clinical trial. *Journal of the American Academy of Child and Adolescent Psychiatry, 37,* 412–419.

Gillespie, K., Duffy, M., Hackmann, A., & Clark, D. M. (2002). Community based cognitive therapy in the treatment of posttraumatic stress disorder following the Omagh bomb. *Behaviour Research and Therapy, 40,* 345–357.

Greenberg, L. S., & Malcolm, W. (2002). Resolving unfinished business: Relating process to outcome. *Journal of Consulting and Clinical Psychology, 70,* 406–416.

Hill, D. (2004). Hazlitt quotation. "Wish I'd Said That!" Retrieved December 2004 from http://www.wist.info/

Hilsenroth, M., Ackerman, S., Blagys, M., Baity, M., & Mooney, M. (2003). Short-term psychodynamic psychotherapy for depression: An evaluation of statistical, clinically significant, and technique specific change. *Journal of Nervous and Mental Disease, 191,* 349–357.

Hofmann, S. G., Barlow, D. H., Papp, L. A., Detweiler, M. F., Ray, S. E., Shear, M. K., et al. (1998). Pretreatment attrition in a comparative treatment outcome study on panic disorder. *American Journal of Psychiatry, 155,* 43–47.

Hollon, S. D., DeRubeis, R. J., Evans, M. D., Wiemer, M. J., Garvey, M. J., Grove, W. M., et al. (1992). Cognitive therapy and pharmacotherapy for depression: Singly and in combination. *Archives of General Psychiatry, 49,* 774–781.

Humphreys, K., & Weisner, C. (2000). Use of exclusion criteria in selecting research subjects and its effects on the generalizability of alcohol treatment outcome studies. *American Journal of Psychiatry, 157,* 588–594.

Huppert, J. D., & Abramowitz, J. S. (2003). Going beyond the manual: Insights from experienced clinicians. *Cognitive and Behavioral Practice, 10,* 1–2.

Huppert, J. D., Franklin, M. E., Foa, E. B., & Davidson, J. R. T. (2003). Study refusal and exclusion from a randomized treatment study of generalized social phobia. *Journal of Anxiety Disorders, 17,* 683–693.

Kearney, C. A., & Albano, A. M. (2000). *When children refuse school: A cognitive–behavioral therapy approach. Parent workbook.* San Antonio, TX: The Psychological Corporation.

Kendall, P. C., Chu, B., Gifford, A., Hayes, C., & Nauta, M. (1998). Breathing life into a manual: Flexibility and creativity with manual-based treatments. *Cognitive and Behavioral Practice, 5,* 177–198.

Kozak, M. J., Liebowitz, M. R., & Foa, E. B. (2000). Cognitive behavior therapy and pharmacotherapy for OCD: The NIMH-Sponsored Collaborative Study. In W. Goodman, M. Rudorfer, & J. Maser (Eds.), *Obsessive compulsive disorder: Contemporary issues in treatment* (pp. 501–530). Mahwah, NJ: Erlbaum.

Krueger, R. F., & Piasecki, T. M. (2002). Toward a dimensional and psychometrically-informed approach to conceptualizing psychopathology. *Behaviour Research and Therapy, 40,* 485–499.

Lindsay, M., Crino, R., & Andrews, G. (1997). Controlled trial of exposure and response prevention in obsessive–compulsive disorder. *British Journal of Psychiatry, 171,* 135–139.

Luborsky, L., & Crits-Christoph, P. (1990). *Understanding transference: The core conflictual relationship theme method.* New York: Basic Books.

March, J. S., Mulle, K., & Herbel, B. (1994). Behavioral psychotherapy for children and adolescents with obsessive–compulsive disorder: An open trial of a new protocol-driven treatment package. *Journal of the American Academy of Child and Adolescent Psychiatry, 33,* 333–341.

Marks, I., Hodgson, R., & Rachman, S. (1975). Treatment of chronic obsessive–compulsive neurosis by *in vivo* exposure. *British Journal of Psychiatry, 127,* 349–364.

McLean, P. L., Whittal, M. L., Thordarson, D. S., Taylor, S., Sochting, I., Koch, W. J., et al. (2001). Cognitive versus behavior therapy in the group treatment of obsessive–compulsive disorder. *Journal of Consulting and Clinical Psychology, 69,* 205–214.

Meyer, V. (1966). Modification of expectations in cases with obsessional rituals. *Behaviour Research and Therapy, 4,* 273–280.

Mitchell, J. E., Maki, D. D., Adson, D. E., Ruskin, B. S., & Crow, S. J. (1997). The selectivity of inclusion and exclusion criteria in bulimia nervosa treatment studies. *International Journal of Eating Disorders, 22,* 243–252.

Orlinsky, D. E., Ronnestad, M. H., & Willutzski, U. (2004). Fifty years of psychotherapy process-outcome research: Continuity and change. In M. Lambert (Ed.), *Bergin and Garfield's handbook of psychotherapy and behavior change* (5th ed., pp. 307–389). New York: Wiley.

Pediatric OCD Treatment Study Team. (2004). Cognitive–behavioral therapy, sertraline, and their combination for children and adolescents with obsessive–

compulsive disorder: The Pediatric OCD Treatment Study (POTS) randomized controlled trial. *Journal of the American Medical Association, 292,* 1969–1976.

Persons, J. B., & Silberschatz, G. (1998). Are results of randomized controlled trials useful to psychotherapists? *Journal of Consulting and Clinical Psychology, 66,* 126–135.

Piacentini, J., Bergman, R. L., Jacobs, C., McCracken, J. T., & Kretchman, J. (2002). Open trial of cognitive behavior therapy for childhood obsessive–compulsive disorder. *Journal of Anxiety Disorders, 16,* 207–219.

Price, J. L., Hilsenroth, M., Callahan, K., Petretic-Jackson, P. A., & Bonge, D. (in press). A pilot study of psychodynamic psychotherapy for adult survivors of childhood sexual abuse. *Clinical Psychology and Psychotherapy.*

Rosen, G. M., & Davison, G. C. (2003). Psychology should list empirically supported principles of change (ESPs) and not credential trademarked therapies or other treatment packages. *Behavior Modification, 27,* 300–312.

Rothbaum, B. O., & Shahar, F. (2000). Behavioral treatment of obsessive–compulsive disorder in a naturalistic setting. *Cognitive and Behavioral Practice, 7,* 262–270.

Rush, A. J., Beck, A. T., Kovacs, M., & Hollon, S. D. (1977). Comparative efficacy of cognitive therapy and pharmacotherapy in the treatment of depressed outpatients. *Cognitive Therapy and Research, 1,* 17–37.

Smith, M., & Glass, G. (1977). Meta-analysis of psychotherapy outcome studies. *American Psychologist, 32,* 752–760.

Stirman, S. W., Crits-Christoph, P., & DeRubeis, R. J. (2004). Achieving successful dissemination of empirically supported psychotherapies: A synthesis of dissemination theory. *Clinical Psychology: Science and Practice, 11,* 343–359.

Stirman, S. W., DeRubeis, R. J., Crits-Christoph, P., & Brody, P. E. (2003). Are samples in randomized controlled trials of psychotherapy representative of community outpatients? A new methodology and initial findings. *Journal of Consulting and Clinical Psychology, 71,* 963–972.

Strupp, H., & Binder, J. (1984). *Psychotherapy in a new key: A guide to time-limited dynamic psychotherapy.* New York: Basic Books.

Stuart, G. L., Wade, W. A., & Treat, T. A. (2000). Effectiveness of an empirically based treatment for panic disorder delivered in a service clinic setting: 1-year follow-up. *Journal of Consulting and Clinical Psychology, 68,* 506–512.

Taylor, T. K., Schmidt, F., Pepler, D., & Hodgins, C. (1998). A comparison of eclectic treatment with Webster–Stratton's parents and children series in a children's mental health setting: A randomized controlled trial. *Behavior Therapy, 29,* 221–240.

Thompson-Brenner, H., & Westen, D. (in press). A naturalistic study of psychotherapy for bulimia nervosa, Part 1: Comorbidity and therapeutic outcome. *Journal of Nervous and Mental Disorders.*

Valderhaug, R., Gotestam, K. G., Larsson, B., & Piacentini, J. C. (2004, May). *An open clinical trial of cognitive behaviour therapy for childhood obsessive–compulsive disorder in regular outpatient clinics.* Paper presented at the SOGN Centre Conference on Pediatric Anxiety Disorders in Children and Adolescents, Oslo, Norway.

van Balkom, A. J. L. M., de Haan, E., van Oppen, P., Spinhoven, P., Hoogduin, K. A. L., Vermeulen, A. W. A., et al. (1998). Cognitive and behavioral therapies alone and in combination with fluvoxamine in the treatment of obsessive compulsive disorder. *Journal of Nervous and Mental Disease, 186*, 492–499.

Wade, W. A., Treat, T. A., & Stuart, G. L. (1998). Transporting an empirically supported treatment for panic disorder to a service clinic setting: A benchmarking strategy. *Journal of Consulting and Clinical Psychology, 66*, 231–239.

Wampold, B. E. (2001). *The great psychotherapy debate: Models, methods, and findings.* Mahwah, NJ: Erlbaum.

Warren, R., & Thomas, J. C. (2001). Cognitive–behavior therapy of obsessive–compulsive disorder in private practice: An effectiveness study. *Journal of Anxiety Disorders, 15*, 277–285.

Weersing, V. R., & Weisz, J. R. (2002). Community clinic treatment of depressed youth: Benchmarking usual care against CBT clinical trials. *Journal of Consulting and Clinical Psychology, 70*, 299–310.

Weinberger, J. (2000). *Why can't psychotherapists and psychotherapy researchers get along?: Underlying causes of the EST-effectiveness controversy.* Unpublished manuscript, Adelphi University.

Weisz, J. R., Weersing, V. R., & Henggeler, S. W. (in press). Jousting with straw men: Comment on Westen, Novotny, and Thompson-Brenner (2004). *Psychological Bulletin.*

Westen, D., & Morrison, K. (2001). A multidimensional meta-analysis of treatments for depression, panic, and generalized anxiety disorder: An empirical examination of the status of empirically supported therapies. *Journal of Consulting and Clinical Psychology, 69*, 875–899.

Westen, D., Novotny, C. M., & Thomson-Brenner, H. (2004a). The empirical status of empirically supported psychotherapies: Assumptions, findings, and reporting in controlled clinical trials. *Psychological Bulletin, 130*, 631–663.

Westen, D., Novotny, C., & Thompson-Brenner, H. (2004b). The next generation of psychotherapy research. *Psychological Bulletin, 130*, 677–683.

Westen, D., Novotny, C., & Thompson-Brenner, H. (in press). EBP ≠ EST: Reply to Crits-Christoph, Wilson, and Hollon (2005) and Weisz, Weersing, and Henggeler (2005). *Psychological Bulletin.*

Wever, C., & Rey, J. M. (1997). Juvenile obsessive compulsive disorder. *Australian and New Zealand Journal of Psychiatry, 31*, 105–113.

EPILOGUE

JOHN C. NORCROSS, LARRY E. BEUTLER, AND RONALD F. LEVANT

Mental health professionals comprise a nation of differences. Those differences do not necessarily make us weak; differences can serve as sources of creativity, strength, and progress if constructively harnessed. In the view of Feyerabend, a philosopher of science, the interplay between tenacity and proliferation is an essential feature in the development of science. It is not the puzzle-solving activity that is responsible for the growth of our knowledge, but the active interplay of various tenaciously held views. In the words of Dante (*Paradiso*, Canto VI), "Of diverse voices is sweet music made." But diverse voices can also sound like nails on a blackboard if they are dissynchronous and out of harmony.

In this volume, we have tried to constructively harness the active interplay of these various tenaciously held views, to find the harmony among these diverse voices on evidence-based practices (EBPs) in mental health. Proponents of divergent, even opposing, perspectives on fundamental EBP questions have generously contributed position papers, followed by commentaries featuring their respective points of contention and convergence. In this brief epilogue, we summarize the take-home, consensus messages of our book without minimizing the salient differences that remain among us.

EVIDENCE-BASED PRACTICES IN GENERAL

The call for accountability in health care is here to stay. All mental health professions will need to respond to the clarion call for EBPs by demonstrating the safety, efficacy, and efficiency of their work. In fact, the demands for evidence from various constituencies will escalate in the future. No amount of kvetching, howling at the moon, or passing resolutions will alter that reality.

EBPs have profound implications for mental health practice, training, and policy. What is designated or privileged as "evidence-based" will determine in part what therapies and tests are conducted, what is reimbursed, what is taught, and what is researched.

As a consequence, EBPs are ripe for misuse or abuse. If not watched, third-party payers could selectively use research findings as cost-containment devices as opposed to quality-improvement methods. If not checked, certain parties could restrict the definition of "evidence" and commandeer the entire discussion. If not careful, trainers committed to a particular theoretical orientation could unfairly impose it onto all students and situations. The definition, identification, and implementation of EBPs are high-stakes endeavors.

At the same time, most mental health treatments have already been empirically established as effective and as safe as other health care and educational interventions. Psychology, in particular, has always striven to be an evidence-based profession. We can do better and more of course, but we begin from a solid research tradition and a strong empirical base.

Given their dual proficiency in practice and science (the scientists among the clinicians *and* the clinicians among the scientists), psychologists are in an ideal position to proclaim the strong empirical base for psychological interventions and to provide incisive critiques of the fundamental questions underlying EBPs. Moreover, psychologists can advocate for more inclusive conceptualizations of EBPs that prize individual differences, the human relationship, and cultural context. Psychology can proactively shape EBPs.

EVIDENCE-BASED PRACTICES IN PARTICULAR

Reading only the position papers in the preceding nine chapters might lead one to conclude that rampant professional discord exists about EBPs. And there is. The clash of colliding worlds may generate confusion about what conclusions are warranted and may engender despair that consensus will never be achieved. However, reading the subsequent dialogue commentaries will probably lead one to recognize the impressive convergence in the field. And there is.

Here we explicate the major points of convergence we encountered in each chapter:

- Evidence is variously sought in clinical expertise, patient values, and scientific research. Although partisans disagree about the relative validity and importance of the three, a consensual definition of EBPs will probably involve all three bases (chap. 1).

One of us (LEB) disagrees with including patient values as a basis of evidence but views it as serving an important role in the development of hypotheses that can be tested for empirical value.

- Scientific research is the bedrock of EBPs, and such research consists of a variety of methodologies and designs, depending on the purpose of the study and its context. We should embrace all research designs, including case studies, single-participant designs, qualitative research, process studies, effectiveness research, and randomized clinical trials (RCTs), that help us to identify and understand the success of interventions. RCTs possess superior control and rigor for making causal statements but will never be the only suitable design for determining EBPs (chap. 2).

- Psychotherapy manuals are helpful for training and research. In particular, they enhance the internal validity of comparative outcome studies, facilitate treatment integrity, ensure the possibility of replication, and provide a systematic way of training and supervising therapists. At the same time, manuals are also associated with some untold negative effects. There is no conclusive evidence that manuals improve treatment outcomes or that they should be required in practice (chap. 3).

- Although earlier RCTs screened out more complex and difficult patients, that is less the case today. Some evidence exists to suggest that patients enrolled in clinical trials of psychotherapy are representative, especially in recent years, but the degree to which we can confidently generalize from laboratory to clinic remains a source of fierce debate (chap. 4).

- The treatment method, the individual therapist, the therapy relationship, and the patient are vital contributors to the success of psychotherapy and all must be studied. Further, principles of change might generate more parsimony and consensus. Comprehensive EBPs will consider all these determinants and their optimal combinations. For practical and reimbursement purposes, however, specific treatment and assessment methods will continue to be the focus of most professional and policy attention (chap. 5).

- The production, dissemination, and interpretation of research are inherently human endeavors; there is no purely "objective" or "unbiased" pursuit of truth. In particular, the researcher's theoretical allegiance, funding sources, and conventional wisdom regularly influence the results of published research findings, on which EBPs are heavily based (chap. 6).

- The available research demonstrates that psychological treatments designated as empirically supported or evidence based are superior to no treatment and placebo treatment. However, it remains unclear and controversial whether ESTs outperform structurally equivalent therapies not designated as ESTs (chap. 7).
- Neither EBPs nor treatments as usual (TAUs) satisfactorily address various dimensions of human diversity in mental health. Race–ethnicity, gender, sexual orientation, and disability status have largely been ignored to date (chap. 8).
- Efficacious laboratory-validated treatments can transport to other practice settings and situations, but not necessarily. Something, but surely not everything, is lost in transport from lab to practice (chap. 9).

TWO FINAL COMMENTS

In bringing this volume to a close, we would collegially offer two comments, one process and one outcome. First, in terms of process, informed dialogue and respectful debate are surely the ways to progress. Methodological pluralism and diverse values are essential; "of diverse voices is sweet music made." And progress we must; patient access to care, reimbursement decisions, professional livelihoods, and clinical training are all at stake. Let's keep the dialogue alive.

Second, in terms of outcome, we should remember that the overarching goal of EBPs, however defined and disseminated, is to enhance the effectiveness of patient services and to improve public health. Debate and dialogue we should, but let's keep our eye on the goal: happier and healthier people.

AUTHOR INDEX

Numbers in italics refer to listings in the reference sections.

Brill, P. L., 147, *156*
Brody, B. A., *127*
Brody, N., 301, *323*
Brody, P. E., 173, 183, *187*, 386, *401*
Brom, D., 260, 283, 288
Bromley, D. B., 321, *324*
Brooks, G. R., 342, *368*
Brooks, G. W., *250*
Brown, A. L., 22, 48
Brown, G. S., 204, 206, 207, 238, 240, 249, 256
Brown, J., 142, 146, 147, *155*, *158*, 238, 252
Brown, L. S., 119, 342, 350, 353, *368*
Brown, T. A., 166, *184*, 260, 273, 287, 384, 398
Brown, W. A., 270, *292*, *298*
Browne, G., 264, *288*
Bruce, M., 183, *184*
Brunette, M. F., 392, *398*
Bryant, R. A., 35, *51*
Buchanan, J. A., 7, *12*
Bufka, L. F., 50, *250*
Buitelaar, J. K., 379, *398*
Burdick, E., *290*
Burlingame, G. M., 211, *247*
Burns, D. D., *120*, 273, 287
Busseri, M. A., 222, *247*
Butler, G., 259, 260, *288*, 303, *323*
Butler, S. F., 63, *123*, *129*, 134, 144, 150, *154*, *156*
Byrne, C., *288*
Bystritsky, A., 314, *323*

Cacciola, J., *293*
Cahill, S. P., 382, *398*
Calhoun, K. S., *11*, 38, *53*, 120, *323*, *368*
Calhoun, L. G., 222, *255*
Callaham, M. L., 269, *288*
Callahan, K., 396, *401*
Calvert, S. J., 228, *247*
Campbell, D. T., 60, 63, 95, 97, 99, 103, 108, 113, *120*, *121*, *128*
Campbell, E. G., 269, *288*
Campbell, J. M., 73, *120*
Campeas, R., *399*
Cantor, N., 219, 220, *247*
Carey, L. A., *290*
Carozzoni, P., *123*
Carpinello, S. E., 16, 48
Carroll, K. M., 139, 145, *155*, *158*, 176, *184*, 248
Carter, J. A., 14, 48
Carter, M. M., 183, *185*
Carter, S., *254*

Casacalenda, N., 264, *288*
Cashman, L. A., *399*
Caspi, A., 175, *187*
Castonguay, L. G., 22, 48, *51*, 87, 90, 91, 93, 95, *120*, *126*, *127*, 134, 136, 144, 150, *155*, 212, 227, 228, 231, 244, *247*, *251*, 320, *322*
Catalan, J., *185*
Catell, D., 272, *291*
Causino, N., 269, *288*
Cech, T. R., 269, *288*
Cerny, J. A., 304, *322*
Chalk, M. B., 146, 148, *158*
Chalmers, I., 269, *289*
Chambers, A., *322*
Chambless, D. L., 5, *11*, *12*, 16, 18, 25, 27, 48, 64, 65, 69, 91, *120*, *121*, 149, *155*, 175, *185*, 192, 194, 195, 197, 227, 236, *247*, 248, 275, 278, 289, 299, 301, 302, 304, 305, 310, 311, *323*, 331, 338, 340, *368*, 382, *398*
Chan, A., 271, *289*
Chang, E., 264, *295*
Charbonneau-Powis, M., 260, *298*
Cheavens, J. S., 220, *255*
Chen, C. P., 337, *369*
Chen, W., 269, 287
Cheung, F., 333, *371*
Chevron, E. S., 60, *125*, 135, *157*, 315, *325*
Chlebowski, R. T., 17, *48*, 99, *121*
Cho, M. K., 270, *288*
Choate, M. L., 181, *184*
Chopra, S. S., 269, *289*
Chorpita, B. F., 16, 48, 166, *184*
Choudhry, N. K., 270, *289*
Christensen, D. M., *373*
Christie, J. E., 261, *288*
Chu, B., 133, *157*, 380, *400*
Chung, J., *187*
Clark, D. M., *187*, 303, *323*, 382, *399*
Clark, O., 269, *293*
Clarke, G. N., 91, 95, *121*
Clarkin, J. F., 39, *48*, 135, *154*, 230, 244, 246
Coady, C. A. J., 242, *248*
Cochran, S. D., 347, *369*
Cochran, S. V., 342, *372*
Cocking, R. R., 22, 48
Cogar, M. M., 76, *124*
Cohen, J., 28, *48*, 178, *185*
Cohen, L. R., *298*
Cohen, P., 178, *185*
Cohen, R. A., 15, 48
Cole, B., 65, *124*

Coles, M. E., 399
Colins, J., 290
Collins, I. F., 249
Collins, J. F., 49, 121, 185, 187, 324
Comtois, K., 186
Condeluci, A., 358, 369
Connolly Gibbons, M. B., 198, 246, 248
Connors, G. J., 145, 155
Constantino, M. J., 93, 120
Consumer Reports, 48
Cook, A., 15, 52
Cook, T. D., 95, 103, 121, 128
Coon, D. W., 264, 297
Cooney, N. L., 228, 248
Cooper, Z., 166, 181, 185
Corbett, M. M., 76, 124
Corbin, J., 74, 129
Corey, P. N., 268, 293
Costello, E., 236, 247, 314, 318, 322
Cottraux, J., 175, 185, 305, 324, 377, 398
Cox, A., 106, 121
Crago, M., 228, 247
Craighead, W. E., 280, 291
Craske, M. G., 133, 135, 155, 304, 310, 314,
        318, 322, 323
Crawford, I., 355, 367
Creed, P. A., 183, 185
Crino, R., 377, 400
Cristol, A. H., 213, 255, 296
Crits-Christoph, P., 11, 48, 120, 146, 155,
        156, 173–175, 183, 185, 187, 188,
        196, 198, 201, 203, 234–236, 246,
        248, 251, 283, 293, 301, 305, 306,
        313, 315, 319, 323, 368, 384, 386,
        396, 400, 401
Cronbach, L. J., 103, 121
Crosbie, J., 73, 121
Cross, D. G., 224, 248, 260, 289
Crow, S. J., 390, 400
Cucherat, M., 305, 324
Cummings, E. E., 373
Curfman, G. D., 271, 289
Curry, J., 186
Curtis, J. T., 87, 128

Daiuto, A., 323, 368
Daldrup, R. J., 246
Dame, L. A., 296
Dancu, C. V., 398
Dansky, B., 176, 184

Danton, W. G., 267, 273, 287
Dardennes, R. M., 274, 290
Darwin, C., 58, 121
Dattilio, F. M., 321, 324
Davidoff, F., 24, 48, 269, 289
Davidson, E. B., 376
Davidson, J. R. T., 399
Davidson, K. W., 17, 30, 48, 185, 186, 188
Davies, D., 47
Davies, S. O., 399
Daviet, C., 26, 51
Davis, K. M., 145, 158
Davis, L., 119
Davis, M. K., 38, 52, 197, 228, 251, 285, 294
Davis, T. E., III, 321, 325
Davis, T. L., 123
Davison, G. C., 30, 53, 55, 148, 155, 384, 401
Dawes, R. M., 136, 155
DeAngelis, C. D., 269, 274, 285, 289, 290
Deaux, K., 340, 369
Debellis, K., 291
DeBord, K. A., 347, 348, 372
Deci, E. L., 222, 248
Defares, P. B., 260, 288
de Haan, E., 379, 398, 401
DeLeon, P. H., 37, 51
Dellario, D. J., 355, 372
DeLoach, C., 356, 369
DeMichele, J. T., 214, 253
Demler, O., 50
DeNelsky, G. Y., 273, 287
Denman, D. W., III, 76, 124
Dent, J., 185
Denzin, N. K., 74, 121
Department of Health, 6, 12
DeRubeis, R. J., 19, 48, 50, 104, 121, 124,
        132, 158, 172–176, 183, 185, 187,
        188, 215, 235, 248, 249, 291, 315,
        323, 384, 386, 398, 399, 401
Detsky, A. S., 270, 289
Detweiler, M. F., 399
Devereaux, P. J., 22, 49
Deyo, R. A., 268, 289
Dickersin, K., 274, 289
DiClemente, C. C., 145, 155, 222, 253
Dierberger, A. E., 139, 158, 178, 187
Dies, R. R., 52
Diguer, L., 52, 126, 186, 251, 293, 294, 325
DiGuiseppe, R., 264, 289
DiMascio, A., 261, 289, 303, 323
Dimeff, L., 186
Division 32 Task Force, 248

Fox, K. R., *129*
Fox, P. D., 28, *49*
Foxx, R., 70, *119, 122*
Frank, A., 150, *158*
Frank, E., *297*
Frank, J. D., 30, *49, 53,* 277, 286, *290*
Frank, M., 150, *156, 157, 159*
Franklin, M. E., 150, *156,* 179, *186,* 376, 377, 379, 384, *397, 399*
Franko, D. L., 133, *156*
Frantz-Renshaw, S., *119*
French, M., 344, *369*
French, N. H., 314, *325*
Fretter, P. B., 87, *128*
Freud, S., 61, *122*
Freund, B., 264, *291*
Friedman, E. S., *297*
Friedman, R. A., 268, *290*
Friedson, E., 45, *49*
Frijda, N. H., *122*
Frizelle, F. A., *289*
Fuhriman, A., 211, *247*
Furr, J. M., 377, *397*
Fydrich, T., 175, *185*

Gaffan, E. A., 258, *290,* 305, *324*
Gafni, A., *288*
Gallagher, D., 212, *249,* 259, 260, 283, *290,* 297
Gallagher-Thompson, D., 229, 231, *246, 251,* 264, *297*
Gallop, R., 198, *248*
Gandhi, T. K., 268, *290*
Garb, H. N., 21, 29, *49,* 55, 192, *249*
Garcia, A., 175, *185*
Garfield, S. L., 25, *49,* 133, 142, *156, 157,* 196, 209, *249*
Garmazy, N., 222, *252*
Garske, J. P., 38, *52,* 145, *158,* 197, 228, *251,* 285, *294*
Garvey, M. J., *291, 398, 399*
Gass, M., 48, *121*
Gaston, L., 212, *249*
Gawande, A., 20, *49*
Gelder, M., 260, 288, 303, *323*
Gelenberg, A. J., *50,* 292
Gelfand, L. A., 215, 235, *249*
Gelso, C. J., 77, 81, *122,* 287
Gendlin, E. T., 87, *125*
Gershefski, J. J., 214, *249*
Gething, L., 356, *369*

Getter, H., *248*
Ghahramanlou, M., 264, 265, *290*
Ghinassi, F., *158*
Gibbons, M. B. C., *156*
Gibbons, R. D., *324*
Gifford, A., 133, *157,* 380, *400*
Gilbody, S. M., 269, *290*
Gill, M. M., *53*
Gillespie, K., 382, *399*
Ginsburg, G. S., 183, *186, 255*
Giorgi, A., *122*
Gladis, L., *246*
Glaser, B., 74, 76, *122*
Glass, C. R., 214, 237, 245, 249, 277, *296*
Glass, G. V., 24, 25, *54, 72, 122,* 194, *255,* 300, *326,* 395, *401*
Gleitman, H., 30, *49*
Glen, A. I. M., 261, *288*
Glick, I., *292*
Gloaguen, V., 305, *324*
Gluud, C., 269, *287*
Goebel-Fabbri, A. E., 133, *156*
Goin, M. K., 213, *249*
Gold, J. R., 224, *249,* 276–278, *291, 296*
Goldberg, J., 78, *124, 125*
Goldfried, M. R., 22, 48, 87, *120, 126, 128,* 134, 140, 144, 150, *155, 156,* 247, 287, 336, *371*
Goldin, J. C., 260, *298*
Goldman, R. N., 86–88, *122, 124,* 127
Goldsmith, B., *293*
Goldstein, A., 175, *185,* 377, *398*
Goldstein, M., *48*
Gollan, J., *157*
Gollan, J. K., *124, 325*
Good, G. E., 342, 344, 368, 372, *373*
Goodheart, C. D., 20, 22, 23, 32, *49*
Goodrich, T. J., 342, 344, *373*
Goodwin, F. K., *53*
Goodyer, I., 175, *186*
Gordon, H. G., 22, *49*
Gordon, J. S., 273, *287*
Gordon, L. B., *130,* 264, 298, 306, 315, *328*
Gore, K. L., 183, *185*
Gorman, J. M., 5, *12,* 16, 17, 47, *50, 53,* 69, 127, 227, 231, *250, 252,* 312, *322*
Gotesman, K. G., 379, *401*
Gottman, J., 72, *122*
Gotzsche, P. C., 272, *289*
Gould, M., 273, *297*
Gould, R. A., *295*
Gracely, E., 175, *185*

Gram, L. F., 270, *291*
Grawe, K., 219, *253*
Gray, M. J., 35, *51*
Grayson, B., 377, *399*
Green, B., *187*
Green, C. E., *287*
Green, M. F., 21, *54*
Greenberg, L. S., 83–88, 113, *119, 122–124,*
    127, 128, 130, 192, 211, 222, *247,*
    250, 253, 264, 265, 273, 290, 305,
    315, *324,* 351, *368, 396, 399*
Greenberg, M. D., 273, *291*
Greenberg, R. P., 210, 249, 273, *287, 291*
Greene, J., 167, *184*
Greer, B. G., 356, *369*
Gregoire, T., 73, *126*
Gregory, J., 193, *250*
Grissom, R. J., 301, *324*
Gross, C.P., 267, *287*
Grove, W. M., *398, 399*
Gurin, J., 26, *51,* 222, *249*
Gurwitz, J. H., 268, *291*
Gusfield, J. R., 15, *49*
Guyll, M., 332, *369*

Haaga, D. A. F., 106, *123,* 313, *324*
Haahr, M., 272, *289*
Haas, E., 210, 240, *250*
Hackmann, A., *323,* 382, *399*
Haddock, G., *184*
Hahlweg, K., 150, *156, 157*
Hakstian, A. R., 303, 304, *325*
Haldeman, D. C., 349, *370*
Hall, G. N., 167, *189,* 331, 333, 334, 361,
    370, 374
Hall, J., 303, *326*
Halstead, T. S., 310, *326*
Han, S. S., *328*
Hansen, N. B., 147, *156,* 207, 238, *251*
Harding, C., 222, *250*
Hardtke, K., *119*
Hardy, G., 106, *123*
Hardy, R., 273, *295*
Hare-Mustin, R. T., 342, *370*
Harp, J. S., *123*
Harrold, L. R., *291*
Harwood, T. M., 47, *120, 154,* 231, 238, 246,
    250, 277, *287*
Hatgis, C., 144, 150, *153, 154, 322*
Haug, C., *289*
Haug, T. T., *398*

Hawkins, E. J., *157, 160*
Hawley, K. M., 164, *188*
Hayes, A. M., 22, 48, 66, 87, *120,* 134, 144,
    150, *155, 247*
Hayes, C., 133, *157,* 380, *400*
Hayes, J. A., 77, *123*
Hayes, S. C., 66, 68, 70, 71, *119, 123*
Haynes, B. P., 22, 24, 48, *49*
Haynes, R. B., 24, *53, 54,* 191, *254,* 320, *326*
Heagerty, P., *186*
Healy, D., 268, 269, 272, *291*
Heard, H. L., 311, *325*
Heindreich, T., *187*
Hellstrom, B., 304, *326*
Hellstrom, K., *326, 398*
Helmreich, R. L., 343, *373*
Hembree, E. A., 133, *156,* 382, *398*
Hendricks, M. N., 85, *123*
Hendrickse, W., *47*
Hendrix, S. L., 48, *121*
Henggeler, S. W., 132, *156,* 389, *402*
Henry, W. P., *123,* 134, 144, 150, *154, 156,*
    300, *324*
Herbel, B., 379, *400*
Herbert, J. D., 30, *52,* 175, *186*
Herek, G., 350, *370*
Herron, W. G., *298*
Hersh, A. L., 17, *50*
Hershenson, D. B., 355, *374*
Hess, S. A., 77, 78, *123, 125*
Hibbert, G. A., 311, *327*
Hibbs, E., 90, *124*
Hicks, R. E., 183, *185*
Hill, C. E., 22, *53,* 74, 76–79, 93, *122–126,*
    128, 287, 353, *370*
Hill, D., 395, *399*
Hill, R., 210, *250*
Hilsenroth, M. J., 38, *47,* 396, *399, 401*
Himmelstein, D. U., *293*
Hirschfeld, R., 264, *291*
Hirshoren, A., 193, *250*
Hitt, J., 23, 24, 41, *50*
Hoagwood, K., 90, 91, *124*
Hodgins, C., 310, *327,* 382, *401*
Hodgson, R., 377, *400*
Hoey, J., *289*
Hoffman, M. A., *124*
Hofmann, S. G., 376, *399*
Hohmann, A. A., 334, *370*
Hojgaard, L., *289*
Holbrook, D., 106, *121*
Hole, A. V., *293*

Keller, M. B., 17, 50, 264, 271, 292
Kelley, M., 72, 122
Kelly, A., 76, 125
Kemp-Wheeler, S. M., 258, 290, 305, 324
Kendall, P. C., 133, 157, 194, 250, 380, 400
Kendler, K. S., 181, 186
Kennedy, P., 354, 356, 369, 370
Kenny, D. A., 103, 119
Kessler, R. C., 19, 42, 50
Kewman, D. G., 209, 254
Khan, A., 260, 270, 292
Khan, S., 270, 292
Kiesler, C., 152, 157
Kiesler, D. J., 87, 125
Kihlstrom, J. F., 25, 28–31, 50–52
Kihlstrom, L. C., 25, 51
Kim, D. M., 201–203, 250, 307, 325
King, N. J., 69, 127, 311, 318, 319, 325
Kingdon, D., 150, 159
Kipnis, D., 194, 250
Kirsch, I., 210, 250, 270, 271, 273, 274, 284, 292
Kjaergard, L. L., 269, 287
Kleber, R. J., 260, 283, 288
Klein, D. F., 256, 260, 273, 274, 283, 292, 298
Klein, D. N., 22, 50, 51, 197, 216, 251, 291, 292
Klein, G., 22, 51
Klein, M. H., 87, 125
Kleinman, A., 219, 251
Klerman, G. L., 60, 125, 135, 139, 157, 160, 289, 315, 323, 325
Klosko, J. S., 304, 322
Knapen, J., 129
Knapp, M., 188
Knatterud, G. L., 48
Knepp, D., 355, 367
Knolls, M. L., 354, 368
Knox, S., 77, 78, 123, 125, 353, 370
Koch, W. J., 400
Koerner, K., 124, 134, 136, 157, 159, 325
Kohlenberg, B., 274, 295
Kohn, L. P., 183, 186
Koin, D., 264, 297
Kolchakian, M. R., 123
Kopp, A., 292
Kopte, S. M., 147, 156
Koran, L. M., 291
Kornstein, S. G., 291
Kosciulek, J. F., 358, 370
Kotkin, M., 26, 51
Kovacs, M., 96, 128, 261, 296, 401

Kozak, M. J., 150, 156, 186, 377, 378, 398–400
Kraemer, H. C., 93, 125, 264, 287
Krasnow, A. D., 138, 150, 153, 154, 177, 184, 322
Kratochwill, T., 65, 72, 125
Krause, E. D., 52, 126, 186, 293, 325
Krause, M. S., 147, 156
Krauss, D. R., 94, 126
Kretchman, J., 379, 401
Krimsky, S., 270, 272, 292
Krueger, R. F., 166, 181, 186, 386, 400
Krupnick, J. L., 145, 157, 187, 212, 216, 251
Krzyzanowska, M. E., 269, 292
Kuch, K., 294
Kühnlein, I., 223, 251
Kunzel, R., 144, 159
Kurcias, J. S., 155, 248
Kurtines, W. M., 255
Kuykendall, D. H., 127
Kyle, G., 270, 292

Ladany, N., 78, 123, 126
Lakoff, G., 242, 251
Lambert, M. J., 28, 53, 76, 93, 123, 126, 129, 141, 142, 144, 146, 147, 154, 156, 157, 160, 207, 208, 210, 218, 221, 226, 238, 240, 249–251, 257, 265, 293, 358, 370
Lampert, N., 310, 327
Lampropoulos, G. K., 16, 51, 126
Lane, D., 48, 121
Lane, J. S., 350, 369
Lang, P. J., 140, 157
Langer, K. G., 356, 370
Langer, R. D., 48, 121
Lantz, J., 73, 126
Largo-Marsh, L., 264, 293
Larkin, K., 254
Larssom, B., 379, 401
Lasovik, A. D., 140, 157
Lasser, K. E., 268, 293
Lasser, N. L., 52, 126
Latimer, P., 377, 399
Laughren, T. P., 270, 293
Laupacis, A., 292
Lauterback, W., 187
Lazarou, J., 268, 293
Lazarus, A. A., 277, 293
Leavitt, D., 183, 186
Leff, H. S., 4, 12
Leibing, E., 319, 325

Morrow, S. L., 74, *127*, 352, *371*
Morrow-Bradley, C., 63, *127*
Moseley, J. B., 104, *127*
Moses, H., 269, *295*
Moyer, J., *251*
Moyher, J., *157*
Moynihan, D. P., 27, *52*
Muenz, L. R., 228, *246*
Mueser, K. T., 392, *398*
Muir-Gray, J. A., 24, *53*, 320, *326*
Mulle, K., 379, *400*
Mulsant, B., *184*
Muñoz, R. F., 17, *52*, 183, *186*, 260, *298*
Murphy, G. E., 261, *295*
Murphy, J. J., 226, *252*
Murphy, P. M., 213, *252*
Murphy, T., *324*
Myers, J., 181, *186*
Nace, D. K., 142, *155*
Nachmias, J., 30, *49*
Najavits, L. M., 139, *158*, 176, 178, *187*, 189, 213, *252*
Nakayama, E. Y., *123*
Narducci, J., 198, *248*
Narrow, W. E., *52*, *53*
Nasby, W., 29, *51*, *52*
Nathan, D. G., 268, *295*
Nathan, P. E., 5, *12*, 16, 17, *53*, 69, *127*, 227, 231, *252*
National Institutes of Health, 16, *53*
Nau, S. D., 301, *323*
Nauta, A., 133, *157*
Nauta, M. C. E., *327*, 380, *400*
Navarro, A. M., 144, *159*
Neale, M. C., 181, *186*
Neimeyer, R. A., 258, *296*, 305, *326*
Neisser, U., 30, *49*
Nelson, A. R., 334, *373*
Nelson-Gray, R. O., 66, 72, 109, *119*, 121, *123*, *322*
Nemec, P. B., 359, *371*
Nestoros, J. N., *126*
Nettles, R., 355, *370*
Neu, C., 289, *323*
Newman, D., 175, *187*
Newman, F., 83, 95, *123*
Newman, M. G., 95, *120*, *127*
Newman, R., 6, *12*
Nezworski, M. T., 29, *55*
Ni, H., 15, *48*
Nicholls, M. G., 270, 284, *289*
Nicholls, S. S., *292*
Nielsen, S. L., *157*, *160*

Nierenberg, A. A., 274, *295*
Nietzel, M. T., 303, *327*
Nisbett, R. E., 21, *53*, 102, 117, *127*
Noble, S., *47*, *154*, *246*
Nofzinger, E. A., *297*
Norcross, J. C., 5, *12*, 22, 32, 39, *53*, 84, 85, *127*, 146, *158*, 206, 209, 211, 214, 215, 217, 222, 227, 228, 231, 240, *252*, *253*, 277, 280, *295*, *296*, 336, 345, 348, *371*
Norman, S. M., *292*
Noshirvani, H., *294*
Note, B., *185*
Note, I., *185*
Novotny, C., 18, 26, 41, *55*, 135, *160*, 162, 180, 181, *188*, *189*, 204, 256, 300, *328*, 389, *402*
Nunez, J., 167, *189*, 331, 361, *374*
Nunn, R., 70, *119*
Nury, A. M., *398*
Nutt, R. L., 342, *371*

O'Brien, C., *298*
O'Brien, K., 78, 79, *123*, *126*
O'Brien, R., *184*
Oden, T., 183, *186*
O'Donohue, W., 7, *12*, 193, *253*
Ogles, B., 28, *53*, 141, 142, 144, *157*, 209, 226, *251*, *253*
O'Leary, K. D., 301, *325*
Olkin, R., 354, 355, 357, 358, *371*, *372*
Ollendick, T. H., 25, 27, 48, 69, 91, *121*, *127*, *155*, 192, 195, 227, 236, *248*, 275, 278, 289, 310, 311, 316, 318, 319, 321, *323*, *325*, *328*, 340, 368, 382, *398*
Olmsted, M., *254*
O'Malley, K., *127*
Omenn, G. S., 268, *289*
O'Neil, J. M., 344, *372*
Onghena, P., *129*
O'Reardon, J. P., *50*, *124*, 172, *185*
Orleans, C. T., *48*
Orlinsky, D. E., 85, 87, *127*, 145, 147, *156*, *158*, 214, 219–221, 226, 241, *253*, 396, *400*
Orne, M. T., *49*
Öst, L. G., 303, 304, *326*
O'Sullivan, G., *294*
Otto, M. W., 264, 274, *295*
Otto-Salaj, L., 194, *250*

418   AUTHOR INDEX

Schafer, J., 377, *398*
Schafer, R., *53*
Schamberger, M., 198, *248*
Scharrón-Del Río, M. R., 331, 333, 346, *368*
Scher, M., 342, *373*
Schmidt, F., 310, *327*, 382, *401*
Schmidt, U., *185, 186, 188*
Schoenwald, S., 132, *156*
Scholinski, D., 348, *373*
Schön, D. A., 220, *254*
Schottenbauer, M. A., 277, 278, 281, *296*
Schulberg, H., *184*
Schulman, K. A., 269, 275, *296*
Schulte, D., 144, *159*
Schulte-Bahrenberg, T., 144, *159*
Schulz, K. F., 272, *294*
Schuman, W., 310, *327*
Schut, A. J., 93, *120*
Schwager, M., 16, *48*
Schwartz, J. E., *51, 251*
Schwartz, S. A., 377, *397*
Sciarra, D., 74, 77, *128*
Scoboria, A., 270, 284, *292*
Scott, J., 152, *159*
Secher, S., *175, 186*
Sechrest, L., 29, *54*, 136, *160*
Segal, Z. V., *120*
Seger, A. C., 290, *291*
Seidman, S. N., 273, *297*
Seils, D. M., *296*
Seligman, D. A., *52*, 94, *126, 186*, 293, 294, *325*
Seligman, M. E. P., 18, 26, *54*, 90, 99, *128*, 179, *187*
Seltzer, M., 176, *188*
Serafini, L. T., *255*
Serlin, R. C., 201, 202, 204, *254*, 256, 306–307, *328*
Shadish, W. R., 95, *128*, 144, *159*
Shaffer, D. R., 226, *254*
Shafran, R., 166, 181, *185*
Shahar, F., 379, *401*
Shaner, A., 21, *54*
Shapiro, D. A., 82, 107, *129*, 265, 296, 300, *326*
Shapiro, S. J., 237, *245*
Shaw, B. F., 134, *154, 155*, 197, 206, 235, 246, *254*, 265, 278, 287, *296*
Shaw, S. R., 139, *158*, 178, *187*
Shea, M. T., 49, *121*, 175, *185, 187*, 249, 290, *324*
Shear, M. K., 17, 47, *50, 250*, 312, *322, 399*
Sheehan, P. W., 224, 248, 260, *289*

Shelton, R. C., 48, *50, 121, 124*
Shepherd, M., 301, *326*
Sherman, J. J., 306, *326*
Sherwood, A., 356, *371*
Shirk, S. R., 211, *255*
Shoham, V., *11, 48*, 265, 296, *368*
Shroeder, B., 150, *156, 157*
Shull, R., 73, *128*
Siddique, J., *187*
Siemer, M., 201, 202, *255*
Sigouin, C. S., *119*
Silberschatz, G., 87, *128*, 376, *400*
Silva, P., *175, 187*
Silva, S., *186*
Silverman, J., 213, *249*
Silverman, W. H., 133, *159*
Silverman, W. K., 224, *255*
Silverstein, L. B., 339, 342, 344, 345, *371, 373*
Simmens, S., *157*
Simmons, S., *251*
Simon, G., 268, *289*
Simon, R., 152, *159*
Simons, A. D., 261, *295*
Simpson, R. J., 261, *295*
Singer, B. H., 25, *52*, 82, 101, *126*, 142, 149, *158*
Singh, A., 73, *128*
Siobud-Dorocant, E., 274, *290*
Siqueland, L., *158, 246*
Sisenwein, F., *298*
Sloan, W. W., Jr., 86, *129*
Sloane, R., 213, *255*, 260, *296*
Slovic, P., 102, *125*
Sluys, M., *398*
Sluzki, C., 335, *373*
Smart, D., *157, 160*
Smedley, B. D., 334, *373*
Smith, L., *297*
Smith, M. L., 24, 25, *54*, 74, *127*, 194, *255*, 300, 326, 333, *371*, 395, *401*
Smith R., 24, *48*
Sneed, T., *119*
Snyder, C. R., 220, 222, *255*
Snyder, M., 195, *255*
Sochting, I., *400*
Society of Clinical Psychology, 338, *367*
Solis, H. L., *373*
Sommer, B. R., 264, *297*
Song, F., 269, *290*
Sorrell, R., 146–148, *158*
Sotsky, S. M., 49, *121, 157, 185, 187*, 249, 290, *324*
Soysa, C., *154*

SUBJECT INDEX

Blindness assessment, 274
Borderline personality disorder, 311
Brady, J. V., 100
British Psychological Society, 6
BTs. *See* Behavioral therapies
Bulimia, 167

Campbell Collaboration, 6
Case formulation, 387
Case studies, 57–64
    advantages/disadvantages of, 63–64
    application of, to theory, 62–63
    statistical hypothesis-testing strategy vs., 59–61
    triangulation used in, 61–62
Causal inference, 97–99
CBTs. *See* Cognitive–behavioral therapies
Center for Cognitive Therapy, 380
Center for the Treatment and Study of Anxiety (CTSA), 377, 378
Cervantes, Saavedra Miguel de, 147
Change, principles of, 226–234, 316, 317
    and curative factors, 228–230
    and integration of factors, 229–230
    and participant factors, 228–229
    participant-related, 232–233
    and relationship factors, 228
    relationship-related, 232
    systematic treatment selection, 230–231
    therapeutic, 231–232
    and treatment factors, 229
    treatment-model-related, 233
Change processes, 85–87
Change process research, 81–89
    designs for, 87
    example of, 87–89
    importance of, 81–83
    methods of, 86–87
Changing criterion design, 67, 69
Child and adolescent treatments
    clinic-based, 310–311
    for depression, 163–164
    effectiveness of, 314–315
    in EX–RP, 379
    transportability studies of, 382, 389–391
Class strain, 340
Client-centered therapy, 315
Client factors, 336
Client reports, 213–214
Client resistance, 214–215

Clients
    active, 218–226
    differential processes of, 84–85
    perspective of, 75–76
Clinical expertise, 13–23, 40–41
    definition of, 20
    depth of, 22
    devaluation of, 16–18
    and EBP as public idea, 14–16
    need for data-based reassertion of importance of, 18–23
    treatment manuals vs., 146
    usefulness of, 20
Clinical practice
    qualitative research findings useful to, 77–78
    S-P design in, 70–71
    treatment manuals used to improve outcomes in, 135–137
Clinical trials
    assessment/treatment in, 176–179
    interpretation/presentation of results of, 162–164
    as not representative of clinical practice, 161–171
    patient characteristics in, 172–176
    representativeness of length of treatments in, 170
    representativeness of treatments selected for, 168–170
    as representative of clinical practice, 171–179
    sampling decisions and generalizability in, 165–167
"Clinic therapy," 310–311
CMHC. *See* Community mental health center
Cochrane Collaboration, 6
Cognitive analytic therapy, 281
Cognitive–behavioral treatments (CBTs), 7, 18, 25
    for children/adolescents, 314–315
    for depression, 104–105, 304, 311
    effectiveness of, 303, 304
    ERP vs., 305–306
    impact of theoretical allegiance on, 265
    for LGB clients, 347
    outcome measurement of, 281
    for panic disorder, 143–144, 311–312
    as theoretically integrated treatment, 278
    transportability studies of, 382

Cognitive therapy (CT), 19, 25
    for depression, 380–381
    effectiveness of IPT vs., 315
    impact of theoretical allegiance on, 259, 260, 262–264
    systematic desensitization vs., 300–301
Committee on Quality of Health Care in America, 321
Common factors approach, 85, 277–278, 385–386
Community mental health center (CMHC), 179, 181, 380, 389–391
Comorbidity
    and differential outcomes, 175–176
    and length of treatment, 178
    and sampling decisions, 165–167
    and transportability of treatment, 385–390
Comprehensive process analysis, 86–87
Conduct disorder, 390
Conflicts of interest in research, 269–272
Consensual qualitative research (CQR), 74, 75, 79
Consolidated Standards of Reporting Trials (CONSORT) statement, 272–274
Construct validity, 102–103
Consumer Reports, 26–27
Contract research organizations (CROs), 271
Core assessment battery, 93, 94
Countertransference, 358
CQR. See Consensual qualitative research
Crits-Christoph, P., 313–314
CROs (contract research organizations), 271
CT. See Cognitive therapy
Cultural competence, 335–337, 347–353
Cultural gender role ideology, 343
Culturally sensitive therapies, 333–334
Cummings, Elijah E., 334
Current Controlled Trials Meta-Register, 274

Data withholding and delay, 269–270
DBT. See Dialectical behavior therapy
Decision-making, clinical, 21–22
Department of Health and Human Services (DHHS), 16, 334, 335
Depression, 19
    CBT for, 311
    in children/adolescents, 314–315
    ESTs for, 302–305
    in LGBT clients, 347
    manuals for, 385

in people with disabilities, 354, 356
sampling decisions for RCT of, 167
transportability of treatment for, 380–381
Design of studies
    in EX–RP, 378–379
    for process-outcome, 87
    in RCTs, 376
Diagnoses, 21–22
    and client characteristics, 39
    limitations of, 32
    in practice vs. trial, 176–177
    and transportability, 386–388
Diagnostic and Statistical Manual of Mental Disorders (DSM–IV), 21–22, 349, 386
Diagnostic criteria, gender bias in, 341
Dialectical behavior therapy (DBT), 281, 311
Different treatments, assignment to, 279–280
Disabilities, models of, 355
Disabilities, people with
    assessment measures for, 357
    availability of research to, 357
    and countertransference, 358
    and EBPs, 356–359
    flexibility of research for, 357
    heterogeneity among, 354
    lack of training for treating, 355–356
    mistakes in treating, 356
Disability strain, 340
Disclosure of conflicts of interest, 271, 272
Discovery-oriented research, 333
Discrepancy strain, 343–344
Diversity issues
    for ethnic minority populations, 329–337
    with gender, 338–345
    for LGBT clients, 346–353
    for people with disabilities, 353–359
Dodo Bird effect, 141–142, 300
Double blind tests, 274
Dream treatment, 79–80
Drug reactions, adverse, 268
DSM–IV. See Diagnostic and Statistical Manual of Mental Disorders
Dynamic therapies, 259, 260, 262–264
Dysfunction strain, 344

EBPs. See Evidence-based practices
Eclectic–integrative orientation, 276, 277
Effectiveness research, 26–27, 89–96
Effect sizes, theoretical allegiance and, 264, 265

Efficacy research, 19, 26–27
  biases in misperceptions of, 102
  effectiveness research vs., 90
  evidence behind, 30–31
EMDR. *See* Eye Movement Desensitization
    and Reprocessing
Empathy, 345, 351
Empirically supported relationships (ESRs), 5
Empirically supported treatments (ESTs),
    5–7. *See also* EST vs. non-EST
    effectiveness
  for depression/anxiety, 302–306
  designation as, 299–300
  effectiveness of non-EST therapies vs.,
    299–322
  and ethnic minority populations, 331
  meta-analyses of, 300–301
  nonsupported vs., 193–195
  number of designated, 310
  placebos vs., 301–302
  and psychotherapy integration, 275–282
  for specific disorders, 313–315
  transportability of, 277
Empowerment models of treatment, 358
Empty-chair dialogues, 84
"Equivalent outcomes paradox," 265
ERPs. *See* Exposure and response prevention
ESRs (empirically supported relationships), 5
ESTs. *See* Empirically supported treatments
EST vs. non-EST effectiveness, 299–322
  in community practice settings, 310–313
  criteria for establishing, 307–308
  for depression/anxiety, 302–306
  meta-analyses of, 300–301
  methodological issues with, 306–307
  placebos, 301–302
Ethnicity strain, 340
Ethnic minority populations, 329–337
  cultural competency research with,
    335–337
  disparities in treatment of, 332
  lack of research on, 330–332
  political considerations in research
    with, 334–335
  research methodology for, 333–335
Evaluation of interventions
  principles for, 320
  standards for, 28
Evidence-Based Medicine Notebook, 22
Evidence-based practices (EBPs), 3, 320
  clinical scientists and support for, 16–17
  controversies surrounding, 7–9
  definition of, 13–14
  efficacy vs. effectiveness of, 25–27
  and ethnic minority populations,
    329–337
  fundamental questions about, 9–11
  and gender, 338–345
  in general, 403–404
  health professionals' resistance to, 16
  historical background, 4–5
  and LGBT clients, 346–353
  and managed care, 15–17
  organizations providing lists of, 6
  in particular, 404–406
  and people with disabilities, 353–359
  as public idea, 14–16
  resistance to demand for, 26
  scientific background for, 23–25
  standards for, 27–29
  and treatment manuals, 134
  as worldwide movement, 6
Experiential therapies
  for GAD, 306
  impact of theoretical allegiance on, 265
Expert knowledge, 22
Explicit theories, 58
Exposure and response prevention (ERP),
    303, 305–306
Exposure and response prevention (EX–RP),
    377–379
Exposure therapy
  for phobias, 303, 304
  transportability studies of, 382
External validity, 91, 97
Eye Movement Desensitization and
    Reprocessing (EMDR), 30, 281,
    306
Eysenck, Hans J., 24, 101, 309, 310, 318

FDA. *See* Food and Drug Administration
Feminist therapies, 345
Flexibility
  of S-P design, 71–72
  and treatment manual use, 133–134
  of treatments, 379–380, 387
Flexner Report, 4
Food and Drug Administration (FDA), 4–5
  antidepressant database of, 270, 274
  standards of, 27
Franklin Commission, 30
Funding source, impact of, 267–275
  and conflicts of interest, 269–272

and potential methodological biases, 272–274

and research safeguards, 274–275

GAD. *See* Generalized anxiety disorder

Gay, Lesbian, Bisexual, Transgendered (GLBT) clients. *See* Lesbian, gay, bisexual, and transgendered clients

Gender, 338–345

    EBP and, 344–345

    role strain paradigm for, 342–344

    studies of, 340–342

Gender Identity Disorder, 349

Gender Role Conflict, 343–344

Gender Role Identity Paradigm, 338, 342–344

Gender Role Strain Paradigm, 338, 342–344

Gender studies, 340–342

Generalizability of treatments, 78–79, 375, 391

    and interpretation/presentation of results, 162–164

    lack of, in efficacy research, 90

    and sampling decisions, 165–167

Generalized anxiety disorder (GAD), 306, 307

    effectiveness of treatments for, 314

    sampling decisions for RCT of, 167

Glass, Gene V., 25, 318

GLBT clients. *See* Lesbian, gay, bisexual, and transgendered clients

Goal consensus, 345

Gold standard (for evidence), 275

Goodall, Jane, 103

Guidelines for Psychotherapy With Lesbian, Gay, and Bisexual Clients (APA), 349–352

Guidelines on Multicultural Education, Training, Research, Practice and Organizational Change for Psychologists (APA), 338

Habit reversal and control, 70

Health care. *See also* Managed care

    definition of quality, 31–32

    inadequacy of U.S., 15

Healy, David, 269

Heterosexism, 349, 350–351

Heuristics, 102

HHS. *See* Department of Health and Human Services

Hispanics, 334

Hollon, Steven D., 380–381

Homophobia, 349, 350

Homosexuality, 349

Honda, Michael M., 334–335

Hormone replacement therapy (HRT), 17, 99–100

Human Affairs International, 142

Huxley, Thomas Henry, 141

Hypothesis-testing strategy, 59–61

Imipramine, 24, 28

Impact of funding source on published research, 267–275

Institute of Medicine, 31, 321

Institutional Review Board, 274

Integration

    assimilative, 278

    theoretical, 278

Integrative psychotherapies, 260, 276–278

Internal validity, 90, 91, 97, 98–99

Interpersonal therapy (IPT), 18

    for depression, 60, 104

    effectiveness of, 303, 315

James, William, 11

Job loss, 35

Journal of Clinical Psychology, 63

Journal of Consulting and Clinical Psychology, 389

Journal of the American Medical Association, 375

Journals

    and conflicts of interest, 271

    CONSORT statement adopted by, 273

    pharmaceutical industry ties with, 272

review of studies in, 274

Koch, Robert, 24

Kraeplin, Emil, 4

Laboratory-validated treatments

    as not necessarily transportable to clinical practice, 383–393

    as transportable to clinical practice, 375–383

Latinos, 331

Lesbian, gay, bisexual, and transgendered (LGBT) clients, 340, 346–353

    cultural competence with, 349–353

    as frequent users of psychotherapy, 347

    lack of legal protections for, 364

stigma of, 346
treatment as usual for, 348
Levitt, E. E., 309
LGBT clients. *See* Lesbian, gay, bisexual, and transgendered clients
Little Albert case example, 61

Major depressive disorder (MDD), 162, 163, 175, 302, 381
Managed care, 42
demands of, 25
and EBP, 15–17
Manual-based treatments, 134
Manualized treatments
common factors approach to, 385–386
criticisms of, 379
for depression, 385
explosion of, 141
revision of, for subpopulations, 385
Marketing departments, 271, 272
Marks, I. M., 268–269
Medical disability model, 355
Medical model of psychotherapy, 220–221
Mesmer, Franz, 30–31
Meta-analysis, 24
Methodological issues, 306–307
Methodological biases, potential, 272–274
Methodology for ethnic minority populations, 333–335
Mexican Americans, 336
"Minority stress," 339
Moral disability model, 355
Multiple baseline design, 68, 69

Narcissism, 39
National Association of Social Workers, 6
National Institute of Health (NIH), 334
National Institute of Medicine, 334
National Institute of Mental Health (NIMH), 16, 140, 306, 331
National Register of Health Service Providers, 276
Nefazadone, 271
Nicotine patch, 269–270
Nietzsche, Friedrich, 148
NIH (National Institute of Health), 334
NIMH. *See* National Institute of Mental Health
Nondirective therapy
for agoraphobia, 304

for GAD, 314
North American Society for Psychotherapy Research (NASPR), 231
Null hypothesis, 28, 307

Observation, 58–59
Obsessive–compulsive disorder (OCD), 302, 303
ESTs for, 305–306
patient variables in treatment of, 196–197
sampling decisions for RCT of, 167
and Tourette Syndrome, 35
transportability of treatment for, 377–380
Oppositional–defiant disorder, 382, 390
Oppression, impact of, 338–339
Outcome measurement, 29, 280–281
Outcome-oriented approaches, 276

Pacific Islanders, 334
Panic control therapy (PCT), 311–312
Panic disorders, 303, 304
CBT for, 143–144, 311–312
sampling decisions for RCT of, 167
transportability studies of treatments for, 382
Panic disorder with agoraphobia, 268–269
Participants. *See also* Clients
change principles related to, 232–233
perspective of, 75–76
Pasteur, Louis, 23–24
Patient response and feedback, 376
Patient screening, 375, 377–378, 385
Patient values and practices, 31–40
case examples of, 33–39
definition of, 31–32
and limitations of diagnoses, 32
Patient variables, 195–197, 209–210
Pennsylvania Psychological Association, 94
Permeability, 59, 62
Pharmaceutical industry
and adverse drug reactions, 268
annual revenue of, 267
changing research funding patterns in, 271
and conflicts of interest in research, 269–272
financial ties of, 268–269
impact on research of funding by, 267–268
research design biases in, 271–272
research publication restrictions by, 272

Pharmacotherapy, 19, 259, 261–264
Phenothiazines, 24
Phobias, 303, 304
Placebo control, 284, 308
    difficulties in implementing, 27–28
    ESTs vs., 301–302
Placebo washout, 273, 274
Pleck, Joseph, 342, 343
PMR (progressive muscle relaxation), 314
Political considerations, 334–335
Popper, Karl, 102
Posttraumatic stress disorder (PTSD), 306
    case examples of, 33–39
    in LGBT clients, 347, 352
    in people with disabilities, 354
    sampling decisions for RCT of, 167
    transportability studies of treatments for,
        382
Practice-based evidence, 147–148
Practice research networks (PRNs), 93–95
Pragmatic Case Studies in Psychotherapy, 63
Prescriptive psychotherapy, 281
President's New Freedom Commission on
    Mental Health, 321, 337
Principles of change. *See* Change, principles of
PRNs. *See* Practice research networks
Procedural evidence, 75
"Procedural slippage," 336
Process–experiential therapy (PET)
    effectiveness of, 315
    impact of theoretical allegiance on, 265
Process-outcome research
    designs for, 87
    examples of, 87–89
Pro-feminist therapies, 345
Progressive muscle relaxation (PMR), 314
Prozac, 163
Psychotherapies
    impact of theoretical allegiance on, 259,
        261–264
    medical model of, 220–221
Psychotherapist, validation of, 200–208
Psychotherapists
    characteristics/actions of, 206–207
    and confounded variables, 205–206
    and methodological considerations,
        201–202
    and outcome data, 207
    sources of outcome variability for, 201
    validating, 205–208
    variability in outcomes due to, 202–205

Psychotherapy integration *See also*
    Integration Models
    approaches to, 277–278
    and ESTs, 275–282
    outcome measurement of, 281
Psychotherapy manuals. *See* Treatment
    manuals
Psychotherapy research, goal of, 91–93
Psychotropic drugs, 24, 25, 333
Public idea, evidence-based practice as, 14–16
Public registry of clinical trials, 274

Qualitative research, 74–81
    advantages/disadvantages of, 75–79
    defining evidence in, 75
    example of, 79–80
    variations in, 74
Quality health care, 31–32

Race strain, 340
Random assignment, 279, 330–331
Randomized clinical trials (RCTs), 17–22,
    27, 96–105, 274
    assumptions of, 279–281
    consequences of failing to use, 99–101
    construct validity and limitations of,
        102–103
    and heuristics/biases, 102
    and internal validity/threats to causal
        inference, 98–99
    problems with, 83–85
    processes of change, 81–82
    specificity in, 103–104
RCTs. *See* Randomized clinical trials
Relaxation
    applied, 303, 304
    for depression, 303, 304
    for panic disorder, 303, 304
Representativeness
    of patient characteristics in clinical trials,
        172–176
    of treatment length in clinical trials, 170
    of treatments selected for testing, 168–170
Reprint measure, 258–261, 263, 264
Research. *See also* Case studies
    change process, 81–89
    conflicts of interest in, 269–272
    effectiveness, 89–96
    qualitative, 74–81

single-participant design, 64–73
and theoretical allegiance, 257–267
use of, by managed care, 16–17
Research contracts, 275
Research protocols, 274–275
Research safeguards, 274–275
Responsiveness, 83–84, 106–107
Reversal (ABA/ABAB) design, 66
Review of data, independent, 274
Rezulin, 268
Rogers, C. R., 350
Role strain, 339
Rosenzweig, Saul, 142
Rush, Benjamin, 4, 101

Sa'di, 145
SAMHSA. *See* Substance Abuse and Mental Health Services Administration
Sampling decisions, 165–167
Saxe, John Godfrey, 61
Schizophrenia, 82
Science, theory as main product of, 58–59
Scientific research, 23–31, 57
and controversy over evidence-based medicine, 23–25
and "efficacy" vs. "effectiveness" research, 25–27
and managed care, 25
and standards for EBP, 27–29
theory behind, 30–31
Sechrest, Lee, 97
Selective Serotonin Reuptake Inhibitors (SSRIs)
in PTSD treatment, 34, 37
suicidal behavior linked to, 269
Self-directed exposure for specific phobia, 303, 304
Self-disclosure, 353
Self-healing, 218–226
client's role in active, 219–220
evidence for, 221–222
and medical model, 220–221
techniques of, 222–225
Self-report measures
patient-rated vs. clinician-rated, 274
of theoretical allegiance, 259–262, 264
September 11, 2001 terrorist attacks, 35–39
SES. *See* Socioeconomic status
Sexist bias, 341
Sexual orientation strain, 340
Sexual victimization, 347

Simple baseline (AB) design, 65–67
Single-participant (S-P) design, 64–73
advantages of, in clinical practice, 70–71
advantages of, in research, 71–72
core feature of, 65
data analysis from, 72–73
examples of, 69–70
types of, 65–69
Site–management organizations (SMOs), 271
Smith, M. L., 25
Social anxiety disorder, 382
Social disability model, 355, 358
Social phobia, 306
Social skill training, 306
Society of Clinical Psychology, 5, 27, 231, 309
See also APA Division 12
Socioeconomic status (SES), 384, 389, 390
"Soft constraints" approach, 395–396
S-P design. *See* Single-participant design
Specificity, 103–104
Spontaneous remission, 194–195
SSRIs. *See* Selective Serotonin Reuptake Inhibitors
Standards
for EBP, 27–29
S-P design assists clinician in meeting, 71
Statistical hypothesis-testing strategy, 59–61
Steketee, Gail, 397
Stress inoculation, 303
STS. *See* Systematic Treatment Selection
Substance Abuse and Mental Health Services Administration (SAMHSA), 6, 16, 331
Substance abuse disorders, 347
Suicidal behavior, 164, 269
Systematic desensitization, 30, 300–301
Systematic Treatment Selection (STS), 230–231

TADS. *See* Treatment of Adolescent Depression Study
Task analysis, 86
Task Force Report on Promotion and Dissemination of Psychological Procedures, 308, 310
TAU. *See* Treatment as usual
TDCRP. *See* Treatment of Depression Collaborative Research Program
Theory (as main product of science), 58–59
Therapeutic alliance, 38, 88
empathy in, 345

treatment manuals vs., 145

Therapeutic relationship

    change principles related to, 232

    for people with disabilities, 358

    treatment method vs., 197–198

Therapist differences, 306–307

Therapist factors, 198, 336–337

Therapy relationship

    challenges in validating, 215–217

    client reports of effective, 213–214

    evidence for power of, 210–214

    evidence for relational matchmaking in, 214–215

    individual outcome studies of, 212–213

    meta-analyses of, 210–211

    sources of outcome variability for, 209–210

    validation of, 208–218

Third-party payers, 29, 140

Thompson, Tommy, 335

Time-limited dynamic psychotherapy (TLDP), 144

Tourette Syndrome (TS), 34–36

Training

    of graduate students, 195

    manuals used for, 144

Training clinics, 94–95

Transgendered persons, 349

Transportability of laboratory-validated treatments, 375–383

    data clarity in, 388–392

    for depression, 380–381

    diagnosis defined in, 386–388

    for OCD, 377–380

    unit of treatment package defined in, 384–386

Transtheoretical therapy, 281

Trauma strain, 344

Treatment as usual (TAU), 169, 171, 309–313, 316, 318–319, 321, 348

Treatment context, 146

Treatment manuals

    advantages/disadvantages of, 141

    clinical outcomes improved from use of, 135–137

    debate over, 137–139

    and EBPs/manual-based treatments, 134

    evolution of, 132–134

    ineffectiveness of, 140–149

    practice-based evidence vs., 147–148

    in practice vs. trial, 177–178

    and sources of variance, 145–147

and specific effects, 141–143

transportability of, 143–144

Treatment methods, 191–200

    defining, 192

    empirically supported vs. nonsupported, 193–195

    patient variables vs., 195–197

    principles vs., 199

    relationship variables vs., 197–198

    therapist factors vs., 198

Treatment of Adolescent Depression Study (TADS), 163, 169

Treatment of Depression Collaborative Research Program (TDCRP), 28, 59–60, 145–146, 175, 203, 206, 212–213, 306, 315

Treatment setting, 337

Triangulation, 61–63

TS. *See* Tourette Syndrome

"Unequal Treatment" (Smedley, Stith, & Nelson), 334

Unfinished business, 84–85

U.S. Surgeon General, 331, 332, 337

Upjohn, 268–269

Validation

    of active client, 218–226

    of principles of change, 226–234

    of psychotherapist, 200–208

    of therapy relationship, 208–218

    of treatment method, 191–200

Validity, internal vs. external, 97

Victimization, 347

Wait-list controls, 308

Wampold, B. E., 313–314

Washington, George, 101

Weiss, Jay, 100

"White privilege," 336

Wundt, Wilhelm, 4

Xanax, 268–269